Drugs in Sport

Fifth Edition

Edited by David R. Mottram

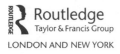

Routledge
Taylor & Francis Group

LONDON AND NEW YORK

362.29088796
MOT
3029394

First published 1988
Second edition 1996
Third edition 2003
Fourth edition 2005
Fifth edition 2011
by Routledge
2 Park Square, Milton Park, Abingdon, Oxon OX14 4RN

LEEDS TRINITY UNIVERSITY

Simultaneously published in the USA and Canada
by Routledge
711 Third Avenue, New York, NY10017

Routledge is an imprint of the Taylor & Francis Group

© 1988, 1996, 2003, 2005, and 2011 David R. Mottram
for selection and editorial matter; individual chapters the
contributors

The right of David Mottram to be identified as author of the
editorial material, and of the authors for their individual chapters
has been asserted in accordance with sections 77 and 78 of the
Copyright, Designs and Patents Act 1988.

Typeset in Times by Glyph International Ltd.

British Library Cataloguing in Publication Data
A catalogue record for this book is available from the
British Library

Library of Congress Cataloging in Publication Data
Drugs in sport / edited by David Mottram. — 5th ed.
    p. cm.
Includes bibliographical references and index.
1. Doping in sports. I. Mottram, D. R. (David R.), 1944–
[DNLM: 1. Doping in Sports. 2. Sports Medicine.
3. Substance-Related Disorders. QT 261 D7944 2011]
RC1230.D786 2011
362.29—dc22   2010017015

ISBN 978-0-415-55086-4(hbk)
ISBN 978-0-415-55087-1(pbk)
ISBN 978-0-203-87382-3(ebk)

This edition of *Drugs in Sport* is dedicated to Tom Reilly who died in June 2009. Tom was the first Professor of Sports Science in the UK and had an exemplary record in teaching and research. He had been a contributor to this book since its first edition in 1988. Tom is sadly missed by his colleagues.

Contents

17 Beta blockers   235

DAVID R. MOTTRAM

SECTION 3
Substances and methods permitted in sport   245

18 Supplements for high intensity exercise: creatine
and other ergogenic aids   247

DON MACLAREN

19 Supplement use in sport   262

DAVID R. MOTTRAM

20 Caffeine   274

NEIL CHESTER

21 Over-the-counter stimulants and herbal preparations   294

NEIL CHESTER

22 Non-steroidal anti-inflammatory drugs   317

PETER N. ELLIOTT

Contributors

David J. Armstrong
Peter N. Elliott
David R. Mottram
School of Pharmacy and Biomolecular Sciences
Liverpool John Moores University
Byrom Street
Liverpool
L3 3AF
UK

Neil Chester
Don MacLaren
Thomas Reilly
Jim Waterhouse
Centre for Sport and Exercise Science
Liverpool John Moores University
Byrom Street
Liverpool
L3 3AF
UK

Mark Stuart
International Forum on Quality and Safety in Health Care
BMJ Group Ltd.
BMA House
Tavistock Square
London
WC1H 9JR

Dominic J. Wells
Gene Targeting Group, Department of Cellular and Molecular Neuroscience
Division of Neuroscience and Mental Health
Imperial College London
Hammersmith Hospital Campus
160, Du Cane Road
London
W12 0NN

Section I

The basis for and regulation of drug use in sport

Chapter 1

An introduction to drugs and their use in sport

David R. Mottram

1.1   Definition of a drug

Drugs are chemical substances that, by interaction with biological targets, can alter the biochemical systems of the body. The branch of science investigating drug action is known as pharmacology. Interactions may be mediated through a variety of target tissues within the body. For example, effects on cardiac muscle by drugs such as ephedrine can be an increase in the force and rate of beating of the heart; stimulation of nerve endings in the central nervous system by drugs such as amphetamine can produce changes in mood and behaviour; interaction with metabolic processes with drugs such as insulin can be used in the treatment of disorders such as diabetes.

In this chapter, frequent reference is made to drugs on the World Anti-Doping Agency (WADA) Prohibited List. The 2010 version of this list is presented in Table 1.1.

1.2   Classification and description of drug names

Drugs are variously classified and described by their:

- generic name (international non-proprietary name, INN)
- proprietary name (manufacturer's name)
- mechanism of action.

The generic name (INN) is the internationally recognised name of the drug and should normally be used when describing the drug.

When a pharmaceutical company first develops a new drug, it patents the drug under a proprietary name. When the patent expires, other pharmaceutical companies may produce the same drug but they give the drug their own proprietary name to distinguish their version of the drug from that of other companies. Examples of the classification and names of drugs subject to restrictions in sport are presented in Table 1.2.

Table 1.1 WADA prohibited list, January 2010

SUBSTANCES AND METHODS PROHIBITED AT ALL TIMES (IN AND OUT OF COMPETITION)

Prohibited substances
S.1   Anabolic agents
S.2   Peptide hormones, growth factors, and related substances
S.3   Beta-2 agonists
S.4   Hormone antagonists and modulators
S.5   Diuretics and other masking agents

Prohibited methods
M.1   Enhancement of oxygen transfer
M.2   Chemical and physical manipulation
M.3   Gene doping

SUBSTANCES AND METHODS PROHIBITED IN COMPETITION
Categories S.1 to S.5 and M.1 to M.3 and:

S.6   Stimulants
S.7   Narcotics
S.8   Cannabinoids
S.9   Glucocorticosteroids

SUBSTANCES PROHIBITED IN PARTICULAR SPORTS

P.1   Alcohol
P.2   Beta blockers

Source: www.wada-ama.org (October 2009).

Table 1.2 Examples of the classification and description of drugs by their names

Class of drug	Generic name	Proprietary name
Androgenic anabolic steroids	Nandrolone	Deca-Durabolin
Diuretics	Furosemide	Lasix
Beta-2 Agonists	Salbutamol	Ventolin
Narcotics	Morphine	Sevredol
Beta blockers	Atenolol	Tenormin
Human growth hormone	Somatropin	Humotrope

The mechanism of action describes the pharmacology of the drug and the therapeutic use for which the drug is designed. Examples are given in Table 1.3.

1.3   Development of new drugs

Over the centuries, herbalists and apothecaries have extracted drugs from plant and animal sources. A few drugs are still derived from natural sources. For example, morphine is extracted from the opium poppy (*Papaver somniferum*) and digoxin is derived from the foxglove plant (*Digitalis purpurea*). However, the

Table 1.3 Examples of the classification of drugs by their mechanism of action and use

Class of drug	Pharmacological action	Therapeutic use in
Diuretics	Prevention of re-absorption of water from the kidneys	Heart failure Hypertension
Beta-2 Agonists	Bronchodilation through stimulation of β_2-adrenoreceptors	Asthma Chronic obstructive pulmonary disease
Morphine	Agonist on opioid μ receptors	Severe pain
Beta blockers	Antagonists on β-adrenoreceptors	Angina Hypertension Cardiac arrhythmias Anxiety

majority of drugs are produced by pharmaceutical companies through chemical synthesis. Current research into gene technology is revolutionising the development of new drugs.

The development of new drugs is monitored by government agencies who evaluate data on the activity and safety of new drugs before awarding a product licence. The product licence states the therapeutic purpose(s) for which the drug may be used. The development of a new drug can take between 10 and 12 years and at a cost of several hundred million dollars.

1.4   Dosage forms for drug delivery to the body

There are many different dosage forms through which drugs can be delivered to the body. Examples for drugs subject to restrictions in sport are presented in Table 1.4.

Table 1.4 Examples of dosage forms for drugs used in sport

Generic drug name	Dosage forms
Testosterone (androgenic anabolic steroid)	Oral capsules Intramuscular injection Transdermal patches
Terbutaline (bronchodilator)	Aerosol inhaler Oral tablets Syrup Injection
Hydrocortisone (glucocorticosteroid)	Oral tablets Injection Ear/eye drops Cream/ointment
Pethidine (narcotic analgesic)	Oral tablets Injection

The selection of the most appropriate dosage form depends on a number of factors:

- Speed of action
  - Oral preparations are slow to be absorbed from the gastrointestinal tract Modified release tablets can slow this process even more, to give a longer duration of action.
  - Injections, particularly intravenous, are very rapid.
  - Aerosol inhalers provide rapid effects on the airways.
  - Transdermal patches provide a slow sustained delivery by absorption through the skin.
- Site of action
  - Oral and most injection preparations lead to extensive distribution of the drug around the body.
  - Creams/ointments/ear drops/eye drops/aerosol inhalers are each delivered to the site where they are specifically needed.
- Reduction of side effects
  - Generally, the more widely distributed the drug is in the body the greater the chance of side effects. Therefore, topical administration has advantages over systemic delivery by mouth or by injection.

1.5   The absorption, distribution, metabolism and elimination of drugs

For a drug to exert its effect it must reach its site of action. This will involve its passage from the site of administration to the cells of the target tissue or organ. The principal factors that can influence this process are absorption, distribution, metabolism and elimination. Consideration of these factors is known as the *pharmacokinetics* of drug action.

Absorption

The absorption of a drug is, in part, dependent upon its route of administration. Most drugs must enter the bloodstream in order to reach their site of action and the most common route of administration for this purpose is orally, in either liquid or tablet form. Absorption from the gut can be affected by:

- lipid solubility of the drug (strong acids or bases are generally poorly absorbed)
- gastrointestinal motility
- gastrointestinal pH (acidity)
- physico-chemical interaction with the contents of the gut (enzymes, food, other drugs).

Where a drug is required to act more rapidly, or is susceptible to breakdown in the gastrointestinal tract, the preferred route of administration is by injection. There are a number of routes through which drugs are injected and the main ones are subcutaneous (under the skin), intramuscular (into a muscle) and intravenous (directly into the bloodstream via a vein).

Many drugs can be applied topically for a localised response. This may be done by applying a cream, ointment or lotion to an area of skin for treatment of abrasions, lesions, infections or other such dermatological conditions. Topical applications may also involve applying drops to the eye, ear or nose.

Drugs administered by a topical route are not normally absorbed into the body to the same extent as drugs administered orally. Consequently, the WADA regulations regarding certain drugs are complex and are summarised in Table 1.5.

Distribution

Apart from topical administration, a significant proportion of a drug will reach the bloodstream. Most drugs are then dissolved in the water phase of the blood plasma. Within this phase some of the drug molecules may bind to proteins and thus may not be freely diffusible out of the plasma. This will affect the amount of drug reaching its target receptors.

An additional obstruction to the passage of drugs occurs at the 'blood-brain barrier', which comprises a layer of cells that covers the capillary walls of the vessels supplying the brain. This barrier effectively excludes molecules that are poorly lipid soluble. The blood-brain barrier is an important factor to consider in drug design because a drug's ability to cross this barrier can influence its potential for centrally mediated side effects.

Metabolism

The body has a very efficient system for transforming chemicals into safer molecules that can then be excreted by the various routes of elimination. This process

Table 1.5 WADA regulations regarding the route of administration for drugs that are subject to restrictions

Drug class	Prohibited	Allowed subject to therapeutic use	Permitted exemption
Beta-2 Agonists (selected drugs)	Oral Systemic injections	Inhalation	
Glucocorticosteroids	Oral	Inhalation	Topical (anal, aural, nasal, skin, eye)
	Systemic injections	Local injection routes	
	Rectal		

is known as metabolism and many drugs that enter the body undergo metabolic change.

There are several enzyme systems that are responsible for producing metabolic transformations. These enzymes are principally located in the cells of the liver but may also be found in other cells. They produce simple chemical alterations of the drug molecules by processes such as oxidation, reduction, hydrolysis, acetylation and alkylation.

The consequences of drug metabolism may be seen in a number of ways:

1   An active drug is changed into an inactive compound. This is the most common means for the termination of a drug's activity.
2   An active drug can be metabolised into another active compound. The metabolite may have the same pharmacological action as the parent drug or it may differ in terms of higher or lower potency or a different pharmacological effect.
3   An active drug can be changed into a toxic metabolite.
4   An inactive drug can be converted into pharmacologically active metabolites. This mechanism can occasionally be used for beneficial purposes where a drug is susceptible to rapid breakdown before it reaches its site of action. In this case a 'prodrug' can be synthesised, which is resistant to breakdown but which will be metabolised to the active drug on arrival at its target tissue.

Generally speaking, the metabolism of drugs results in the conversion of lipid-soluble drugs into more water-soluble metabolites. This change affects distribution, in that less lipid-soluble compounds are unable to penetrate cell membranes. The kidneys are able to excrete water-soluble compounds more readily than lipid-soluble molecules because the latter can be reabsorbed in the kidney tubules and therefore can re-enter the plasma.

Metabolism is a very important factor in determining a drug's activity because it can alter the drug's intrinsic activity, its ability to reach its site of action and its rate of elimination from the body.

Many drugs are completely metabolised before being excreted in the urine. *The WADA testing procedures in doping control detect both the parent drug and its metabolite(s), where appropriate.*

Elimination

There are many routes through which drugs can be eliminated from the body:

- kidneys (urine)
- salivary glands (saliva)
- sweat glands (sweat)
- pulmonary epithelium (exhaled gases)

- mammary glands (mammary milk)
- rectum (faeces).

The most important route for drug excretion is through the kidneys into the urine. *Urine sampling is the principal method used in dope testing.* The methods available for detecting drugs and their metabolites are extremely sensitive and capable of determining both the nature and the concentration of the drug/metabolite present.

Pharmacological means have been used in an attempt to mask drug-taking activities. These have included the concomitant use of drugs such as Probenecid, whose therapeutic use is in the treatment of gout. Probenecid has also been used for many years in combination with certain antibiotics, as it will delay the excretion of these antibiotics and therefore prolong their antibacterial effect within the body. This property of Probenecid has been used by competitors to try to delay the excretion of banned drugs such as anabolic steroids and thereby avoid detection. However, this effect is not absolute and the testing procedures are sophisticated enough to detect minute quantities of drugs in the urine. Probenecid itself has been on the IOC/WADA list of banned substances since 1987. Diuretics have also been used as masking agents by accelerating urine excretion.

1.6   Effect of exercise on pharmacokinetics

Under most circumstances exercise does not affect the pharmacokinetics of drug action. During severe or prolonged exercise, blood flow within the body will be altered, with a decrease in blood supply to the gastrointestinal tract and to the kidneys. However, there is little documentary evidence to suggest that such changes significantly affect the pharmacokinetics of the majority of drugs.

1.7   Drugs and their targets

Ideally, a drug should interact with a single target to produce the desired effect within the body. However, all drugs possess varying degrees of side effects, largely dependent on the extent to which they interact with sites other than their primary target. During their development, drugs undergo a rigorous evaluation in order to maximise therapeutic effects and minimise side effects. "Designer" drugs, produced by "back-street" laboratories to supply the illicit sport market, will not have undergone rigorous testing for safety.

Drugs can interact with enzymes, carrier molecules and ion channels in cell walls to produce their pharmacological effects. However, the sites through which most drug molecules interact are known as receptors. These receptors are normally specific areas within the structure of cells. They may be located intracellularly but most receptor sites are found on cell membranes. Receptors are present within cells to enable naturally occurring substances, such as neurotransmitters, to induce their biochemical and physiological functions within the body.

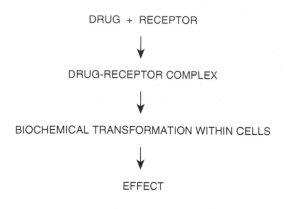

DRUG + RECEPTOR

↓

DRUG-RECEPTOR COMPLEX

↓

BIOCHEMICAL TRANSFORMATION WITHIN CELLS

↓

EFFECT

Figure 1.1 The drug-receptor process.

We exploit the fact that receptors exist, by designing drugs to stimulate (agonists) or block (antagonists) (see section 1.8) these receptors and thereby intensify or reduce biochemical processes within the body.

The interaction between a drug (ligand) and a receptor is the first step in a series of events that eventually leads to a biological effect. This process is illustrated in Figure 1.1. The drug receptor interaction can therefore be thought of as a trigger mechanism.

There are many different receptor sites within the body; each site possesses its own specific arrangement of recognition sites. Drugs are designed to interact with the recognition sites of particular receptors, thereby inducing an effect in the tissue within which the receptors lie. The more closely a drug can fit into its recognition site the greater the triggering response, and therefore the greater the potency of the drug on that tissue. In designing drugs it is sometimes necessary to sacrifice some degree of potency on the target receptor site in order to decrease the side effects.

1.8   Agonists and antagonists

A drug that mimics the action of an endogenous biochemical substance (i.e., one that occurs naturally in the body) is said to be an *agonist*. The potency of agonists depends on two parameters:

- *affinity*: The ability to bind to receptors.
- *efficacy*: The ability, once bound to the receptor, to initiate changes that lead to effects.

Another group of drugs used in therapeutics is known as *antagonists*. They also have the ability to interact with receptor sites but, unlike agonists, do not

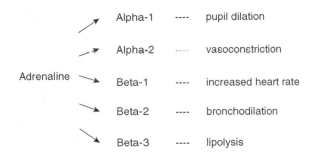

Figure 1.2 Some physiological effects of adrenaline mediated through the five principal classes of adrenergic receptors.

trigger the series of events leading to a response. Their pharmacological effect is produced by preventing the body's own biochemical agents from interacting with the receptors and therefore inhibiting particular physiological processes.

A typical example of this can be seen with beta blockers. They exert their pharmacological effect by occupying beta receptors without stimulating a response but, by doing this, they then prevent the neurotransmitter, noradrenaline (norepinephrine) and the hormone, adrenaline (epinephrine), from interacting with these receptors. Beta blockers therefore reduce the heart rate in exercise or under stress conditions.

Many receptor classes can be subclassified. This can be illustrated by looking at the effect of adrenaline (epinephrine) on adrenergic receptors. We know that there are at least five subclasses of adrenergic receptors, known as alpha-1 (α_1) alpha-2 (α_2) beta-1 (β_1) beta-2 (β_2) and beta-3 (β_3). Adrenaline can interact with all of these receptors, producing a variety of physiological effects, some of which are shown in Figure 1.2. The drug Salbutamol was developed to have a selective effect on beta-2 receptors. It therefore produces bronchodilation, without the other effects associated with adrenaline. As such it is a first-line drug in the treatment of asthma. The selective nature of Salbutamol is recognised by the WADA, who permit its use in sport while other less selective sympathomimetics are banned.

1.9   Side effects of drugs

All drugs produce side effects. Some side effects occur at normal, therapeutic dose levels while other side effects are experienced only at higher dose levels. It should be remembered that, in many instances, athletes take drugs in doses far in excess of those required for therapeutic purposes and in so doing they increase the risk of side effects. Side effects associated with some of the drugs that are commonly misused in sport are shown in Table 1.6.

The side effects of drugs are usually well documented as a result of extensive toxicity studies during the development of the drug and from adverse reaction

Table 1.6 Side effects associated with some drugs that are commonly misused in sport

Class of drugs	Side effects
Amphetamines	Restlessness; irritability; tremor; insomnia; cardiac arrhythmias; aggression; addiction (Knopp, Wang et al., 1997)
Beta-2 agonists	Tremor; tachycardia; cardiac arrhythmias; insomnia; headache (Prather, Brown et al., 1995)
Narcotic analgesics	Constipation; respiratory depression; addiction
Anabolic androgenic steroids	Acne; hypertension; mania; depression; aggression; liver and kidney tumours In females: masculinisation; cliteromegaly In males: testicular atrophy; gynaecomastia (Tucker, 1997)
Diuretics	Dehydration; muscular cramp (Caldwell, 1987)
Human growth hormone	In children: gigantism In adults: acromegaly (hypertension; diabetes; muscular weakness; thickening of the skin) (Healy and Russell-Jones, 1997)
Erythropoietin	Flu-like symptoms; hypertension; thromboses (Drug and Therapeutics Bulletin, 1992)

reporting once the drug is on the market. These predictable toxic effects are more pronounced when the drug is taken in overdose. Accidental toxicity can easily occur with athletes who self-medicate themselves without appreciating the full implications of their actions. The naive philosophy that if one tablet produces a particular desired effect then three tablets must be three times as good frequently prevails in these circumstances.

Non-predictable toxicity can also occur following the administration of therapeutic or even sub-therapeutic doses of drugs. An example of this is *idiosyncrasy,* where a drug produces an unusual reaction within an individual. This effect is normally genetically determined and is often due to a biochemical deficiency, resulting in the patient's over-reaction to the drug. This may be due to the person's inability to metabolise the drug.

A second type of non-predictable toxicity is *drug allergy*. This is an acquired qualitatively altered reaction of the body to a drug. It differs from normal toxicity to drugs in that patients will only exhibit the reaction if they have been previously exposed to the drug or a closely related chemical. This initial exposure to the drug, or its metabolite, sensitises the patient by inducing an allergic response. The drug combines with a protein within the body to produce an antigen, which in turn leads to the formation of other proteins called antibodies. This reaction in itself does not induce toxic effects. However, subsequent exposure to the drug will initiate an antigen-antibody reaction. This allergic reaction can manifest itself in a variety of ways. An acute reaction is known as anaphylaxis and normally occurs within one hour of taking the drug. This response frequently involves the respiratory and cardiovascular systems and is often fatal. Sub-acute allergic reactions usually occur between 1 and 24 hours after the drug is taken and the most common manifestations involve skin reactions, blood dyscrasias, fever and dysfunctions of the respiratory, kidney, liver and cardiovascular systems. Examples of drugs known to produce such allergic responses are aspirin and some antibiotics, including penicillins and cephalosporins.

1.10   Complex drug reactions

Complex reactions may occur during long-term usage of a drug or where more than one drug is being taken simultaneously.

If the frequency of administration exceeds the elimination rate of a drug, then *drug cumulation* occurs, thereby increasing the likelihood of toxic reactions. The reason for a slow elimination may be related to a slow metabolism, a strong tendency to plasma protein binding or an inhibition of excretion, which occurs in patients with kidney disease.

The opposite response to cumulation is seen in patients with *drug resistance*. This drug resistance may be genetically inherited or acquired. The former type of resistance is not common in humans, though it is an increasing problem in antibacterial therapy where pathogenic microbes can develop genetic changes in their structure or biochemistry, which renders them resistant to antibiotic drugs. Acquired resistance to drugs, also known as *tolerance*, can develop with repeated administration of a drug. Where tolerance occurs, more of the drug is needed to produce the same pharmacological response.

A very rapidly developing tolerance is known as *tachyphylaxis* and is seen when a drug is repeatedly administered with a decreasing response to each administration. This is usually caused by a slow rate of detachment of the drug from its receptor sites, so that subsequent doses of the drug are unable to form the drug-receptor complexes that are required to produce an effect.

A number of drugs acting on the central nervous system, particularly the group known as the narcotic analgesics, produce tolerance, which is accompanied by *physical dependence*. This is a state in which an abrupt termination of the administration of the drug produces a series of unpleasant symptoms known as the abstinence syndrome. These symptoms are rapidly reversed after the readministration of the drug. A further manifestation of this problem involves psychogenic dependence in which the drug taker experiences an irreversible craving, or compulsion, to take the drug for pleasure or for relief of discomfort.

Where more than one drug is being taken, there is a possibility for a *drug interaction* to occur. Less commonly, drugs may interact with certain foodstuffs, particularly milk products in which the calcium can bind to certain drugs and limit their absorption. The interactions are, in the main, well documented (BNF, 2009). Their effects can range from minor toxicity to potential fatality.

Table 1.7 Drug interactions between drugs that may be misused in sport

Interacting drugs	Nature of the interaction
Corticosteroids: Human growth hormone	The growth-promoting effect may be inhibited by corticosteroids.
Corticosteroids: Diuretics	Corticosteroids antagonise the diuretic effect. Plasma potassium levels may be decreased (hypokalaemia)
Corticosteroids: β_2-agonists	High doses of these drugs increase the risk of hypokalaemia
Diuretics: Beta blockers	These can enhance a reduction in blood pressure (hypotension)
Diuretics: NSAIDs[+]	Diuretics increase the risk of kidney disease (nephrotoxicity) due to NSAIDs
Diuretics: β_2-agonists	There is an increased risk of hypokalaemia if certain diuretics are taken with β_2-stimulants
NSAIDs[+]: Beta blockers	NSAIDs antagonise the hypotensive effect of beta blockers

[+] NSAIDs (non-steroidal anti-inflammatory drugs) are used commonly for the treatment of sporting injuries and are permitted in sport by WADA.

Interactions involving more than one drug that may be misused in sport are shown in Table 1.7.

1.11   Drugs and the law

The manufacture and supply of drugs is subject to legal control. This legislation may vary from country to country but the principles are the same.

The definition of a medicinal product

A Medicinal product means any substance that is manufactured, sold, supplied, imported or exported for use in either or both of the following ways:

(a) administered to human beings or animals for medicinal purposes
(b) as an ingredient in the preparation of substances administered to human beings or animals for medicinal purposes.

"Medicinal purpose" means any one or more of the following:

(a) treating or preventing disease
(b) diagnosing of disease or physiological condition
(c) providing contraception

(d) inducing anaesthesia
(e) otherwise preventing or interfering with the normal operation of physiological function.

Classes of medicinal products

In many countries, there are three classes of medicinal products:

(1) general sale list medicines (GSL)
(2) pharmacy medicines (P)
(3) prescription-only medicines (POM).

The law of the country dictates which medicines may be purchased and which can only be obtained through a prescription. In general these laws are similar from country to country but exceptions do occur. Most drugs can be obtained, legally or illegally, through internet sources.

Doctors may normally only prescribe drugs or medicines to patients for their licensed therapeutic use. Patients can obtain these *prescription-only medicines* (POMs) from medical practitioners in a hospital, clinic or community practice. Prescriptions are then dispensed by a pharmacist or, in some cases, by a dispensing doctor. Once the prescription has been dispensed, the medicine becomes the property of the patient.

Over-the-counter (OTC) medicines are available for purchase by the general public, without a prescription. These medicines are normally only available from a pharmacy (P medicines) although some medicines, such as aspirin and other analgesics, may be obtained in small pack sizes from other retail outlets (GSL medicines). OTC drugs pose particular problems for athletes, because a number of drugs subject to WADA regulations are available in OTC preparations.

Controlled drugs (CDs), normally those drugs with addictive properties, are subject to further legal restrictions. In most countries CDs include:

• hallucinogenic drugs (e.g. LSD and marijuana)
• opiates (narcotic analgesics, e.g. morphine, heroin)
• amphetamines
• cocaine.

For these drugs, the law states that it is illegal to possess such drugs, except where the user is a registered addict and has obtained their drug legally on prescription.

In some countries anabolic steroids, clenbuterol and some polypeptide hormones are classed as CDs as a further deterrent to their misuse in sport and in body building.

1.12   Why drugs are used in sport

Although there may be many reasons why sportsmen and women use drugs, four main reasons can be identified:

- legitimate therapeutic use (prescription drug or self-medication)
- performance continuation (treatment of sports injuries)
- recreational/social use (legal and illegal)
- performance enhancement.

In each of the above categories there are drugs that appear in the WADA list of banned substances.

Inevitably, clear distinctions cannot always be made between these uses. It would be easy to say that athletes should avoid taking drugs, for any reason, particularly at the time of a competition. However, there are many circumstances when drug taking is advisable, if not imperative for the general health and well-being of the athlete. Therefore it would be prudent for athletes to consider the specific need for taking drugs and the full implications of their action.

Legitimate therapeutic use of drugs

Like any other person, an athlete is liable to suffer from a major or minor illness that requires treatment with drugs. A typical example might involve a bacterial or fungal infection necessitating the use of an antibiotic or antifungal agent. Apart from side effects such treatment would be unlikely to affect an athlete's performance. A less common but more serious medical condition would be epilepsy or diabetes. Under these circumstances it would be inconceivable for an athlete to consider participating in sport without regular treatment with drugs.

For many minor illnesses, such as coughs, colds, gastrointestinal upsets and hay fever, it is possible to obtain medications without visiting the doctor. There is a wide range of preparations available for the treatment of minor illnesses, which can be purchased from a pharmacy without a prescription. Athletes should carefully scrutinise the labels on such medication to ensure that a banned substance such as ephedrine, methylephedrine or cathine is not included in the medicine.

It is in the athlete's interest, in the event of visiting a medical practitioner, to discuss the nature of any drug treatment and to avoid the prescribing of prohibited substances wherever possible.

Performance continuation

Athletes frequently experience injuries involving muscles, ligaments and tendons. Provided that the injury is not too serious, it is common for the athlete to take palliative treatment in the form of analgesic and anti-inflammatory drugs.

This enables the athlete to continue to train and even compete during the period of recovery from the injury. The wisdom of such action is perhaps open to question but the use of analgesics under these circumstances is unlikely to confer an unfair advantage.

The doping regulations restrict the type of analgesics that can be used and control the methods of administration for drugs such as glucocorticosteroids. In weighing up the consequences of giving a pain-killing injection, a doctor would probably take into account the time available before the athlete is in competition and the extent of the injury. The inappropriate injection of glucocorticosteroids could have deleterious effects on joints (Fredberg, 1997) and systemic complications are not uncommon (Leadbetter, 1990). Even non-steroidal anti-inflammatory drugs (NSAIDs), such as aspirin, though widely used, are liable to produce adverse effects such as gastrointestinal bleeding and ulceration (Weiler, 1992; Leadbetter, 1995). Hertel (1997) has suggested that NSAIDs may not hasten the return of injured athletes back to competition.

Recreational/social use

Many cultures, throughout the ages, have used the drugs listed in Table 1.8 for social and recreational purposes. These substances range from caffeine, a constituent of beverages frequently consumed in many societies, through generally socially tolerated drugs such as alcohol and cannabinoids, to the hard, addictive drugs such as the narcotic analgesics related to heroin and morphine and the psychomotor stimulants such as cocaine. The use of these drugs, particularly in Western cultures, has grown in recent years. This has been reflected in the increasing numbers of positive test results, particularly for cannabinoids, from WADA-accredited laboratories.

Although these drugs may be taken in a social or recreational setting, they can all affect performance, hence they are subject to WADA regulations.

Amphetamines

In the UK, it has been estimated that 10 per cent of 16- to 59-year-olds, rising to 20 per cent of 16- to 29-year-olds have tried amphetamine (Anon, 2000).

Table 1.8 Drugs used socially or recreationally that are subject to WADA regulations

Drug	WADA regulation
Amphetamines	Prohibited class S6 (stimulants)
Cocaine	Prohibited class S6 (stimulants)
Narcotics	Prohibited class S7
Alcohol	Prohibited in particular sports class P1
Cannabinoids	Prohibited class S8

Amphetamines are used socially to produce alertness and energy. However, they also impair judgement and concentration and heavy use leads to depression and anxiety. There is a risk of addiction with regular use of amphetamine (Knopp, Wang *et al.*, 1997).

Cocaine

Cocaine is a powerful stimulant. It is usually inhaled as a powder but a crystalline ("crack") form of cocaine is smoked as a vapour. The complex pharmacology of cocaine leads to a wide spectrum of adverse effects, including a negative effect on glycogenolysis, paranoid psychosis, seizures, hypertension and myocardial toxicity, which could lead to ischaemia, arrhythmias and sudden death, especially following intense exercise (Conlee, 1991; Eichner, 1993). Smoked "crack" cocaine is more dangerous as the rate of absorption is greater, leading to a more intense effect on the cardiovascular system (Ghaphery, 1995). After regular use, addictive cravings for cocaine can persist for a period of months.

Some bizarre fatalities have been linked to concomitant use of cocaine with alcohol and anabolic steroids, which may have resulted in the production of a novel, cardiotoxic metabolite, norcocaine (Welder and Melchert, 1993).

Caffeine

Perhaps the most widely used social drug is caffeine, which is present in many of the beverages that we consume daily. Caffeine was on the IOC-banned list but was removed by WADA in January 2004. However, it is still on the WADA monitoring list.

Narcotics

Narcotics are potent drugs whose effects are primarily on the central nervous system. The discovery of opiate receptors within the brain has helped in understanding the mode of action of morphine, heroin and other related narcotic analgesics. They appear to mimic the effect of certain endogenous opiates, known as endorphins and enkephalin. Narcotics are renowned for their ability to cause tolerance and dependence in the regular user.

Alcohol

Alcohol is the most commonly used drug in Britain, with only 7 per cent of males and 13 per cent of females describing themselves as non-drinkers (Anon, 2000). Though taken for recreational purposes, the effects of alcohol may well be manifested in the field of sport. Some sporting events even take place in an environment where alcohol is freely available both to the spectator and the performer. Alcohol suppresses inhibitions but also impairs judgement and reflexes. Alcohol is prohibited in certain sports.

Cannabinoids

The precise mode of action of cannabinoids is not fully understood but the effects produced are principally euphoria and elation accompanied by a loss of perception of time and space. Although unlikely to be used as a performance-enhancing substance in sport, events in recent years have shown that marijuana is used as part of the lifestyle of many athletes. Cannabinoids are prohibited, by WADA, in all sports.

Performance enhancement

Drug use for potential performance enhancement is the most serious threat to the credibility of competitive sport and has become subject to doping control regulations. It concerns the deliberate, illegitimate use of drugs in an attempt to gain an unfair advantage over fellow competitors.

Trying to define performance enhancement may actually obscure the fundamental principle, as explained by Sir Arthur Porritt, first Chairman of the IOC Medical Commission. "[T]o define doping is, if not impossible, at best extremely difficult, and yet everyone who takes part in competitive sport or who administers it knows exactly what it means. The definition lies not in words but in integrity of character" (Porritt, 1965). In essence, it encompasses the principle of cheating, defined in the antidoping regulations of individual sports. The issue of doping is one that will continue to attract extensive media attention at major sporting events.

The remaining chapters of this book provide a detailed analysis of the substances and methods that are used for performance enhancement in sport and the past and present attempts at doping control.

1.13   References

Anon. (2000). *Drugs: Dilemmas, choices and the law*. Joseph Rowntree Foundation, York, England.

British National Formulary (BNF). (2009). *Appendix 1. Drug Interactions*. British Medical Association and Royal Pharmaceutical Society of Great Britain, London.

Caldwell, J.E. (1987). Diuretic therapy and exercise performance. *Sports Medicine* **4**, 290–304.

Conlee, R.K. (1991). *Amphetamine, caffeine and cocaine: Perspectives in exercise science and sports medicine*. Brown and Benchmark, New York. 285–328.

Drug and Therapeutics Bulletin. (1992). Epoetin. An important advance. *Drug and Therapeutics Bulletin* **30**, 29–32.

Eichner, E.R. (1993). Ergolytic drugs in medicine and sports. *American Journal of Medicine* **94**, 205–211.

Fredberg, U. (1997). Local corticosteroid injection in sport: Review of literature and guidelines for treatment. *Scandinavian Journal of Medicine and Science in Sports* **7**, 131–139.

Ghaphery, N.A. (1995). Performance-enhancing drugs. *Orthopedic Clinics of North America* **26**, 433–442.

Healy, M.L. and D. Russell-Jones. (1997). Growth hormone and sport: Abuse, potential benefits, and difficulties in detection. *British Journal of Sports Medicine* **31**, 267–268.

Hertel, J. (1997). The role of nonsteroidal anti-inflammatory drugs in the treatment of acute soft tissue injury. *Journal of Athletic Training* **32**, 350–358.

Knopp, W.D., Wang, T.W., and Bacch, B.R. Jr. (1997). Ergogenic drugs in sports. *Clinics in Sports Medicine* **16**, 375–392.

Leadbetter, W.B. (1990). *Corticosteroid injection therapy in sports injuries: Sports-induced inflammation.* American Academy of Orthopaedic Surgeons, Park Ridge, Illinois. 527–545.

Leadbetter, W.B. (1995). Anti-inflammatory therapy in sports injury: The role of nonsteroidal drugs and corticosteroid injection. *Clinics in Sports Medicine* **14**, 353–410.

Porritt, A. (1965). Doping. *The Journal of Sports Medicine and Physical Fitness* **5(3)**, 166–168.

Prather, I.D., Brown, D.E., North, P. *et al.* (1995). Clenbuterol: a substitute of anabolic steroids? *Medicine and Science in Sports & Exercise* **27**, 1118–1121.

Tucker, R. (1997). Abuse of anabolic-androgenic steroids by athletes and body builders: A review. *Pharmaceutical Journal* **259**, 171–179.

Weiler, J.M. (1992). Medical modifiers of sports injury: The use of nonsteroidal anti-inflammatory drugs (NSAIDs) in sports soft-tissue injury. *Clinics in Sports Medicine* **11**, 625–644.

Welder, A.A. and Melchert, R.B. (1993). Cardiotoxic effects of cocaine and anabolic-androgenic steroids in the athlete. *Journal of Pharmacological and Toxicological Methods* **29**, 61–68.

Chapter 2

A historical perspective of doping and anti-doping in sport

David R. Mottram

2.1 Introduction

The history of organised sport dates back to ancient Greece. By the seventh century BC, religion, culture and sport were all an integral part of Greek society and this tradition continued through to the Roman era. There is little documented evidence for organised sport between the fall of the Roman Empire and the mid-nineteenth century. At this time, sport comprised recreational activities associated with religious, cultural and seasonal events (Anon, 2001). By the end of the nineteenth century, urbanisation and industrialisation had transformed sport into a more organised activity with associated rules and the formation of sporting clubs and institutions. As the twentieth century progressed, participation in sport increased. More people became spectators and commercial interests developed.

After the Second World War, international pharmaceutical companies expanded the armoury of medicines available to tackle ill health. Drugs that had hitherto been derived principally from plant and animal sources were now manufactured in the laboratory. Athletes turned to these new, potent drugs to enhance performance.

Attempts to control substance misuse in sport began around the nineteen fifties. However, ignorance of the extent of the problem, a lack of sophistication of testing procedures and uncoordinated systems for legislating against doping meant that those intent on introducing anti-doping measures were initially playing catch-up. It was not until the beginning of the twenty-first century, with the formation of the World Anti-Doping Agency (WADA), that the anti-doping movement gained the upper hand.

Figure 2.1 shows a time-line for significant events related to sport, doping and anti-doping, from the ancient Olympics to the current time. These events are described in more detail in the rest of this chapter.

2.2 The ancient Olympic and Roman games

The Ancient Olympic Games began in 776 BC and were the most important of the Panhellenic Games. Initially, the Games were composed of just running events.

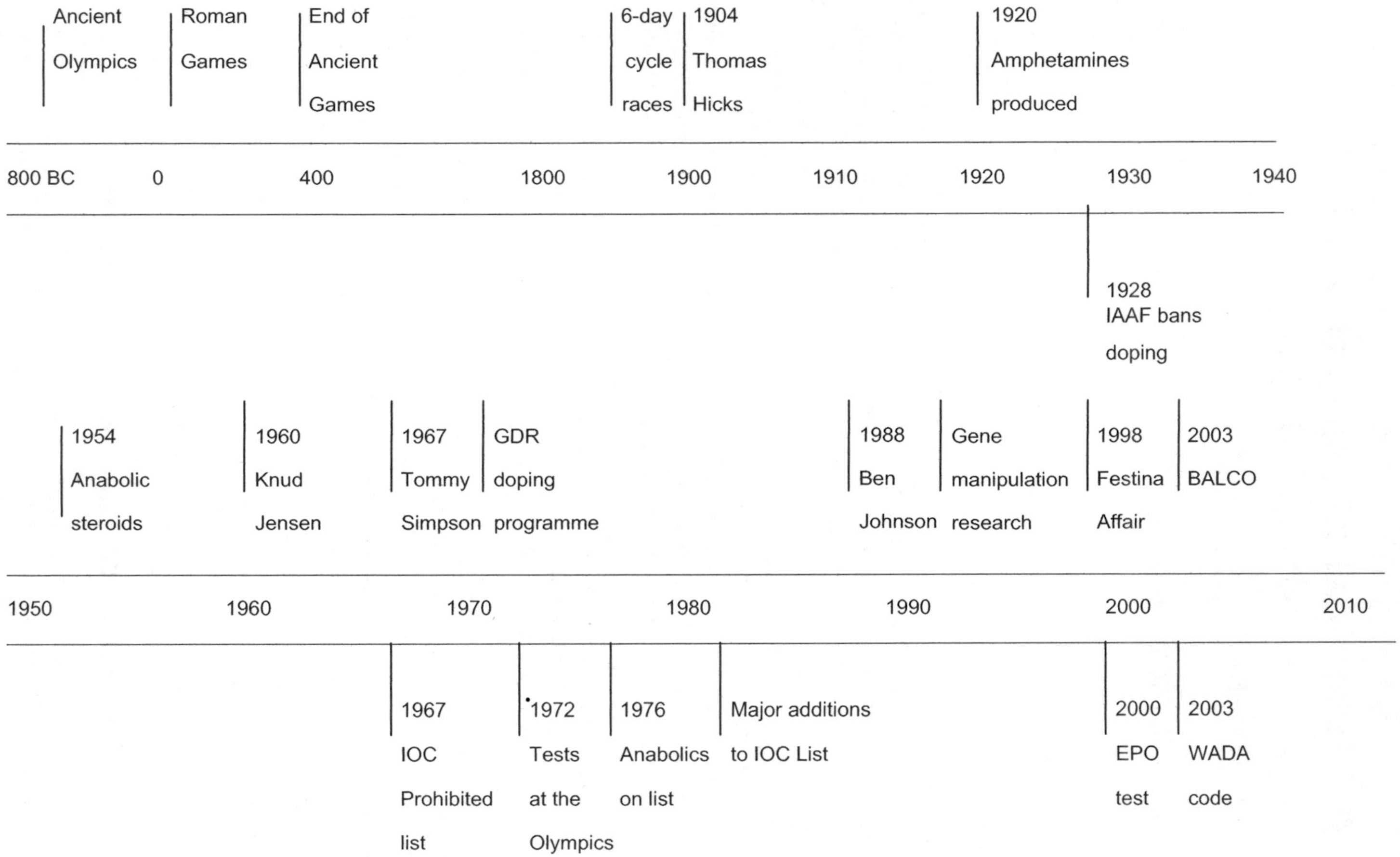

Figure 2.1 Time-line for significant events related to sport, doping and anti-doping.

Over the centuries other sports, such as wrestling, boxing, chariot racing, long jump, javelin and discus throwing were introduced. Participants represented their city-states and the victors were rewarded with rich prizes and high esteem. Even in those days athletes resorted to cheating in order to reap the rewards of victory.

2.3   Nineteenth century

At the beginning of the nineteenth century sport reflected a rural way of life, including boxing, races, football and sports involving animals, such as cockfighting (Anon, 2001). The increasing industrialisation of society altered people's lifestyles. Transport systems improved and leisure time increased along with people's disposable income. All these factors had an impact on the development of sport, which became more organised, with clubs and societies being formed. Some sports became more professional and stadia were built where spectators could pay to watch their heroes.

Most drugs were still extracted from plant and animal sources. Those used by athletes included stimulants such as caffeine (from tea and coffee), strychnine (from the seeds of *Strychnos nux vomica*) and cocaine (from the leaves of the coca plant). The analgesic morphine (from the opium poppy) and the depressant alcohol (brewed and/or distilled from a variety of sources) were also used. It is widely accepted that the word "doping" derives from "dop", an alcoholic beverage made from grape skins that was used in South Africa and exported by the Dutch in the nineteenth century.

Few reports of drug use in sport were recorded, although cycle racing, a sport long associated with substance misuse, had its roots in the late nineteenth century when gruelling six-day cycle races took place in Europe and involved cyclists taking cocktails of the types of drugs mentioned above.

2.4   Early twentieth century

The first recorded instance of drug use in the modern Olympics occurred in the 1904 Games in St. Louis, where the marathon runner, Thomas Hicks, received doses of strychnine and brandy during the closing stages of the race. Drugs were still crude products, the international pharmaceutical companies having not yet been developed.

Amphetamine, in 1920, was one of the earliest drugs to be produced synthetically in the laboratory. In 1935 it was used to treat narcolepsy, depression, anxiety and hyperactivity in children (George, 2005). Athletes were free to access what substances were available as there was little regulation in sport. The first International Sport Federation to ban the use of doping (stimulants) was the International Amateur Athletic Federation, in 1928, although restrictions remained ineffective because no tests were made (Fraser, 2004).

2.5   Nineteen forties and nineteen fifties

Amphetamine was used widely in society to enhance mental awareness, a property that was exploited during the Second World War to delay fatigue in combat troops and air crew. This non-therapeutic use of drugs was then mirrored in sport, where athletes experimented with amphetamines to enhance performance (Verroken, 1996).

The use of anabolic steroids in sport dates back to the nineteen fifties. Dr. John Ziegler, a physician to the American weightlifting team, suspected the Soviet team of using testosterone at the 1954 World Weightlifting Championships in Vienna (Hoberman, 1992). Dianabol was synthesized in 1958 and was used by the American weightlifters at the 1962 World Championships.

In the nineteen fifties, multinational drug companies evolved and invested huge sums of money on research into new classes of drugs for the treatment of diseases. It was not long before athletes tapped into this rich source of potential performance-enhancing drugs.

2.6   Nineteen sixties

Several major new classes of drugs, developed by the pharmaceutical industry in the nineteen fifties, were marketed in the nineteen sixties. These included oral contraceptives, corticosteroids, beta blockers, tranquilizers and antidepressants. The nineteen sixties heralded the era of experimentation into the non-therapeutic use of drugs both socially and in sport.

Although it is difficult to attribute mortality and morbidity directly to drug use, as there may be other contributory factors, there were a number of deaths of athletes directly associated with drug taking during the nineteen sixties. The cyclist Knud Jensen died in the 100-km team time trial at the 1960 Rome Olympic Games and Tommy Simpson perished during the 1967 Tour de France. Both deaths were associated with amphetamine use but both occurred under exceptional conditions of heat and exhaustion (George, 2005).

The fear of bringing sport into disrepute meant that many sporting authorities denied the possibility that doping took place, therefore, anti-doping testing was, at best, haphazard. The international federations for football (FIFA) and cycling (UCI) introduced doping tests into their respective world championships in 1966. In 1967, the International Olympic Committee (IOC) instituted its Medical Commission and set up a list of prohibited substances (Table 2.1). The first mandatory tests at Olympic events were in 1968 at the Winter Olympics in Grenoble and at the Summer Games in Mexico (Fraser, 2004).

2.7   Nineteen seventies

The paper by Franke and Berendonk (1997), written after the reunification of Germany, provides a startling account of state-controlled doping by the German

Table 2.1 Major changes to the IOC Prohibited List, 1967–2003

Year	Classes of substances and methods prohibited	Major changes
1967	1. Central nervous system stimulants 2. Psychomotor stimulants 3. Sympathomimetic amines 4. Narcotic analgesics	
1976		• Anabolic steroids added
1985		• Beta blockers and diuretics added • Prohibited methods added, including blood doping and pharmacological, chemical and physical manipulation
1987		• Probenecid and other masking agents added
1988	I *Doping classes* Stimulants Narcotic analgesics Anabolic steroids Beta blockers Diuretics II *Doping methods* Blood doping Pharmacological, chemical and physical manipulation III *Classes of drugs subject to certain restrictions* Alcohol Local anaesthetics corticosteroids	• CNS and psychomotor stimulants and sympathomimetics grouped under stimulants • Classes of drugs subject to certain restrictions added
1989		• Peptide hormones and analogues added
1993		• Beta blockers moved to "drugs subject to certain restrictions" • Anabolic steroid class re-named as anabolic agents to incorporate clenbuterol • Codeine removed from the list
2000		• Oxygen carriers and plasma expanders added • Erythropoietin added to peptide hormones

(continued)

Table 2.1 (Cont'd)

Year	Classes of substances and methods prohibited	Major changes
2003	I *Prohibited classes of substances* Stimulants Narcotics Anabolic agents Diuretics Peptide hormones, mimetics and analogues Agents with anti-oestrogenic activity Masking agents II *Prohibited methods* Enhancement of oxygen transfer Pharmacological, chemical and physical manipulation Gene doping III *Classes of prohibited substances in certain sports* Alcohol Cannabinoids Local anaesthetics Glucocorticosteroids Beta blockers	• The IOC and WADA produce a joint prohibited list • Agents with anti-oestrogenic activity added • A separate class of masking agents added • Gene doping added as a prohibited method • Enhancement of oxygen transfer added to include blood doping and the administration of products that enhance the uptake, transport or delivery of oxygen • The title of Section III changed • Marijuana changed to cannabinoids

Democratic Republic during the late sixties and nineteen seventies. Scientists and physicians undertook research into systematic doping of thousands of athletes, with particular emphasis on the use of anabolic steroid administration to adult women and adolescent girls, despite documentation of serious side effects.

Most international sports federations had introduced systems for drug testing by the nineteen seventies. However, the IOC prohibited list only contained narcotic analgesics and three classes of stimulants (sympathomimetic amines, psychomotor stimulants and central nervous system stimulants). The first comprehensive testing at an Olympic games took place in Munich in 1972. Nine positive results for stimulants were detected from more than 2000 tests.

The use of anabolic steroids was known to be widespread but a reliable method for testing was not available in the early nineteen seventies. The IOC added anabolic steroids to the prohibited list in 1976, as testing improved.

Whilst anti-doping measures to control stimulants and anabolic steroids was beginning to have an impact, the nineteen seventies witnessed the use of blood doping as a method to increase the oxygen-carrying capacity of the blood.

2.8   Nineteen eighties

The nineteen eighties was a turbulent time for sport, with political differences being manifested through boycotts at the Olympic Games of 1980 in Moscow and 1984 in Los Angeles. In addition, there were accusations of a cover-up at the 1983 World Track and Field Championships and the withdrawal of athletes from the Pan American Games when word got through that drug testing was to be included (Hunt, 2008).

Blood doping, in 1985, was the first doping method to be added to the IOC prohibited list, following reports of its use by the US cycling team at the 1984 Los Angeles Olympics. In 1985, the IOC amended the prohibited list to include beta blockers and diuretics as doping agents and pharmacological, chemical and physical manipulation as prohibited methods. Despite this, in 1988 at the Tour de France the cyclist Pedro Delgado tested positive for probenecid, a masking agent that was banned according to the IOC prohibited list but was not on the banned list for the International Cycling Union. This inconsistency between sporting authorities meant that Delgado was not disqualified and eventually won the race.

During the late nineteen eighties, a number of countries, particularly in Scandinavia, developed national anti-doping organisations (NADOs) in an attempt to strengthen anti-doping activity across the boundaries of individual sports (Vance, 2007).

The most significant event of the nineteen eighties occurred at the Seoul Olympic Games in 1988, when Ben Johnson tested positive for the anabolic steroid stanazolol. This was significant for a number of reasons. It showed that athletes in disciplines other than pure strength events were using steroids and that athletes who thought that they could avoid detection were vulnerable to testing regimes. The Ben Johnson affair drew the attention of the world to the issue of doping in sport.

2.9   Nineteen nineties

The incidence of high-profile doping cases continued into the nineteen nineties. Many of these illustrated the inconsistencies that existed between the IOC and individual sports federations regarding their respective prohibited lists and the application of regulations.

Evidence for the use of the hormone erythropoietin (EPO) to enhance oxygen transport, by increasing red blood cell production, led to the addition of EPO to the IOC prohibited list, despite the absence of a validated test.

In 1992, the sprinter Diane Modahl received a four-year ban when she tested positive for testosterone during an event in Portugal. However, after a protracted appeal her suspension was lifted, the laboratory having failed to follow the accredited procedures for testing.

The pre-testing of two British weightlifters, prior to the 1992 Olympic Games in Barcelona, led to their ban for using clenbuterol. This drug is (beta-2 agonist), classed under stimulants. However, clenbuterol was being used for anabolic effects, a secondary pharmacological property that a number of β_2-agonists possess. The chemical nature of β_2-agonists does not permit their classification as anabolic steroids. Consequently, in 1993, the IOC changed its prohibited list to include the class of anabolic agents, which include anabolic steroids and other agents with anabolic properties, principally the β_2-agonists.

The culture of athletes taking substances to enhance performance has meant that the majority of athletes use legal supplements. These may be nutritional, such as vitamins, or ergogenic, such as protein supplements. However, the production and marketing of supplements is not always robust. In the late nineteen nineties, a spate of positive dope tests for the anabolic steroid nandrolone occurred, which, it was claimed, had been taken inadvertently in supplements. This was substantiated by a study showing that many supplements do contain hormone-based constituents that may lead to athletes testing positive (Schänzer, 2002).

In 1963, the French government had enacted national anti-doping legislation. This allowed the French police to undertake a raid during the 1998 Tour de France in which they recovered a large number of prohibited substances. This became known as the "Festina Affair" (Armstrong, 2005).

By the end of the nineteen nineties, questions were being asked as to whether the IOC prohibited list needed updating (Mottram, 1999). More significantly, the whole question of the harmonization of doping control was called into question. The IOC convened the World Conference on Doping in Sport in February 1999 resulting in the establishment of WADA in November 1999 (Anon, 2008). The main reasons for WADA being created were that different international sport federations and national anti-doping organisations were operating different rules, leading to doping cases being contested in courts. There was a lack of a coordinated research policy, particularly with respect to new analytical methods; little had been done to promote anti-doping activities internationally (Catlin *et al.*, 2008).

2.10   Two thousand and beyond

The first decade of the new millennium heralded a number of significant events associated with doping and anti-doping.

A validated test for EPO was introduced at the 2000 Olympic Games in Sydney (Lasne and Ceaurriz, 2000). Despite this, many athletes continued to use EPO, particularly in the sport of cycling.

With the increasing robustness and sensitivity of testing procedures, illicit drug suppliers were attempting to produce "designer" drugs that were ostensibly "undetectable". The most notorious of these was tetrahydrogestrinone (THG), produced by the Bay Area Laboratory Co-operative (BALCO). This drug was eventually identified, resulting in the widespread sanctioning of a large number of high-profile athletes.

The use by athletes of over-the-counter (OTC) medicines to treat minor conditions has created serious problems. Many of these products contain minor stimulants such as ephedrine. A number of high-profile athletes tested positive, including Andreea Raducan, a gymnast who lost her gold medal from the Sydney Olympics in 2000 for using pseudoephedrine and Alain Baxter, the skier who tested positive for methamphetamine at the 2002 Winter Olympics in Salt Lake City (Armstrong and Chester, 2005). These and other cases led to the removal of most of these OTC drugs from the first prohibited list produced by WADA in 2004. These drugs were placed on a monitoring list and their use is still recorded by some WADA laboratories. Recent evidence, however, has suggested that some of these drugs are now perceived as a fair target for performance enhancement (Mottram et al., 2008), leading WADA to reconsider their prohibited status. In January 2010, WADA re-introduced pseudoephedrine to the prohibited list, where an adverse analytical finding is recorded if a urinary threshold of 150 microgram/ml is exceeded.

Research into gene technology had been undertaken to develop non-drug-based prevention and treatment of disease. Such technology was also being used to improve drug design by more precisely targeting drugs to their therapeutic site of action. In anticipation of this technology being applied to enhance sporting performance, the IOC and WADA added gene doping to the prohibited list in 2003. However, by the end of the decade, it was suggested that although gene transfer in humans could theoretically lead to gene doping the prospect remained theoretical (Wells, 2008). Monitoring technological advances in this field remains imperative.

WADA produced the World Anti-Doping Code in 2003 and became responsible for its prohibited list in January 2004 (Table 2.2). WADA invited all stakeholders to comply with the code. This included athletes and their supporters, sports federations, the Olympic movement and governments. The World Anti-Doping Code was implemented for the first time at the Olympic Games in Athens in 2004. By the end of the decade, most sports, apart from some professional sports in the United States, had declared their support for WADA and many governments had signed up in support of the UNESCO International Convention against Doping in Sport. Furthermore, since 2006, WADA had been working closely with international enforcement agencies to uncover doping activities such as trafficking, which would not come to light through the athlete testing procedures (Vance, 2007). This was exemplified by the US Enforcement Administration's operation, called Raw Deal, which involved 10 countries and resulted in 124 arrests and the seizure of large quantities of steroids from 56 laboratories across the US, mainly supplied from companies in China (Vance, 2007).

A further strengthening of the testing procedures was implemented through athletes having to declare their whereabouts for periods during the week in order to facilitate no-notice, out-of-competition testing with penalties for missed tests. Testing authorities increased their use of "intelligence" testing where, instead of

Table 2.2 Major changes to the WADA prohibited list, 2004–2010

Year	Classes of substances and methods prohibited	Major changes
2004	*I Substances and methods prohibited in competition* S1 Stimulants S2 Narcotics S3 Cannabinoids S4 Anabolic agents S5 Peptide hormones S6 β_2-agonists S7 Agents with anti-oestrogenic activity S8 Masking agents S9 Glucocorticosteroids M1 Enhancement of oxygen transfer M2 Pharmacological, chemical and physical manipulation M3 Gene doping *II Substances and methods prohibited in and out of competition* Sections S4 to S8 and M1 to M3 above *III Substances prohibited in particular sports* P1 Alcohol P2 Beta blockers P3 Diuretics *IV Specified substances*	• β_2-agonists now a separate class • Diuretics included in S8 as masking agents but also prohibited in sports (P3) when used to reduce weight • Most OTC stimulants (e.g. caffeine, pseudoephedrine) removed but placed on a monitoring list • Therapeutic Use Exemption introduced for some classes such as β_2-agonists and glucocorticosteroids • Specified substances added where some classes or specific substances within classes are subject to reduced sanctions if taken inadvertently • Glucocorticosteroids now prohibited in all sports
2005	*I Substances and methods prohibited at all times (in and out of competition)* S1 Anabolic agents S2 Hormones and related substances S3 β_2-agonists S4 Agents with anti-oestrogenic activity S5 Diuretics and other masking agents M1 Enhancement of oxygen transfer M2 Chemical and physical manipulation M3 Gene doping *II Substances and methods prohibited in competition* All categories in Section I plus S6 Stimulants S7 Narcotics S8 Cannabinoids S9 Glucocorticosteroids *III Substances prohibited in particular sports* P1 Alcohol P2 Beta blockers *IV Specified substances*	• Re-arrangement of how substances and methods prohibited in competition and out of competition were presented • β_2-agonists now prohibited in and out of competition • Diuretics removed from Section III and specifically mentioned with masking agents

Table 2.2 (Cont'd)

Year	Classes of substances and methods prohibited	Major changes
2008		• Class S4 changed to hormone antagonists and modulators to include other groups of drugs that affect endogenous hormones • Selective androgen receptor modulators added to S1 anabolic agents
2009		• The Section IV specified substances removed as the definition was changed • Abbreviated TUEs removed
2010		• Class S2 changed to peptide hormones, growth factors and related substances • Salbutamol and salmeterol no longer require a TUE • Pseudoephedrine returned to the list

randomly testing athletes, resources are more focused on athletes who are either in higher risk sports and/or by their own behaviour or biological profile (athlete passports) trigger an element of suspicion (Vance, 2007).

WADA undertakes an annual review of the prohibited list, major changes to which are presented in Table 2.2.

2.11   The race between doping and anti-doping

As stated at the beginning of this chapter, taking substances in order to enhance performance in sport dates back to the ancient games. The criteria on which this behaviour is founded are multiple and complex. However, three major criteria can be identified:

- a *culture* of using substances to gain an advantage over fellow competitors;
- the *potential* for performance enhancement based on the effectiveness of current substances;
- the *availability* of such substances.

Similarly, the success of anti-doping policies depends on many criteria, including:

- the *determination* of those responsible for sport to combat the problem of doping;
- the *harmonization* of policies and approaches to combat doping;
- the *effectiveness* of systems for testing doping activity.

The extent to which these criteria have impacted on trends in doping and anti-doping over time has been depicted in Figure 2.2.

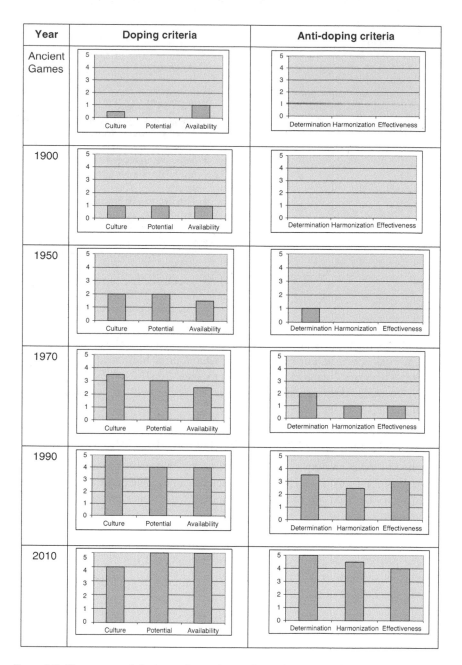

Figure 2.2 The extent of doping and anti-doping from the ancient Games to the present, related to specific criteria.

With respect to *doping,* the *culture* dates back to ancient times. In modern times this culture increased throughout the twentieth century, peaking in the last decade, with a decline by the end of the first decade of the twenty-first century as the impact of WADA became manifest. The *potential* for performance enhancement was virtually non-existent in ancient times, but has again gradually increased over the twentieth century with the development of more potent and selective drugs with fewer side effects. This trend continued into the twenty-first century and is unlikely to recede as drug development techniques improve. With respect to *availability,* those athletes determined to dope have always been able to gain access to doping substances. The advent of internet access in the past few decades has significantly facilitated this access.

Anti-doping has tended to lag several steps behind trends in doping. The *determination* to combat doping was slow to develop. However, doping is now acknowledged as a serious threat to the whole concept of fair play in sport. Those organisations responsible for anti-doping were, for too long, applying different rules and approaches to anti-doping regulation. *Harmonization* only became a reality with the establishment of WADA. However, even at the present time, the World Anti-Doping Code has not been adopted by all stakeholders. The *effectiveness* of testing methods has tended to lag behind the practices of serious dopers and their facilitators, though current testing regimes are highly sophisticated. However, testing regimes still need improving in terms of consistency between nations and a greater emphasis on out-of-competition testing.

In summary, those athletes and their facilitators who have indulged in serious doping activities have so far remained one step ahead of the anti-doping organisations. However, the rapid rise in determination, harmonization and effectiveness of those responsible for anti-doping, including the willingness of all stakeholders to shoulder responsibility, means that the race is now neck-and-neck.

2.12   References

Anon. (2001). *The history of drug use in sport.* Australian Sports Drug Agency. Available at http://www.ausport.gov.au/fulltext/2001/asda/drugsinsporthistory.asp (accessed 20 October 2009).

Anon. (2008). *History of drug-free sport.* World Anti-Doping Agency. Available at http://www.uksport.gov.au/pages/history_of_drug_free_sport/ (accessed 4 November 2009).

Armstrong, D.J. (2005). Blood boosting and sport. In *Drugs in Sport*, 4th ed., ed. D.R. Mottram, Routledge, London.

Armstrong, D.J. and Chester, N. (2005). Drugs used in respiratory tract disorders. In *Drugs in Sport*, 4th ed., ed. D.R. Mottram, Routledge, London.

Catlin, D.H., Fitch, K.D. and Ljungqvist, A. (2008). Medicine and science in the fight against doping in sport. *Journal of Internal Medicine* **264**, 99–114.

Franke, W.W. and Berendonk, B. (1997). Hormonal doping and androgenization of athletes: A secret program of the German Democratic Republic government. *Clinical Chemistry* **43(7)**, 1262–1279.

Fraser, A.D. (2004). Doping control from a global and national perspective. *Therapeutic Drug Monitor* **26**, 171–174.

George, A.J. (2005). CNS stimulants. In *Drugs in sport*, 4th ed., ed. D.R. Mottram, Routledge, London.

Hoberman, J.M. (1992). Faster, higher stronger. A history of doping in sport. In *Mortal engines: The science of performance and dehumanization of sport,* ed. J.M. Hoberman, Maxwell Macmillan Canada, Toronto.

Hunt, T.M. (2008). The lessons of crisis: Olympic doping regulations during the 1980s. *Iron Game History* **10(2)**, 12–25.

Lasne, F. and Ceaurriz, J.D. (2000). Recombinant erythropoietin in urine. *Nature* **405**, 635.

Mottram, D.R. (1999). Banned drugs in sport. Does the International Olympic Committee (IOC) list need updating? *Sports Medicine* **27(1)**, 1–10.

Mottram, D., Chester, N., Atkinson, G. *et al.* (2008). Athletes' knowledge and views on OTC medication. *International Journal of Sports Medicine* **29**, 851–855.

Schänzer, W. (2002). Analysis of non-hormonal nutritional supplements for anabolic-androgenic steroids—An international study. Available at www.olympic.org (accessed 27 September 2009).

Vance, N. (2007). Developments in anti-doping in elite sports. *Journal of Exercise Science and Fitness* **5(2)**, 75–78.

Verroken, M. (1996). Drug use and abuse in sport. In *Drugs in sport*, 2nd ed., ed. D.R. Mottram, E. & F.N. Spon, London.

Wells, D.J. (2008). Gene doping: The hype and the reality. *British Journal of Pharmacology* **154**, 623–631.

Chapter 3

Medicines for Olympic and Commonwealth Games

Mark Stuart

3.1 Introduction

Providing medical services at Olympic, Paralympic and Commonwealth Games is a truly unique challenge, on a scale unrivalled by any other public event. Not only must the medical services cater to the highly specialised therapeutic needs of up to 14,000 athletes during the Olympics and 4,500 athletes of the Paralympic Games, but they must also supply the needs of accredited support staff, team medical units, officials, and media.

For the London 2012 Olympic Games an expected 250,000 accredited people will fall under the care of the Olympic medical services, with around 40,000 people alone living in the Olympic Village. In addition to this, around 9 million tickets will be sold to spectators. London will see a huge population increase during the Games with a possible increased demand on local medical services.

Staffing Olympic and Paralympic medical services is also a huge logistical operation. At the Sydney 2000 Olympic Games, a total of 4500 local medical volunteers provided specialist care at 35 Olympic venues; similarly, 4000 medical volunteers were recruited for the Atlanta 1996 Olympics. In Athens 2004, 400 specialist doctors, 400 nurses and 400 physiotherapists made up the core of the local medical team. For the pharmacy services alone in Beijing 2008, more than 50 pharmacists were required for two Olympic villages in Beijing and Hong Kong. In addition to the local medical workforce, over 1000 doctors also resided in the athlete village to treat each of the teams from around 200 countries.

As well as looking after the athletes' therapeutic sports-medicine requirements, the doctors and pharmacists are also responsible for ensuring that the athletes do not inadvertently take a prohibited substance. In the international games environment, athletes rely heavily on the knowledge and advice of pharmacists, doctors and other medical staff for information on drugs banned in sport, particularly for drugs that are prescribed for the first time in the polyclinic at the Games.

Pharmacists must be familiar with the list of prohibited substances and with the regulations for the provision of drugs that have a restricted status. They must also be aware of drugs that require prior notification through the Therapeutic Use Exemption (TUE) procedure in order to advise athletes appropriately.

There are very tight procedures, and a specific Olympic prescription form is used to ensure that the athletes do not fall afoul of a doping offence. Intensive and specialist training on drugs in sport is provided for healthcare professionals working in the Games environment over the six months before the start of the Games.

An additional responsibility of the Olympic and Commonwealth Games medical services is to ensure that healthcare professionals in the host city have the necessary information to hand should an athlete seek advice or treatment outside of the athlete village environment.

For the Manchester 2002 Commonwealth Games, an education program containing information about drugs in sport was delivered to pharmacies and emergency departments within the vicinity of the Games. For the Beijing 2008 Games, all medical staff working in the city received training to equip them with knowledge about the drugs restricted in sport. Similarly, for the London 2012 Olympic Games, in addition to specific local training, a nationwide education initiative will be implemented to ensure that pharmacists across the UK are prepared to meet the pharmaceutical needs and advice for supporters and spectators, many of whom will be from overseas.

3.2   The Games polyclinic

Within the athlete village at every Olympic and Commonwealth Games is a purpose-built medical centre known as the polyclinic, which is the main medical facility for athletes and team officials.

Medical services offered in the polyclinic are comprehensive and include emergency medical services, sports medicine, general practice, medical imaging, dentistry, eye services (ophthalmologists, opticians, optometrists), physiotherapy, massage therapy, hydrotherapy, podiatry, pathology, medical records, interpreter services, doping control, gender verification and a pharmacy. All of these medical services are provided free to the athletes and team officials for the duration of the Games and are staffed by a dedicated team of expert volunteers. The polyclinic is usually open from 8 AM to 11 PM and is busiest early in the morning and late at night, which coincides with athletes' training and competition schedules.

The Games polyclinic provides an environment unlike any other regular medical practice. On admission, an athlete has immediate access to a multidisciplinary team with expertise in sports medicine, and to the best diagnostic and treatment equipment available. In under an hour an athlete might have a comprehensive specialist consultation, ultrasound or MRI scan interpreted by a radiographer, physiotherapy or nursing intervention, and counselling on prescribed medication by the polyclinic pharmacists.

The polyclinic in the Beijing 2008 Olympic Village contained a fully stocked pharmacy, six dental surgeries, two MRI machines, optometry services dispensing hundreds of pairs of glasses, an emergency medicine department, counselling services, a massive physiotherapy unit with dozens of treatment beds and, for the first time in an Olympic polyclinic, an acupuncture and moxibustion clinic.

Around 20,000 visits over a one-month period were made to the Sydney 2000 polyclinic in the athletes' village. There were 3619 doctor consultations, 2884 physiotherapy treatments and 5622 visits to the pharmacy, making the pharmacy one of the busiest medical services at the Games. In Atlanta in 1996, 2474 athletes and Olympic staff were assessed in the polyclinic.

Dental and eye services are always in high demand at international games. The polyclinic services provide an opportunity for athletes from countries where medical resources are limited to access routine dental and optical treatment. The provision of these services is considered an obligation of the host city. In Atlanta 1996 there were 910 dental appointments resulting in 400 free dental fillings to athletes and team officials. In addition, 620 pairs of spectacles and 50 sets of contact lenses were prescribed and issued. At the Sydney Games, there were around 1800 visits each to dental and optometry services in the polyclinic. Five dental surgeries were kept busy for the duration of the Beijing 2008 Olympics.

A comprehensive interpreter service at the polyclinic ensures that medical staff can communicate effectively with their patients. This is especially important when athletes are being dispensed drugs with restrictions in sport, where they must know the notification procedures and consequences of taking such drugs. At the Sydney 2000 Olympics, 23 interpreters provided 6227 interpretations for the medical team.

At any Games, the polyclinic has close connections with nearby hospitals where patients are referred if they require longer-term or intensive care. In Beijing there were 21 official Olympic hospitals. If an athlete, official or Olympic family member was admitted, their care was coordinated through a 'green passage' process, which meant a speedy and priority service was provided. The designated Olympic hospitals were also able to provide the Olympic pharmacies with any medicines not stocked in the village as needed.

3.3   Medical services at sporting venues

At every Olympic sporting venue, specific medical facilities are provided for athletes and spectators. At the main Olympic stadium, there may be two main athlete medical rooms near the field of play stocked with medicines for sports injuries and emergency drugs. There will also be a number of spectator medical rooms on each spectator level of the stadiums, and additional medical stations in the public areas around the venues.

In Beijing, the medical stations in the Olympic Park area contained a comprehensive selection of drugs for spectator use. These included insulin, glyceryl trinitrate, cardiac emergency drugs, asthma inhalers and intravenous fluids. Single doses of drugs were administered to spectators, who would be referred to a designated hospital if further treatment was required.

The nature of the sporting event also determines how medical services are delivered and the types of drugs that are available for athlete use. For sailing and rowing, medical boats closely follow the competition, and motorbikes carry supplies for the road cycling and marathon events. At the Olympics, the equestrian events carry the most risk of serious trauma injuries. Along the 5.7-km route for the Olympic cross-country events in Hong Kong in 2008, 24 medical teams were stationed at any one time. Each medical team was equipped with a drug suitcase containing over 30 emergency drugs and a variety of medical equipment and first aid consumables.

For the London 2012 Olympic Games, medical services will be provided at 35 spectator competition venues, 41 training venues and 55 non-competition venues across eight UK cities.

3.4   The Games formulary

The main focus of medical treatment at international games is to provide care for newly acquired injuries or disease rather than treating or diagnosing existing complaints. This is reflected in the list of drugs available for prescribing in the polyclinic. The range of medicines stocked in the pharmacy needs to reflect those known and used by the global medical community as well as those frequently used in the host country. The formulary is compiled to reflect the specific drug needs of all the medical specialties including sports medicine, dentistry, physiotherapy, podiatry, optometry and massage therapies.

For each Commonwealth or Olympic Games a list of around 200 different drugs is available for prescribing within the athlete village by local and visiting team doctors, and for supply by doctors at the stadiums near the field of play. All medicines are provided free of charge to athletes and accredited support staff.

Most athletes who are taking long-term medicine for pre-existing conditions will generally bring enough of their own supplies to last for the few weeks of living away from home. In the formulary, there is less emphasis on drugs for long-term or chronic conditions, or those associated with geriatric or paediatric medicine. A limited supply of the most common but necessary medicines used by the general population such as anti-hypertensive drugs are kept, but are only likely to be used for the purpose of assisting a team official who has left his or her regular drugs at home.

A comprehensive range of drugs used in sports medicine, such as anti-inflammatories, is always included. In Manchester, the polyclinic pharmacy was also involved with the supply of diagnostic agents for eye and imaging services, specific dental drugs, and chemicals such as phenol for use by the podiatry team, ultrasound gel and bandage removal solvents for the physiotherapists, and isopropyl alcohol (rubbing alcohol) for the massage therapists.

The Games medicines handbook, which contains the list of drugs on the formulary, also lists the status of each drug according to the World Anti-Doping Agency (WADA) list of prohibited substances as a guide for prescribing physicians and pharmacists. It also contains advice to team doctors about the unique prescribing procedures during the Games.

The formulary for the Turin 2006 Winter Olympics contained a selection of drugs from the most common therapeutic categories. For example, antibiotics available for prescribing were amoxycillin, Augmentin, Cefaclor, ceftazidime, ceftriaxone, ciprofloxacin, doxycycline, erythromycin, imipenem, levofloxacin, metronidazole and Bactrim. NSAIDs, which are the most commonly prescribed group of drugs in sports medicine, included celecoxib, diclofenac, ibuprofen, ketoprofen and aspirin.

The licensed indications for drug use can differ between countries, which may restrict the suitability for some drugs to be included on a particular Games formulary. This was the case at the Manchester 2002 Commonwealth Games, where drugs that selectively inhibit cyclo-oxygenase-2 (including rofecoxib and celecoxib) were not made available, even though they were frequently requested, and visiting foreign athletes were familiar with their use for soft-tissue injury in their home countries. In the UK at the time, they were only licensed for pain and inflammation in osteoarthritis; the initiation of treatment for such conditions would not be expected in the Games environment.

Drugs for the Winter Games versus Summer Games

Planning for a pharmacy at a Winter Olympic Games must take into account unique environmental factors, such as freezing temperatures and high altitude and the medical conditions that can result.

At the 2002 Salt Lake City Winter Olympics there were around 11,000 people, including spectators treated at 35 medical stations located throughout the venues. There were around 2000 medical encounters in the Olympic Village polyclinic. The majority of cases were influenza and respiratory infections, but 43 cases of altitude sickness and 16 cases of frostbite were treated. The relatively moderate altitude of the mountain venues in Italy for the Turin 2006 Winter Olympic Games meant that drugs to treat altitude-related conditions were not considered necessary as a therapeutic group in the Olympic formulary.

Drugs for dental use

Prior to 2004, the use of local anaesthetic drugs was permitted only by the local or intra-articular (into the joint) injection route. For the Manchester 2002 Commonwealth Games it was necessary to notify the Games Medical Commission if they were used, which had implications for their routine use for dental procedures. Although local injection was permitted, dentists at the Manchester Games routinely submitted notification forms for every athlete who required local anaesthetics. Regulations have since changed and local anaesthetics (with the exception of cocaine) are no longer restricted in sport.

Drugs for disasters

Disturbingly, international games have historically been a target for terrorist attacks, and the access to drugs used for a variety of scenarios is seriously considered during the planning of medical services. At the Munich Games in

1972 11 Israeli athletes were killed and the bombing at Centennial Olympic Park in Atlanta in 1996 resulted in 111 injuries and two deaths.

In Atlanta, the possibility of a terrorist attack was recognised in advance and was reflected in the drugs stocked at the Olympic pharmacy. Pralidoxime chloride and atropine were available for the treatment of nerve gas poisoning and decontamination facilities were available in the event of gas or radioactive contamination.

In Manchester, no agents specifically used for treatment of biological or chemical attack were stocked by the polyclinic pharmacy. However, tight links with local public health services meant that in the event of a mass public disaster, medical services would be taken over by the Government National Health Service and patients would be redirected to local hospitals who maintained detailed contingency plans.

Tropical and international medicine

With athletes and support staff from more than 200 countries living in close proximity in the athlete village, the risk of intercontinental disease transmission exists. The medical services must consider having access to drugs for conditions that may not necessarily be endemic or common in the host country.

At the 1996 Atlanta Games, eight cases of malaria were reported, and there was one case of an athlete with malaria and thrombocytopenia who required hospitalisation. There were also three cases of hepatitis and one case of filariasis. Several athletes requested HIV tests with no positive results. At the Manchester Games, a purpose-built observation ward in the polyclinic was used for overnight observation of an athlete with malaria, with the pharmacy promptly obtaining the appropriate anti-malarial treatment. This four-bed ward in the polyclinic would be used to quarantine the athlete from the rest of the team should an infectious disease be diagnosed. At the Melbourne 2006 Commonwealth Games, there was one case of malaria, a condition that is rarely seen in Australia.

Rigorous reporting systems are implemented to notify public health authorities of suspected medical conditions that might pose a threat to public health. In Atlanta these were reported to the state Division of Public Health, so immediate public health interventions could be initiated.

Traditional medicines

The Beijing 2008 Olympics were the first games where traditional medicines were available from the polyclinic. The Beijing and Hong Kong Olympic Village pharmacies stocked four traditional Chinese medicines: Ren Dan and Huoxiang Zhengqi for heatstroke, Tiger Balm ointment for the relief of insect bites and Golden Throat Lozenges, a popular Chinese remedy for sore throats.

Although these traditional medicines were available from the Olympic pharmacy, they were not dispensed to athletes routinely. This was primarily because they were not on the official Olympic formulary and because WADA recommends caution to athletes about the use of herbal preparations, whose composition cannot always be guaranteed.

Quality testing of drugs

For the Beijing 2008 Olympic Games, and for the first time in Game's history, the Chinese government went to admirable lengths to ensure the quality of medicines used in the Beijing Olympic polyclinic. Quality control testing of all batches of drugs used at the Games was undertaken.

The expected quantity of medicines to be used for the Olympic and Paralympic period was estimated, then three times this amount was sent for sample testing to ensure that the composition complied with strict pharmacopoeia standards. This was in addition to the standard Chinese quality assurance testing that the drugs had already passed. The testing ensured that the therapeutic qualities of the drugs were correct and that there were no contaminants in each batch.

3.5   Patterns of drug use

Elite athletes at international games are in peak physical condition and are possibly the fittest and healthiest people on the planet. The patterns of therapeutic drug use at these events are therefore very different to those seen in the average community.

The athletes are most focused in the days before the start of competition. For most, participation at the event will be the culmination of years of intense training and the highlight of their sporting careers. Their anxiety about maintaining perfect health in the days before competition is understandably high, and obsession for a perfect physical state is reflected in the initial demands of the medical services.

In Atlanta, Barcelona and Seoul, medical services began 13 days before the opening ceremonies until three days after the closing ceremony: this was similar for subsequent games and will be the case for London 2012. Patterns of demand for drugs were similar for all three games; drug usage peaked just before the opening ceremony and continued until the end of the first week of competition. After this time there was typically a gradual decline in dispensed prescriptions until the closing ceremony, then a dramatic drop in drug usage occurs as the athletes start to leave the village. Conversely, the demand for MRI and ultrasound imaging increased constantly for the duration of the Games.

In Manchester 2002, antibiotic prescriptions accounted for the majority of the prescriptions dispensed before the start of the competition period. But after the opening ceremony, the daily number of antibiotic prescriptions dropped considerably. This trend might be explained by the possible over-prescribing of antibiotics for either prophylactic measures or for very mild respiratory symptoms.

The high level of antibiotic use very early at these games illustrates the immediate focus of sports medicine at this level. There can be pressure on prescribers from athletes and coaches to act in some way on the most minor of symptoms to ensure that illnesses do not hinder performance. In addition, athletes may be less likely to seek medical attention before their events than after competition, when their anxiety levels are lower.

Anti-inflammatory drugs are by far the most widely used class of drugs at major events, accounting for around 20 per cent of all prescriptions dispensed during the course of these games. Over the last 10 years, diclofenac has always been the most prescribed drug, accounting for about half of all the prescriptions for anti-inflammatory drugs.

The use of injectable local anaesthetics and corticosteroids is common for the treatment of sport injuries affecting the joints. Prescriptions for drugs such as lignocaine and methylprednisolone are commonly dispensed for severe injuries, where they are injected intra-articularly for treatment of acute pain and inflammation. These drugs can be subject to abuse because of their ability to enable otherwise injury-free athletes to exert themselves past natural pain limits. Such use contravenes sporting ethics and can put the athlete at risk of more serious injury.

Antifungal drugs usually account for a significant number of prescriptions at international sporting events. The use of shared training and changing facilities accounts for a high rate of fungal infections such as 'athlete's foot'. The incidence of fungal infections varies with the seasons and Games that are held in warmer, tropical climates typically see a higher demand for antifungal drugs. There was a greater proportion of antifungal drugs prescribed at the Sydney 2000 Games than at the much cooler Manchester 2002 Commonwealth Games.

Local factors can also present unique demands for particular medicines. At the Sydney 2000 Olympics, seasonal allergies were common amongst athletes, given that the Games were held in spring. At the Manchester 2002 Games, a plague of biting insects at the shooting venue meant that antihistamines, topical corticosteroids and anti-itch preparations had to be quickly provided to athletes and spectators. At the Melbourne 2006 Commonwealth Games, around 15 athletes presented at the polyclinic with irritated eyes caused by smoke and ash from the fireworks inside the stadium during the opening ceremony; soothing and anti-inflammatory eye drops were prescribed to them.

3.6   Prescribing procedures

Prescribing and dispensing of drugs in the Games polyclinic is undertaken with great caution to ensure that the prescription falls within the WADA rules. A unique Olympic prescription form is always used at Olympic and Commonwealth Games. These differ from regular prescription orders by the type of information that the IOC specifies must be recorded. Doctors must document the athlete's unique games accreditation number and country. If a restricted drug is prescribed, approval by the IOC must be obtained and shown to the pharmacy. The signatures from the athlete, doctor and pharmacist are obtained before dispensing to indicate the informed consent of the athlete.

As an additional precaution, the pharmacy in the polyclinic will have a bespoke dispensing system, which alerts the pharmacist if a prohibited substance is being supplied. The pharmacist can then ensure that the athlete completes the necessary documentation and obtains the appropriate authorisation from the games Medical Commission to use the drug.

At Commonwealth and Olympic Games, all drugs are issued using a prescription written by a doctor, regardless of whether the drug is available over the counter or not. This enables a safe supply route for the athlete, which is less likely to result in an unintentional doping offence, and it also enables comprehensive medical records to be kept.

If a restricted or prohibited drug is considered necessary for the treatment of an athlete, the doctor and pharmacist inform the athlete about the consequence of taking the drug. The athlete must then sign the prescription to acknowledge understanding of the treatment being prescribed. Restricted drugs may require notification to the Medical Commission, using a Therapeutic Use Exemption (TUE) form, before the athlete competes.

As an additional precaution, all restricted and prohibited drugs are labelled as such at the time of dispensing. They are often also stored separately to drugs that are permitted, further minimising the risk of dispensing them incorrectly.

Failing to submit a TUE form declaring the therapeutic use of a restricted drug could result in a doping violation should the athlete test positive for these substances. However, any drug is permitted to be used in an emergency or life-threatening situation.

Prescribing by team doctors

Each team present at international games usually has at least one accompanying doctor. The laws of the host country will often govern the rights that visiting doctors have in relation to prescribing and supply of drugs to the athletes they are looking after.

For the Sydney Olympics, 1109 visiting team doctors were given prescribing rights in Australia for the period of the Games. This enabled them to prescribe drugs from the Games formulary for members of their own team only.

In Manchester 2002, such prescribing rights were not possible by UK law, so all prescriptions had to be written by doctors registered in the UK. Similarly, at the 1996 Commonwealth Games in Kuala Lumpur, only prescriptions written by doctors registered with the Malaysian Medical Council were honoured. Team physicians were advised to procure temporary registration with the Malaysian Medical Council for the period of the Games.

Importation of drugs for team use

Most large teams bring complete medical kits with them and all teams have allocated space within the athletes' village to set up their own medical clinics.

Around 80 per cent of teams at the Sydney 2000 Games bought their own medical teams and drug supplies.

Guidance is always given to the participating countries by the Games organisers about the legal procedures for importing large quantities of drugs for therapeutic use. The team doctors are usually required to submit detailed lists of imported medicines to the medical services at the Games, and to government customs and importation authorities. The importation of performance-enhancing drugs such as narcotics, psychotropics, growth hormones, anabolic androgenic steroids and erythropoietin is illegal and is monitored closely during the Olympic period.

3.7 Drug information services

The polyclinic pharmacy is the primary point for medicinal information during the Games. Pharmacists are often requested to identify foreign drugs and to provide information on the status of medicines in relation to the WADA rules. Comprehensive international drug references are always available to help identify foreign drug names and determine specific constituents.

At Olympic and Commonwealth Games, the World Anti-Doping Agency usually runs an athlete outreach education centre within the athlete village. This programme teaches athletes about the principles of drug-free sport and the testing procedures that they will inevitably encounter at international games.

A common question asked at the pharmacy by athletes is whether their nutritional supplements are banned or not. Most athletes at international games take a variety of supplements, which are often recommended by coaches and team nutritionists. The advice that must be given to athletes by pharmacists is one of caution, as recent studies have revealed that prohibited substances are found in many commonly available nutritional supplements.

There is variation in the levels of awareness of banned drugs between different sports. This was apparent in the types of pharmacy enquiries at the 2002 Manchester Games. Sports with a lower public profile such as lawn bowls or shooting, compared with more mainstream sports, were generally less aware of the issues around the use of medicines while competing. This may be due to the level of education provided for these sports compared with more high-profile ones. Similarly, athletes from developing countries also seemed to have greatly varying levels of awareness on issues around prohibited substances. From 2004, with all participating countries having to sign up to the WADA code, which outlines standards for doping control, variances in awareness amongst elite athletes is less likely.

3.8 Summary

The scale of Olympic, Paralympic and Commonwealth Games is unrivalled by any other event in the world and the massive task of planning for their medical services begins at least four years before they are held. Supply of medicines for use by athletes within this environment is a truly unique process, both in terms of the types of specialist drugs required and the procedural measures in place to prevent inadvertent doping offences. These games provide a once-in-a-lifetime opportunity and a hugely rewarding clinical, logistical and ethical challenge for healthcare professionals from every specialty.

3.9 References

Anon. (2002). *Thousands treated for medical needs.* Online. Salt Lake City, Utah, KSL Television & Radio. 15 November 2004. Available at http://2002.ksl.com/news-6801i.php?p=1> (accessed 15 June 2009).

Brennan, R.J., Keim, M.E., Sharp, T.W. *et al.* (1997). Medical and public health services at the 1996 Atlanta Olympic Games: An overview. *Medical Journal of Australia* **167**, 595–598.

Clements, A. (2003). Medical support for the Greatest Show on Earth. *The British Travel Health Association Journal* **5**, 52–54.

Eaton, S.B., Woodfin, B.A., Askew, J.L. *et al.* (1997). The polyclinic at the 1996 Atlanta Olympic Village. *Medical Journal of Australia* **167**, 599–602.

London Organising Committee of the Olympic Games and Paralympic Games. (2009). Available at http://www.london2012.com (accessed 14 June 2009).

NSW Health Department. (2000). *NSW Health Services for the Sydney 2000 Olympic and Paralympic Games.* NSW Health Department, Sydney.

Stiel, D., Trethowan, P. and Vance, N. (1997). Medical planning for the Sydney 2000 Olympic and Paralympic Games. *Medical Journal of Australia* **167**, 593–594.

Stuart, M.C. (2005). Pharmacy for elite athletes at international games. In *Sport and exercise medicine for pharmacists*, ed. S.B. Kayne, Pharmaceutical Press, London. 269–296.

Sydney Organising Committee of the Olympic Games, Olympic Co-ordination Authority. (2001). *Official Report of the XXVII Olympiad.* SOCOG, Sydney.

Section 2

Substances and methods prohibited in sport

Chapter 4

Anabolic agents

Alan J. George and David R. Mottram

4.1   Introduction

For centuries, it was popularly believed that symptoms of ageing in men were caused by testicular failure. This stimulated a search for an active principle of the testicles that, when isolated, would restore sexual and mental vigour to ageing men. The testicular principle, we now know, is the male sex hormone testosterone, which was first synthesised in 1935.

Experimental studies in both animals and humans soon showed that testosterone possessed both anabolic and androgenic actions. The androgenic actions of testosterone are those actions involving the development and maintenance of primary and secondary sexual characteristics while the anabolic actions consist of the positive effects of testosterone in inhibiting urinary nitrogen loss and stimulating protein synthesis, particularly in skeletal muscle.

Synthetic anabolic steroids that mimic the effects of testosterone have been manufactured. However, a number of substances possess anabolic activity but are not based on the "steroidal" structure of testosterone. For this reason, the World Anti-Doping Agency (WADA) prohibited list describes the class as anabolic agents, which includes both anabolic steroids and other anabolic agents (Table 4.1). This group of other anabolic agents will be described later in this chapter.

4.2   The testosterone family

Testosterone is a C-19 steroid hormone. The steroid hormones are derived in the body from the substance cholesterol. The structure of testosterone is closely related to the steroid substance androstane and the structure of androstane is used as a reference when naming most of the compounds related to or derived from testosterone (Figure 4.1).

Biosynthesis

In humans, the immediate precursor of testosterone in the biosynthetic sequence from cholesterol is androstenedione, which is converted to testosterone by the

Table 4.1 Class S.1 anabolic agents of the WADA prohibited list (January 2010)

1. Anabolic androgenic steroids (AAS)
   a. Exogenous AAS
   b. Endogenous AAS, when administered exogenously
2. Other anabolic agents, including but not limited to clenbuterol, selective androgen receptor modulators (SARMs), tibolone, zerenol, zilpaterol.

action of the enzyme 17β hydroxysteroid dehydrogenase (Figure 4.2). This enzyme will also act on other steroids with similar structures, such as 19-norandrostenedione, to produce 19-nortestosterone (nandrolone) (Figure 4.2) (Mottram and George, 2000; Wright *et al.*, 2000).

The biochemistry and physiology of testosterone

Testosterone, the most important naturally occurring compound with androgenic and anabolic activity, is formed in the Leydig cells of the testes and also in the adrenal cortex. Adrenocortical testosterone is important in women, as it is responsible for some secondary sexual characteristics such as pubic and axillary hair growth and for its influence on sexuality (Greenblatt *et al.*, 1985). Mean testosterone production in men is approximately 8 mg per day of which 90–95 per cent is produced by the testes and the remainder by the adrenal cortex. When testosterone is synthesised in the body, its isomer epitestosterone is also formed. Epitestosterone has exactly the same number of atoms as testosterone but the -H and OH groups at C^{17} are orientated differently (Figure 4.1). The testes also produce 5-α-dihydrotestosterone (DHT), which is approximately equal in androgenic and anabolic activity to testosterone, and also two compounds with much weaker biological activity: androstenedione and dehydroepiandrosterone. After puberty, plasma testosterone levels are approximately 0.6 mg.dl^{-1} in males and 0.03 mg.dl^{-1} in females. Ninety-five per cent of testosterone in the blood is bound to protein, mainly sex hormone-binding globulin (SHBG).

Mode of action of testosterone

Testosterone produces its principal effect on tissues by altering cellular biochemistry via an interaction with the cell nucleus. Here the testosterone interacts on a particular chromosome with one or more specific binding sites called hormone receptor elements and activates the synthesis of one or more proteins that may be either enzymes or structural proteins. Testosterone and/or anabolic steroids also produce pharmacological effects via androgen receptors (Kicman, 2008). In some tissues testosterone is first converted to DHT, also called androstanolone, by the enzyme 5-α–reductase (Figure 4.2). The DHT is then transported to the nucleus and produces similar biochemical changes to those of testosterone.

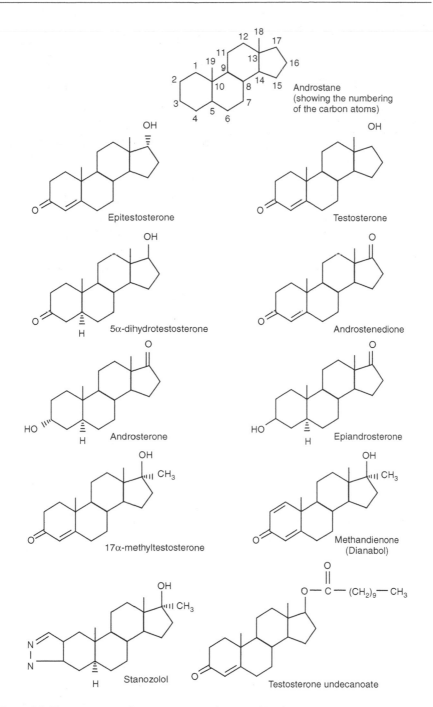

Figure 4.1 The structure of testosterone and some of its derivatives.

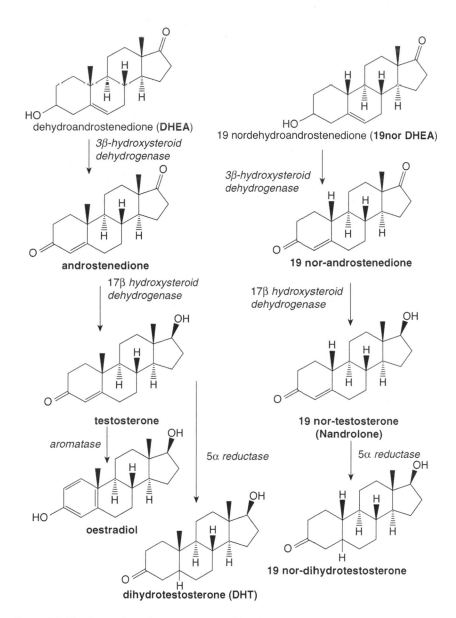

Figure 4.2 The formation of testosterone and its derivatives.

In many testosterone-sensitive tissues, it is thought that the anabolic effects of testosterone are mainly produced by the action of DHT. DHT can be formed from testosterone in the testes, liver, brain, prostate gland and external genitalia, but there is little 5-α–reductase activity and therefore little direct formation of DHT in human skeletal muscle. Generally in the liver, and locally in brain areas such as the hypothalamus, testosterone can be converted by the aromatase enzyme system to oestradiol (Figure 4.2).

The "aromatisation" of testosterone to oestradiol is essential for sexual differentiation of the brain, bone mass consolidation and epiphyseal fusion of the long bones at the end of puberty (Wu, 1997). DHT is primarily androgenic but oestradiol antagonises some androgenic actions while enhancing others. The full details of testosterone synthesis, mode of action and metabolism have been expertly reviewed by Wu (1997), Ueki and Okano (1999) and Kadi (2008).

Metabolism

Apart from conversion to DHT in various tissues, testosterone is metabolised in the liver mainly to DHT, androstenedione and then via the 3-Keto reductive enzymes to either androsterone or one of its two isomers: epiandrosterone or etiocholanolone (Figure 4.3) (Ueki and Okano, 1999; Wright et al., 2000). Androsterone and epiandrosterone have weak androgenic activity, while etiocholanone has none. Some testosterone is converted in the testes to oestradiol. Significant amounts of oestradiol are also thought to be formed from testosterone in the brain.

The physiological role of testosterone

Testosterone and its structurally related analogues possess androgenic and anabolic activity.

Androgenic effects

Testosterone is responsible for the development of primary sexual characteristics in males. Normally in a genetically male foetus (i.e. one with the XY sex chromosome configuration), the embryonic testes begin to differentiate, under the influence of H-Y antigen, the production of which is directed by the Y chromosome. As the male gonad differentiates, Leydig cells are formed, which begin to secrete testosterone. Testosterone and a polypeptide factor MRF (Mullerian Regression Factor) together stimulate the formation of the internal male genitalia, in utero. The external genitalia and prostate develop mainly under the influence of DHT (Wu, 1997). From birth until puberty the Leydig cells, which secrete testosterone, produce small amounts of testosterone and provide a plasma testosterone concentration of up to 2 nmol l^{-1}. From the age of approximately 10 years, in males,

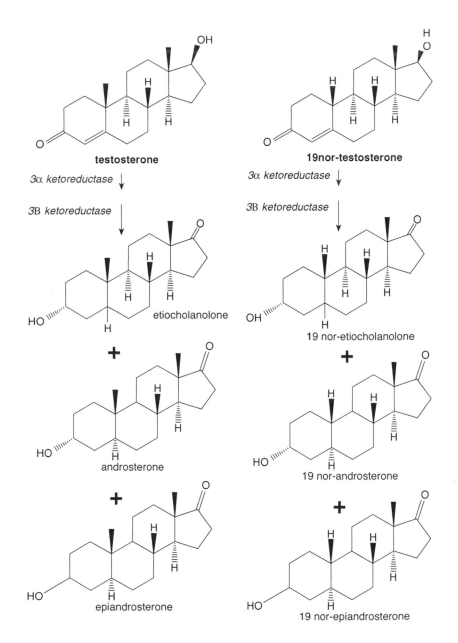

Figure 4.3 The metabolism of testosterone and 19 nor-testosterone.

increased testosterone secretion occurs principally from the testicular Leydig cells. The pubertal changes induced by this increase in testosterone are the secondary sexual characteristics, which include musculo-skeletal configuration, genital size, psychic changes and induction of sperm production. Adult secondary hair growth is stimulated by DHT.

Anabolic effects

The anabolic effects of testosterone and anabolic steroids are usually considered to be those promoting protein synthesis and muscle growth but they also include effects such as stimulation and eventually inhibition of skeletal growth in the young. It should be remembered that though the anabolic action of anabolic steroids may be much greater than testosterone, all anabolic steroids also possess some androgenic activity. There will also be discrete variations in the ratio of androgenic to anabolic activity amongst the family of testosterone derivatives, anabolic steroids and their various metabolites.

4.3   Structural analogues of testosterone: the anabolic steroids

When taken by mouth or by injection, testosterone is rapidly metabolised, mostly to inactive compounds. In the late 1940s medicinal chemists began to develop analogues of testosterone that might be degraded less easily by the body. Forty years of intensive research yielded three major types of testosterone modification, each of which gives rise to a class of anabolic steroids (Figure 4.4). Addition of

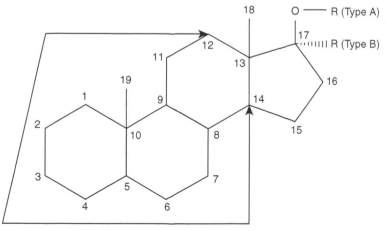

Type C substitution at any point

Figure 4.4 The three major types of testosterone modification (after Wilson, 1988).

an alkyl group at position 17 renders the structure orally inactive (B). A type (A) modification makes the compound suitable for "depot" injection, while type (C) modifications allow oral dosing and sometimes increased potency.

Clinical uses of androgens/anabolic steroids

Replacement therapy in men

Anabolic steroids may be given to stimulate sexual development in cases of delayed puberty. The therapy is then withdrawn gradually once full sexual maturity is reached. They may also be given in cases where the testicles have been surgically removed either because of physical injury or because of a testicular tumour. In this case the replacement therapy must be continued for life.

Replacement therapy in women

Testosterone production is necessary in women as well as in men. In the rare condition known as sexual infantilism, a young female fails to secrete oestradiol, progesterone and testosterone. As a consequence she suffers from amenorrhea, a lack of libido and absence of pubic and axillary hair. Only when she is treated with testosterone does libido appear. Some post-menopausal women suffer from loss of libido. In both these cases administration of testosterone restores sex drive and sexual characteristics (Greenblatt et al., 1985).

Gynaecological disorders

Anabolic steroids are occasionally used to treat gynaecological conditions in women, though long-term usage produces severe side effects such as erratic menstruation and the appearance of male secondary characteristics. Steroids are also sometimes used to combat breast tumours in pre-menopausal women.

Protein anabolism

The initial use of anabolic steroids in the early 1940s was to inhibit the loss of protein and aid muscle regeneration after major surgery, and to stimulate muscle regeneration in debilitating disorders such as muscular dystrophy and diabetes. Many concentration camp survivors owe their early recovery from debilitation to the skilled use of dietary measures coupled with anabolic steroids.

Anaemia

Anabolic steroids are sometimes used in large doses to treat anaemias that have proved resistant to other therapies. This therapy is not recommended in women because of the steroids' masculinising side effects.

Osteoporosis

There is some evidence that combined oestrogen/androgen therapy is able to inhibit bone degeneration in this disorder.

Growth stimulation

Anabolic steroids may be used to increase growth in prepubertal boys who have failed to reach their expected height for their age. The treatment must be carried out under carefully controlled conditions so that early fusion of the epiphyses does not occur.

Side effects of androgens

In females

These include acne, growth of facial hair, hoarsening or deepening of the voice and reduction in body fat. If the dose given is sufficient to suppress gonadotropin secretion then menstrual irregularities will occur. Chronic, or long-term treatment with androgens, as for example, in mammary carcinoma, may produce male pattern baldness, prominent musculature and veins and clitoral hypertrophy. A detailed review of this subject is provided by Elliot and Goldberg (2000).

In children

Administration of androgens can cause stunting of growth, a side effect directly related to the disturbance of normal bone growth and development. The enhancement of epiphyseal closure is a particularly persistent side effect that can be present up to three months after androgen withdrawal.

In males

Spermatogenesis is reduced by testosterone treatment with as little as 25 mg testosterone per day over a six-week period. Anabolic steroids will produce the same effect, since they will suppress natural testosterone secretion. The inhibition of spermatogenesis may persist for many months after anabolic steroid withdrawal.

General side effects

Oedema, or water retention, related to the increased retention of sodium and chloride, is a frequent side effect of short-term androgen administration. This may be the major contribution to the initial weight gain seen in athletes taking these drugs. Significant increases in steroid-induced water retention are likely to produce an increase in blood volume, a result of the simultaneous increase in water retention plus the increased erythropoiesis caused by anabolic steroid administration (Rockhold, 1993).

Jaundice is a frequent side effect of anabolic steroid therapy and is caused mainly by reduced flow and retention of bile in the biliary capillaries of the hepatic lobules. Hepatic cell damage is not usually present. Those anabolic steroids with a 17-α-methyl group are most likely to cause jaundice.

Patients who have received androgens and/or anabolic steroids for prolonged periods may develop hepatic carcinoma, again particularly prevalent with 17-α -methyl testosterone derivatives.

4.4   Anabolic steroids and sport

Ryan (1981) quotes the observation of the ancient Greeks that a high-protein diet was essential for body building and athletic achievement. The Greeks, of course, knew nothing of protein structure or bio-synthesis but they felt that an athlete would gain strength himself by eating the flesh of a strong animal such as the ox.

So, when did anabolic steroids first make their appearance in sport? It is suggested that the Helsinki Olympics of 1952 was the debut for anabolic steroids. Then steroid-filled Russians swept numerous gold medals in the 1954 Vienna Weightlifting Championships. Many early studies on the effect of anabolic steroids involved self-administration and were necessarily anecdotal with no attempt at scientific or controlled investigation of the effect of the steroid drugs. Subsequent studies, many of which were carried out in the late 1960s and early 1970s, were more scientifically based but often entirely contradictory in their results.

Sources, supply and control

In the USA, the major external sources for steroids have been Panama and Mexico while illegal synthesis by "street traders" is another major source. Both these sources provided drugs that are untested, are unstandardised, contained potentially toxic impurities and were not produced in the stringently hygienic conditions of the modern pharmaceutical industry. Catlin et al. (2000) examined seven brands of androstenedione available "over the counter" in US health shops and only one contained the pure compound. In their survey of US college student athletes, Green et al. (2001) found that 32 per cent of anabolic steroid abusers obtained their drugs from a physician not associated with the college team!

All these criminal activities are insignificant in terms of organisation and scale compared to the sponsored and managed promotion and supply of anabolic steroids by the government of the former German Democratic Republic (GDR). Release of State documents following the GDR's collapse indicates the extent of the systematic, programmed dosing of thousands of GDR athletes from 1970 to 1990. A full account of this governmental network of drug supply and administration has been provided by Franke and Berendonk (1997).

In the early part of the twenty-first century, a number of "designer" steroids were produced. These products were not licensed as pharmaceutical preparations or marketed as nutritional supplements (Van Eenoo and Delbeke, 2006). Consequently their safety had not been assessed rigorously. They were sold to athletes as being "undetectable". One of the first was norbolethone (Catlin *et al.*, 2002). Perhaps the most infamous, to date, was tetrahydrogestrinone (THG). This steroid was manufactured and sold to a number of high-profile athletes who were assured that it was undetectable by routine doping control techniques. However, it was identified in 2002 (Catlin *et al.*, 2004). Desoxymethyltestosterone (DMT), also known as madol, was patented in 1961 but never approved for use in patients. It was detected on the illicit black market in 2004 (Sekera *et al.*, 2005).

Patterns of administration and use

Anabolic steroids are broadly available as three types of preparation: oral, injectable oil-based and injectable water-based. The characteristics of these preparations have been described by Graham *et al.* (2008). Oral preparations have a structure resistant to breakdown by stomach acid, can be absorbed by the gastrointestinal tract, tend to withstand total breakdown by lever enzymes but have a short half-life and require frequent dosing. Injectable oil-based preparations have a longer half-life but produce a degree of pain at the injection site and have a slow absorption rate into the bloodstream, so that lower concentrations pass through the liver, thereby reducing liver toxicity. Injectable water-based steroids have a long half-life, though normally less than oil-based preparations, produce less discomfort at the site of injection and can be mixed with other water-based steroids or other drugs.

There are a number of administration regimes in use (Wilson, 1988; Rogol and Yesalis, 1992), though each has its variations and often combinations of regimes may be used concurrently.

Cycling

This is a period of administration followed by a similar period of abstinence before the administration is recommended. Typical cycling patterns are short (6 to 8 weeks on the drug and 6 to 8 weeks of abstinence) or long (6 to 18 weeks on the drug with up to 12 months of abstinence). The rationale here is that the periods of abstinence may reduce the incidence of side effects. This regime is preferred by body builders.

Pyramiding

This is a variation of cycling in which the dose is gradually built up in the cycle to a peak and then gradually reduced again towards the end of the cycle. This regime is said to cause fewer behavioural side effects such as lowered mood, caused by the withdrawal of the drug.

Stacking

This is the use of more than one anabolic steroid at a time. In its simplest form this regime involves the simultaneous use of both an orally administered steroid and an injectable one. More "sophisticated" patterns involve intricate schedules of administration using many different steroids, each with supposedly different pharmacological profiles. The aim of this technique is to avoid *plateauing*, which is the development of tolerance to a particular drug. Exact doses tried by abusers are almost impossible to establish. What is certain is that doses used by weightlifters and body builders have been at least 100 times those indicated for therapeutic use (Rogol and Yesalis, 1992).

The abuse cycles documented above are often followed in males by a dose of human chorionic gonadotropin (hCG), which is used to stimulate endogenous testosterone production that has been suppressed by the chronic administration of testosterone or anabolic steroids (Evans, 1997).

The prevalence of anabolic steroid abuse

There is no doubt, judging by the number of adverse analytical findings from WADA-accredited laboratories, that anabolic steroids remain the most widely misused class of doping agents. Statistical data on this can be found in Chapter 25 of this book.

The prevalence of anabolic steroid abuse in international competition is difficult to judge. At the 1972 (pre-testing) Munich Olympics, 68 per cent of interviewed athletes in middle- or short-distance running or in field events admitted taking steroids. At the 1968 Mexico Olympics, all the US weightlifters admitted taking steroids (Wilson, 1988). Up to 1992, progress in the USA (education programmes, legislation) had encouraged some experts to suggest that the availability and usage of steroids in the USA were decreasing (Catlin *et al.*, 1993). But analysis of US trends (1989–1997) by Yesalis and Bahrke (2000) show that this optimism was unfounded as the abuse figures generally are static and in some surveys may be increasing.

More recent evidence confirms that, in the USA, the use of doping agents is not restricted to competing athletes. Whilst estimates of misuse have to be interpreted cautiously, up to 3 million people (around 1 per cent of the population) are thought to have misused anabolic steroids (Tokish *et al.*, 2004). An estimate of anabolic steroid use in Sweden also arrives at a figure of 1 per cent (Sjöqvist *et al.*, 2008).

Efficacy of anabolic steroids

Anabolic steroids are used, variably, by athletes and others to increase lean body mass, to reduce fat, to enhance performance, to sustain periods of intense training and to improve bodily appearance (Hartgens and Kuipers, 2004).

Effects on muscle

Whether anabolic steroid treatment "works" has been perhaps the most difficult question of all to answer satisfactorily since many of the early investigations which have been carried out were, in the main, poorly designed scientifically, clinically and statistically (see Ryan, 1981 for review). Increases in muscle strength are proportional to increases in the cross-sectional diameter of the muscles being trained but there is no way of showing conclusively, in vivo, that any increase in muscle diameter consists of increased muscle protein rather than increased content of water or fat. Some progress has been made in the analysis of the effects of exercise and drugs on muscle structure (Blazevich and Giorgi 2001).

An important early study on the influence of athletic experience and pre-training on the response of athletes to anabolic steroid treatment was researched by Wright (1980). He noted that inexperienced weightlifters showed no increase in strength or lean muscle mass while simultaneously taking anabolic steroids and protein supplements and undergoing short-term training. In contrast, weightlifters who trained regularly (i.e. to nearly their maximum capacity) did show increased strength compared to their pre-treatment level. However, the presence of a greater initial muscle mass in the trained athletes before anabolic steroid treatment might have been a factor. Another possibility is that trained muscles are different. It is already known that the muscles of trained athletes can increase their uptake of glucose by the production of an endogenous factor, and that regular exercise regimes increase the responsiveness of skeletal muscle to insulin.

Summarising the evidence gained from earlier trials, Haupt and Rovere (1984) concluded that abuse of anabolic steroids will consistently result in a significant increase in strength if all of the following criteria are satisfied:

1   They are given to athletes who have been intensively trained in weightlifting immediately before the start of the steroid regimen and who continue this intensive weightlift training during the steroid regimen.
2   The athletes maintain a high-protein diet.
3   The changes in the athletes' strength are measured by the single repetition-maximal weight technique for those exercises with which the athlete trains.

More sophisticated meta-analysis of 30 of the early studies was carried out by Elashoff et al. in 1991. In addition to the study defects described previously, Elashoff et al. (1991) found marked evidence of poor statistical design and computation in many of the 30 studies examined. Their conclusions were that, in many cases, it must have been obvious to both experimenter and athlete, who was on an active preparation and the athletes would therefore have exhibited the psychopharmacological effects of "being on steroids". As in previous reviews the authors also questioned whether analysis of these studies was worthwhile since the doses of steroids administered were well below the amounts normally misused by dopers.

In a later review, Bhasin *et al.* (2001) concluded that testosterone supplementation increases maximal voluntary strength but that it does not improve specific tension. Thus testosterone would be expected to improve performance in weight-lifting events as these activities are so dependent on maximal voluntary strength.

What changes occur within the muscle itself? Blazevich and Giorgi (2001) have shown that certain changes in muscle architecture commonly associated with high-force production may be induced also by a combination of testosterone and heavy resistance training. Whilst that has little effect on muscle thickness, pennation (the ability of muscle fibre to twist) and the length of muscle fibres were both increased by testosterone. Anabolic steroids might, however, cause hypertrophy in skeletal muscle even without strength training (Sinha-Hikim *et al.*, 2002; Herbst and Bhasin, 2004). Empirical evidence that anabolic steroids enhance performance comes from the fact that world records in power sports seem to reach a steady state once effective doping tests were introduced (Sjöqvist *et al.*, 2008).

Effects on behaviour

Some athletes claim they feel more competitive and aggressive; others may feel they should run faster because they are on anabolic steroids. The increase in body weight and in circumference of leg and arm muscles may improve the athlete's self-image. Whether anabolic steroids enhance aggression or competitiveness is hard to assess. It is difficult to demonstrate conclusively that steroids or indeed testosterone are responsible for aggressiveness since many behaviours are probably learnt. However both male and female sexual behaviour are strongly influenced by androgens. Another possibility is that anabolic steroids may have a placebo effect—abusers may work or train harder because they expect anabolic steroids to work their magic! This has been investigated by Maganaris *et al.* (2000). They demonstrated moderate improvements in performance in athletes who believed they were taking anabolic steroids.

Effects on muscle repair

A further potential advantage conferred on the anabolic steroid taker is that their muscles and associated tissues may have greater reparative powers and so the athlete may be able to undertake more events in a short time. This observation has led to the increased use of steroids by both middle- and long-distance runners and marathon runners. However, a study by Baume *et al.* (2006) found no effect of multiple doses of anabolic steroids on endurance running performance or on bioserum indices of recovery from physical stress.

4.5   Precursors, nandrolone and steroid metabolites

Testosterone is produced naturally in the testes and adrenal cortex by the conversion of dehydroepiandrosterone (DHEA) to androstenedione and then to testosterone. For some years, both these substances were suggested as possible anabolic agents in the knowledge that, when administered, they could be converted to testosterone in the body (Johnson, 1999). Androstenedione was the major substance that Mark McGuire admitted to abusing in his quest for baseball fame in 1997–98. Though several researchers have claimed that androstenedione and DHEA produced increases in serum testosterone concentration of up to 300 per cent in women and 200 per cent in men, this was not correlated with any increases in muscle strength or athletic performance (Johnson, 1999). Despite this, DHEA and androstenedione remain on the WADA prohibited list. Brian Wallace and his colleagues showed in 1999 that, compared with placebo, neither DHEA nor androstenedione was associated with a statistically significant increase in lean body mass, strength or testosterone levels. Since DHEA also disturbs the testosterone/epitestosterone ratio, the ability to cheat with the drug seems much reduced (Johnson, 1999). This lack of androstenedione efficacy may be associated with its rapid conversion to oestrogens in peripheral tissues (Wallace *et al.*, 1999).

5-α-dihydrotestosterone (DHT)

This compound occurs naturally in males and females as a result of the action of the enzyme 5-α-reductase on testosterone (Figure 4.2). DHT is reported to have two to three times the androgenic activity of testosterone (Ueki and Okano, 1999) and its production is necessary for normal male sexual development. As the 5-α–reductase conversion is not readily reversible, the conversion of DHT to oestradiol via the "aromatase" process is minimal, which therefore minimises any possible feminising effects in males, though it increases the likelihood of serious masculinising side effects in females (Ueki and Okano, 1999). It is for this reason that the 19-nor derivative of DHT (formed by the action of 5-α-reductase on nandrolone) has been suggested as a preferred drug of abuse in women, as it has much less androgenic activity than DHT.

Nandrolone

Nandrolone (19-nortestosterone) (Figure 4.2) was introduced as an anabolic steroid in the 1970s. It has structural modifications that allow it to be injected intramuscularly and which also reduce the likelihood of its conversion to oestrogen by aromatase enzymes (Mottram and George, 2000). In addition, nandrolone can be converted by 5-α-reductase to "dihydro-19-nortestosterone" (dihydronandrolone), which has even less androgenic activity and is therefore promoted as a potential "drug of choice" for women athletes. Nandrolone is converted also to the metabolites norandrosterone and noretiocholanone by the same enzyme systems that metabolise testosterone (Figure 4.3) and these components like their respective testosterone metabolites may be detected in urine (Kinze *et al.*, 1999). In 1997, the US Drug Enforcement Agency noticed an increase in the importation of so-called nandrolone precursors norandrostenediol and norandrostenedione into the USA. Research showed that this seemed to be coupled to advertisements on the internet claiming that these two compounds could be converted to nandrolone in humans (Ferstle, 1999a). In theory it should be possible to convert norandrostenedione to 19-nortestosterone (nandrolone) in humans (Wright *et al.*, 2000).

By the mid-1990s, it had been observed that nandrolone metabolites norandosterone and noretiocholanone could be detected in the urine of previously drug-free monkeys (Ferstle, 1999b). Also the progestogen, norethisterone, an ingredient of some oral contraceptives, was shown to increase levels of nandrolone metabolites in urine (Van Eenoo and Delbeke, 2006). It has also been shown that the urinary concentration of norandosterone and noretiocholanone increases in some pregnant women (Mareck-Engelke *et al.*, 2002). Based on this and other analytical evidence the IOC set urinary concentration limits for nandrolone metabolites at 2 ng/ml for men and 5 ng/ml for women. In 2004, WADA lowered the reporting threshold for 19-noradrosterone, for women, from 5 to 2 ng/ml. A large-scale study (Walker *et al.*, 2009) of urine samples from 1202 healthy, non-pregnant women were analysed for 19-noradrosterone. Only one sample exceeded the 2 ng/ml threshold and that from one of the 38 women in the study who were taking norethisterone-containing contraceptives.

Nandrolone metabolites are found in urine from previously drug-free human males and at a concentration below the 2 ng/ml threshold (Dehennin *et al.*, 1999; Le Bizec *et al.*, 2002). Evidence that this is a truly endogenous production comes from the demonstration that nandrolone metabolites levels in male urine can be increased following an injection of human chorionic gonadotropin (hCG), which stimulates androgen release from the testes (Reznik *et al.*, 2001). However, in 1999 Le Bizec *et al.* found that while nandrolone concentrations in half of the 40 samples they tested ranged from 0.05–0.6 ng/ml these values could be increased by a factor of 2–4 after prolonged intense exercise. Could nandrolone and its metabolites be formed in humans in other ways?

There was evidence in the 1980s that methosterone could be converted to a nandrolone metabolite (Ferstle 1999a). Other studies have shown that pregnant women may produce increased amounts of the metabolites because of the action of hCGs on the ovary (Reznik *et al.*, 2001). Other doubts concern the claim that some vitamin and food supplements may contain trace amounts of nandrolone precursors norandrostenedione and norandronstenediol, which are metabolised to nandrolone and then to its metabolites, thus producing a positive test result. To test this, Catlin *et al.* (2000) administered trace amounts of androstenedione or 19-norandrostenedione to 41 healthy men. Twenty of the 24 men receiving androstenedione yielded urine samples containing norandrosterone at a concentration above the IOC limit.

More recently, Ayotte (2006) demonstrated that norsteroid metabolites can be formed in urine by 19-demethylation of urine metabolites.

In October 2000, the IOC commissioned the Institute of Biochemistry in Cologne to investigate nutritional supplementation in sport. The study examined and analysed 634 non-hormonal nutritional supplements obtained from most EU countries and from the USA. Twenty-three samples (24.5 per cent) contained precursors of nandrolone and testosterone, 64 samples (68.1 per cent) contained precursors of testosterone while seven samples contained nandrolone precursors only (Schänzer, 2002). Sample products that tested positive for anabolic steroid precursors originated from the Netherlands (25.8 per cent), Austria (22.7 per cent), UK (18.9 per cent) and the USA (18.8 per cent). Analysis of the positive samples yielded anabolic steroid precursor concentrations of 0.01 $\mu g.g^{-1}$–190 $\mu g.g^{-1}$ (Schänzer, 2002).

In summary:

- nandrolone metabolites and possibly nandrolone are produced naturally in human males and females;
- norandrosterone and norandrostenedione can be converted in humans to nandrolone metabolites (via nandrolone);
- the 2 ng cut off for nandrolone metabolites is fair but further studies need to be done on the effect of prolonged exercise on the urinary concentration of nandrolone metabolites.

4.6   Anabolic steroid side effects with particular reference to athletes

In the introductory section, the general side effects of anabolic steroids were discussed. Of these side effects some are of particular significance to athletes taking steroids.

Cardiovascular

Blood volume

Rockhold (1993) has examined nine studies on the effect of anabolic steroids on blood volume. Eight of these studies were carried out on non-athletes and produced variable results. Some studies showed increases in blood volume while others demonstrated no change. In the single study carried out in athletes, a 15 per cent increase in total blood volume in athletes taking methandienone was recorded. This study did not measure haematocrit and so any effect of the steroid on erythropoiesis could not be determined.

Salt and water retention

Earlier in this chapter, the effect of anabolic steroids on salt and water retention was discussed in relation to steroid-induced gains in body weight and muscle circumference. The increase in salt and water retention responsible for these changes has a deleterious effect on the cardiovascular systems. Sodium ions remain in the extra-cellular fluid and blood unless excreted by the kidney, thus raising osmotic pressure and withdrawing water from the tissues. An expansion of the blood volume then occurs, which imposes an increased workload on the heart. The heart increases its output and the blood pressure rises. The increased sodium concentration may also directly stimulate vasoconstriction, thus enhancing the hypertensive effect of the increased blood volume.

Hypertension

An increased incidence of potentially fatal hypertension in athletes on anabolic steroids was frequently mentioned in early reviews of anabolic steroid abuse in sport (Goldman, 1984; Wright, 1980). According to Rockhold (1993), the evidence for this is equivocal. He mentions three studies—two in athletes, one in healthy men—in which administration of either testosterone or oxandrolone for three months failed to cause an increase in blood pressure. An earlier study by Holma (1979) found a 15 per cent increase in blood volume in men taking methandienone but no increase in blood pressure. However Kuipers et al. (1991) found mean increases in blood pressure of 12 mm Hg in athletes self-administering various anabolic steroids

Ventricular function

Studies in animals of the effect of anabolic steroids on ventricular function and morphology have indicated an association between steroids and ventricular pathology, which may have significance for humans (Lombardo et al., 1991) particularly as the autopsy of an American footballer who was abusing anabolic steroids revealed significant cardiomyopathy. The technique of echocardiography has revolutionised non-invasive investigation of cardiac function and allows clinicians to measure accurately the dimensions of the ventricles during exercise and at rest. A survey of six studies of ventricular function in athletes from different disciplines abusing anabolic steroids has been conducted by Rockhold (1993). The overall conclusion was that in intensely training athletes steroid administration induced left ventricular thickening, increases in end diastolic volume and relaxation index. Nieminen et al. (1996) have reported similar cardiopathology in four young weightlifters with cardiac hypertrophy. Two patients additionally had symptoms of heart failure and one of these had a massive thrombosis in both ventricles. It should be noted that all the above studies were carried out in weightlifters and so may not be relevant to all athletes and it is interesting that while endurance athletes have a significantly greater life expectancy than non-athletes this advantage is not shared by power athletes (Pärssinen and Seppälä, 2002). The effect of anabolic steroids in increasing left ventricular mass may be potentiated by concomitant use of growth hormones (Karila et al., 2003).

Effects on blood lipids and lipoproteins

Anabolic steroids have important adverse effects on the plasma levels of triglycerides, cholesterol and lipoproteins (Thiblin and Petersson, 2005). Lipoproteins are large molecular conglomerates of lipids and specialised proteins called apolipoproteins. Their presence in the blood is to carry water-insoluble lipids from their site of production to tissues where they are utilised or stored. Anabolic steroids have been shown to increase blood triglyceride and cholesterol levels. Effects on blood lipids are particularly associated with the abuse of orally administered steroids (Lombardo et al., 1991).

Steroids decrease the blood levels of high-density lipoproteins (HDL) especially the HDL_2 and HDL_3 fractions, while increasing the level of low-density lipoproteins (LDL). In addition, there is a significant rise in the ratio of free cholesterol to HDL-bound cholesterol following anabolic steroid administration, though the effect is less pronounced with testosterone (Alén and Rahkila, 1988). Costill et al. (1984) have shown that in athletes taking anabolic steroids, HDL fell by 20 per cent after only 102 days of treatment, while cholesterol concentration was unchanged. Rockhold (1993) reports even greater percentage reductions (i.e. HDL down 52 per cent). In normal males 22 per cent of cholesterol is in the form of HDL while in steroid takers only 7.8 per cent of cholesterol is found combined in this way.

The effect on HDL is reversible (i.e. HDL levels return to normal within three to five weeks of cessation of steroid administration) (Lukas, 1993; Rockhold, 1993). A controlled study by Millar (1994), in which moderate doses of anabolic steroids were administered by physicians, reported decreases in HDL and an increase in total cholesterol levels, which returned to normal 6–12 weeks after the end of dosage.

These reductions in HDL levels have been associated with increased incidence of cardiovascular disease (Alén and Rahkila, 1988; Wagner, 1991). Low serum HDL is recognised as a risk factor for cardiac and cerebrovascular disease (Wagner, 1991). There are several well-documented cases of coronary heart disease (CHD) in apparently fit, healthy athletes aged under 40, who have been taking anabolic steroids (Goldman, 1984; Kennedy and Lawrence, 1993; Mark et al., 2005). Street et al. (1996), in their review of anabolic steroid side effects, identified individual cases of serious medical conditions associated with anabolic steroid abuse quoted in medical journals. Although there was only one death due to myocardial infarction, there were several "near misses" including five myocardial infarctions, one stroke, two cases of pulmonary embolism and one cerebral venous thrombosis. The statistics were complicated by the different drug administration regimes used by abusers and complications arising from other risk factors such as smoking.

Blood-clotting

The increased risk of coronary and cerebrovascular disease in anabolic steroid abusers has prompted some physicians to consider whether there is increased risk of platelet aggregation leading to increased blood-clot formation. Animal studies suggest that there is such a relationship but so far there has been only one report of an athlete taking steroids dying of a stroke (Lombardo *et al.* 1991), though Street *et al.* (1996) quote three cases of near deaths from pulmonary embolism and one from venous thrombosis. An association between increased platelet aggregation and age in weightlifters taking steroids has been reported (Lukas, 1993).

Carcinomas

The association between anabolic steroid administration and tumour formation, particularly of the liver and kidney, is now firmly established. Significant changes in liver biochemistry have been found in 80 per cent of otherwise healthy athletes taking anabolic steroids but without any signs of liver disease. In 1965, a detailed case study linked the death of an anabolic steroid-taking athlete with hepatocellular cancer (HC). Since then, 13 other athletes taking anabolic steroids have been demonstrated to have HC and all were taking 17-alkylated androgens.

Anabolic steroids have also been suspected of causing death from Wilm's Tumour of the kidney in at least two adult athletes (Pärsninen and Seppälä, 2002). The tumour is very rare in post-adolescent individuals. In their survey of serious reported anabolic steroid side effects Street *et al.* (1996) could find only one case of prostate carcinoma. Three large case-controlled studies have found a much stronger though not unequivocal link between raised anabolic steroid levels and prostate cancer (Pärssinen and Seppälä, 2002).

Sex-related side effects

Fertility

Administration of anabolic steroids caused inhibition of gonadotropin secretion followed by inhibition of testosterone. Holma (1979) administered 15 mg methandienone to 15 well-trained athletes for two months. During the administration period sperm counts fell by 73 per cent and in three individuals azoospermia (complete absence of sperm) was present. Thus fertility was severely reduced in males in this study, which provides confirmation of many clinical reports of the same phenomena. Many of these effects were however shown to be reversible. Some clinical data suggest that long-term anabolic steroid-induced infertility might be permanent though. In their review of published work up to 1995, Street *et al.* (1996) found no evidence of long-term effects in fertility on young males given anabolic steroids to suppress excessive growth. Similarly, a study on the concomitant abuse of human chorionic gonadotropin and supraphysiological doses of anabolic steroids caused transient impairment on semen quality, although spermatogenesis was maintained (Karila *et al.*, 2004).

Effects on libido

The suppression of testosterone secretion in both males and females may well have effects on libido. Libido in males and females is thought to be influenced, at least in part, by testosterone. Thus, high levels of anabolic steroids in the blood suppress testosterone secretion and reduce libido. However, Yates *et al.* (1999) studied men using doses of testosterone up to 500 mg per week and could find no significant changes in male libido during a 14-week administration period.

Gynaecomastia

This is a paradoxical condition occurring in athletes attempting to increase their muscle mass as it involves the development of mammary tissue. The most common cause of this condition in anabolic steroid abusers is that the agent they are administering is converted by liver aromatase enzymes (see Figure 4.2) to oestradiol, which then induces development of mammary tissue. Thus athletes who abuse anabolic steroids and testosterone (or hCG which releases testosterone) are all at risk from developing gynaecomastia (Friedl and Yesalis, 1989). Concurrent administration of the anti oestrogen, tamoxifen, is thought by many abusers to be an effective antidote to gynaecomastia induced by steroids (Perry *et al.* 1992). Though it is sometimes effective in reducing the pain associated with this condition, tamoxifen seems to have little effect on the size of breast tissue in steroid abusers (Friedl and Yesalis, 1989).

Specific actions in female athletes

Considering the side effects why do female athletes take anabolic steroids? The simple answer is that, according to some reports, the effects of anabolic steroids on muscle strength and bulk in a female athlete are considerably greater than in men. This has been explained by the lower normal circulating level of testosterone in females as compared to men.

In 1996, Korkia *et al.* interviewed 15 female body builders who admitted to anabolic steroid abuse, nine of whom reported deepening of the voice; eight had menstrual problems and seven had clitoral enlargement. Three complained of reduction in breast size while the other side effects mentioned were similar to males. Side effects such as menstrual problems are not necessarily indicative of anabolic steroid abuse, as regular intense endurance exercise is known to induce amenorrhoea as discussed by Warren and Shantha (2000).

Priscilla Choi (1998) described the case of a female body builder who, as a result of chronic anabolic steroid abuse, became permanently masculinised in that eight years after cessation of anabolic steroid abuse, her enlarged clitoris and her deep voice remained and she appeared to be suffering psychologically from a gender identity crisis.

The androgenisation of sportswomen from the former East Germany led to severe adverse effects, such as hirsutism and gynaecological disorders like ovarian cysts and long-term amenorrhoea (Prendergast *et al.*, 2003).

Tendon damage

Researchers have noted the increased incidence of tendon damage in athletes taking anabolic steroids. A summary of the various tendon pathologies associated with anabolic steroid abuse in powerlifters has been provided by Laseter and Russell (1991). These include the quadriceps and rectus femoris tendons and the triceps. This phenomenon has been explained in at least three different ways. First, the increase in muscle strength acquired by a course of steroids, plus training, produces a greater increase in muscle power, whereas anabolic steroids have little or no effect on tendon strength and tendons respond slowly to strength regimes. Second, it is thought that anabolic steroids have, in common with corticosteroids (such as cortisol), the ability to inhibit the formation of collagen, an important constituent of tendons and ligaments. Third, anabolic steroids appear to induce changes in the arrangement and contractility of collagen fibrils in tendons, leading to critical alterations in physical properties known as the "crimp angle". The overall effect is to reduce the plasticity of the tendons. It should be pointed out that tendon ruptures also occur in athletes not abusing steroids. Weightlifters taking anabolic steroids appear to be particularly prone to muscle and tendon injuries. This has been explained by apologists for anabolic steroid abusers as evidence of greater weights being lifted. Sports doctors say it is the biochemical effects of anabolic steroids while others say that the increased aggressiveness and competitiveness induced by anabolic steroid administration causes athletes to attempt more and greater lifts with an increasingly reckless attitude to the actual mechanics of the lifting.

Glucose regulation

Hobbs *et al.* (1996) found that testosterone administered at 300 mg/week had little effect on glucose uptake from the plasma while the same dose of nandrolone enhanced glucose removal from the plasma. These differences were ascribed to the ability of testosterone to undergo aromatisation to an oestrogen.

Behavioural effects and addiction

Since the late 1940s it has been known that anabolic steroids have important influences on behaviour but these have usually been acknowledged to be the stimulatory effects that anabolic steroids have on libido in both males and females (Greenblatt *et al.*, 1985). Studies in the 1980s have suggested that anabolic steroids have reduced the depression symptoms in a number of groups of depressed patients (Williamson and Young, 1992).

A review by Kashkin and Kleber (1989) cites many documented cases of increased aggression and violent behaviour, many of them reported by the abusers themselves. The same authors also report detailed cases of mild to severe psychiatric disturbances occurring in those abusing anabolic steroids ranging from impaired judgement, insomnia and agitation to panic attacks, grandiose ideas and paranoid delusions. Pope and Katz (1988) interviewed 41 body builders and football players who had used anabolic steroids. Nine fulfilled the criteria for mood disorder and five displayed psychotic symptoms associated with steroid use. Williamson and Young (1992) describe several cases of manic episodes in athletes taking anabolic steroids. Kashkin and Kleber (1989) produced evidence of withdrawal symptoms in some individuals who stop taking steroids and cited several studies where steroid withdrawal had resulted in clinical depression. An examination of eight cases of suicide in anabolic steroid abusers by Thiblin *et al.* (2000) showed that depressive symptoms arising after anabolic steroid withdrawal were associated with suicide in five cases while in the remainder depression during anabolic steroid abuse was implicated.

There is also widespread fear, real and imaginary, of what is referred to as "muscle melt down", in those considering or attempting to withdraw from steroid abuse. This appears from the literature to involve feelings of loss of esteem, both social and sexual, if the well-developed torso is seen to "melt away" after steroid withdrawal. Kashkin and Kleber (1989) considered that all the clinical evidence thus far suggested the existence of a "sex steroid hormone dependence disorder", which obeys the following established criteria for addiction:

1   the hormones are used over longer periods than desired;
2   attempts are made to stop without success;
3   substantial time is spent obtaining, using or recovering from the hormones;
4   use continues despite acknowledgement of the significant psychological and toxicological problems caused by the hormones;
5   characteristic withdrawal symptoms occur;
6   hormones (or their supplements) are taken to relieve the withdrawal symptoms.

One of the major reasons proposed by steroid abusers for the use of these drugs in their sport is that it increases their aggression. A number of studies have failed to find any relationship between endogenous testosterone levels and aggression (Archer, 1991). Another review of studies of aggression and hostility in anabolic steroid users versus placebo groups of athletes revealed both positive and equivocal results (Williamson and Young, 1992).

Body builders may suffer from body dysmorphic syndromes (feelings that their body size/shape is inadequate). Pope's research group (1997) thought they could identify a "muscle dysmorphic syndrome" in which affected individuals become "pathologically pre-occupied with their degree of muscularity".

Bahrke (2000) summarised the evidence for anabolic steroid–induced behavioural change and psychiatric disorder. He stated that because a steroid user feels more aggressive and self-reports more aggression, it does not mean that he/she is going to behave violently or develop a mental disorder. His review also emphasises that only a small percentage of anabolic steroid users appear to experience symptoms of mental illness. Of those that do, the majority recover without relapse when the anabolic steroids are withdrawn. In 2006, Pagonis *et al.* concluded that the range and severity of psychiatric side effects associated with anabolic steroid abuse increased with the extent to which they were used singly or in combination.

Long-term risks of anabolic steroid abuse

Exactly how long anabolic steroids have been misused in sport is unknown, but if 50 years is a reasonable estimate then we should now be investigating or realising the long-term effects of their abuse. Mortality studies are notoriously difficult to control and in the case of anabolic steroid abuse the confirmation of abuse and its intensity is difficult to verify. A study of 62 elite power lifters in Finland emphasised the apparent long-term effects of anabolic steroid abuse. These athletes were the prize winners in the Finnish championships (1977–1982) and were followed up for 12 years and compared to a control population. Premature death was 4.6 times higher in the power lifters than in the control population (Pärssinen *et al.*, 2000). As power lifting does not itself cause an increase in mortality the increase in mortality in this group was ascribed to anabolic steroid abuse (Pärssinen and Seppälä, 2002).

Indirect consequences of anabolic steroid abuse

Many athletes use injectable forms of anabolic steroids. This may be due to better awareness of the toxicity of the oral compounds or to the supposedly lower risk of detection with injectable compounds once treatment is stopped. It is surely no coincidence that this switch to injectables appeared to be associated with the appearance of HIV among steroid abusers (Sklarek *et al.*, 1984). There have been several further cases reported subsequently in body builders in the USA (Yesalis *et al.*, 1988). The potential for the spread of HIV by this route in Great Britain has been highlighted by Perry *et al.* (1992), who reported high-risk behaviour (i.e. needle sharing and drug sample sharing) with all the attendant risks of cross contamination of drug supplies and abusers' blood in their sample of body builders in Swansea.

Other related high-risk behaviour such as abuse of other more dangerous drugs, drunk driving, reckless driving behaviour and high-risk sexual activity have been catalogued in anabolic steroid abusers by Middleman and DuRant (1996).

Another unforeseen consequence of anabolic steroid abuse by injection is tissue and organ damage caused by inexperienced and untrained injectors. There are several anecdotal cases reported to me by local GPs of "steroid limp". This condition is characterised by the patient who can only raise his affected leg to walk by using his abdominal adductor muscles. It is caused by damage to the sciatic nerve by injection of anabolic steroids in the buttocks either into or close to the sciatic nerve, resulting usually in permanent neuromuscular impairment.

4.7   Detection of testosterone and anabolic steroids

Tests for anabolic steroids

After the 1950s, testosterone and methandrostenelone (Dianabol) were the most frequently misused steroids in sport. Dianabol was popular as it was potent and orally active due to its 17 α-methyl group, which also rendered methandrostenelone distinguishable from testosterone by the immunoassay (IA) detection method (Catlin et al., 2008). IA screening for anabolic steroids took place at the 1974 European Athletics Championships in Rome, followed by the 1976 Montreal Olympics, with limited success (Dugal et al., 1977). It was shortly after the Montreal Games that the next significant step in detection of anabolic steroids was introduced: this was the use of gas chromatography (GC) and mass spectrometry (MS).

Using this combined method of detection, compounds within the urine are separated by GC, with their chromatographic retention time recorded. The separated compounds are then subjected to MS in which the sample is bombarded with electrons to fragment it into smaller ions whose abundance is recorded according to its mass. A given chemical will always fragment in the same reproducible way; therefore its mass spectrum is characteristic for that compound (Catlin et al., 2008).

Improvements in the sensitivity and reliability of GC-MS continued throughout the 1980s, enabling testers to detect extremely low levels of steroids and their metabolites (Graham et al., 2008).

Liquid chromatography (LC) separates compounds in the liquid phase, as opposed to the GC technique, which requires heat to separate compounds in the gaseous phase. This has the advantage that thermolabile compounds can be separated by LC. Not only anabolic steroids but most substances prohibited in sports are identified by GC-MS or LC-MS. New techniques for detection are constantly under development (Graham et al., 2008).

As detection of synthetic anabolic steroids became easier and more effective, steroid users turned to testosterone and other endogenous steroids, as GC-MS and LC-MS were not capable of distinguishing between endogenous testosterone and other steroids produced in the body and the same steroids produced in the laboratory.

Detection of testosterone misuse

With respect to testosterone, a number of approaches were trialled (Graham *et al.*, 2008). Eventually, it was decided in the early 1980s to use the ratio of testosterone to epitestosterone to detect exogenous testosterone use. Epitestosterone is an isomer of testosterone that has no anabolic effects but which is produced at the same time as testosterone in the body. Both substances are easily detected by GC-MS. Testosterone and epitestosterone appear in the urine in an approximate ratio of 1:1. It was therefore proposed to introduce a testosterone/epitestosterone (T/E) ratio of 6:1 as a cut-off level to determine whether exogenous testosterone had been administered by the athlete.

At the 1984 Los Angeles Olympic Games, all urine samples taken from athletes were screened by GC-MS (Catlin *et al.*, 1987). Sixteen positive results were recorded, of which five had a T/E ratio greater than 6:1.

The T/E ratio method was fraught with difficulties. Some individuals have naturally elevated T/E ratios, while others never exceed the cut-off level due to genetic factors. Some simply use epitestosterone along with testosterone to maintain a "normal" T/E ratio (Graham *et al.*, 2008).

The T/E ratio value, used in doping control to determine testosterone use, has been adjusted on several occasions. The latest WADA regulations specify that exceeding a cut-off level of 4:1 should trigger further investigations.

By the late 1990s, a new testing method for testosterone was introduced, called isotope ratio mass spectromety (IRMS) (Aguilera *et al.*, 2001). The IRMS method relies on the determination of the ratio of carbon-12 (^{12}C) to carbon-13 (^{13}C) within the testosterone isolated from urine samples. Of these isotopes of carbon, ^{13}C possesses an extra neutron in the nucleus of the carbon atoms. Endogenous testosterone is synthesised in the body from cholesterol. Pharmaceutical companies that manufacture testosterone synthesise it from plant materials. Pharmaceutically derived testosterone contains slightly less ^{13}C. Therefore using GC-combustion-IRMS techniques, doping control laboratories can distinguish whether urinary testosterone is natural or synthetic, based on $^{12}C:^{13}C$ ratio (Aguilera *et al.*, 1996).

Current WADA regulations recommend IRMS analysis where urinary samples show a T/E ratio exceeding 4:1, although the level of this threshold continues to generate debate (Saudan *et al.*, 2006; Graham *et al.*, 2008).

Steroid profiling

Another technique for determining the misuse of testosterone and other endogenous steroids is that of steroid profiling. The urinary steroid profile contains concentrations and ratios of various endogenously produced steroidal hormones, their precursors and metabolites. These include testosterone, epitestosterone, dihydrotestosterone, androsterone, etiocholanone, dehydroepiandrosterone, 5α-androstane-3α, 17 β-diol and 5β-androstane-3α, 17 β-diol (Mareck *et al.*, 2008). If the steroid profile of an individual athlete is determined each time a urine sample is taken, any alteration of one or more concentrations or ratios of these parameters raises suspicion of a doping offence. Robust and expert interpretation of steroidal profiling is paramount for its success. Similarly, longitudinal biological profiling of blood tests can be undertaken by WADA laboratories. In future, athletes subjected to the longitudinal studies will have their data recorded on "biological passports".

Cooperation with law enforcement agencies

In recent years, WADA and national anti-doping organisations have cooperated with their respective national law enforcement agencies to combat the illegal supply chains for steroids and other prohibited substances. One of the earliest major investigations was "Operation Gear Grinder", carried out by the US authorities between 2005 and 2007. They uncovered a major trafficking system for steroids from Mexican laboratories, which had received their raw materials from factories in China. Results of this investigation led to a more extensive, worldwide investigation called "Operation Raw Deal". A significant number of clandestine laboratories were shut down as a result of these operations.

Other successful investigations have included "Operación Puerto", set up by the Spanish police, in late 2005, which uncovered large supplies of drugs, including steroids, as well as frozen packs of blood. This investigation implicated a large number of international professional cyclists as well as other athletes. A further investigation directed at cyclists was that of "Operation Quick Step" undertaken by Belgian police in 2007.

WADA is now committed to this approach of using national law enforcement agencies to identify individuals who use prohibited substances and, more importantly, to prevent the supply of such materials to athletes.

4.8   Other anabolic agents

Clenbuterol and other Beta-2 agonists (β_2-agonists)

Just before the start of the Barcelona Olympics in 1992, two British weightlifters, Andrew Saxton and Andrew Davis, tested positive for the drug clenbuterol. During the games the IOC acted swiftly to proscribe the drug.

Clenbuterol is classed as a β_2-agonist; it is structurally related to salbutamol and in some countries is licensed for the treatment of asthma. However, the reason for banning the drug was associated with claims that it increased muscle mass while simultaneously reducing body fat. Clenbuterol does not produce its anabolic effects by interacting with testosterone, growth hormone or insulin (Choo et al., 1992) but via β_2-receptor stimulation. Similarly the fat mobilising action of clenbuterol is also mediated via β_2-receptors.

β_2-agonists can promote normal skeletal muscle growth and experiments with clenbuterol show that it can increase muscle weight in rats by 10–12 per cent after two weeks of treatment (Yang and McElliott, 1989). It has been shown that clenbuterol can reverse experimentally induced muscle fibre atrophy by increasing muscle protein synthesis as well as inhibiting amino acid loss.

Spann and Winter (1995) reviewed clenbuterol experiments. They analysed data from the US Department of Agriculture, which demonstrated increases in muscle mass and lean body mass in steers treated with clenbuterol; this result has also been found in rats, poultry and sheep. Human studies are much more equivocal and show that clenbuterol produces no statistically significant increase in involuntary muscle strength but that certain type II or fast-twitch muscle fibres may benefit from the drug.

Most β_2-agonists possess much weaker anabolic effects than clenbuterol, but the 2010 WADA prohibited list specifically cites two other β_2-agonists, zerenol and zilpaterol, under "other anabolic agents" (see Table 4.1).

Selective androgen receptor modulators (SARMs)

SARMs are non-steroidal compounds that can interact with the androgen receptor. Clinically, they offer a therapeutic advantage over anabolic steroids as they can produce anabolic effects with little or no androgenic activity (Bhasin et al., 2006). This lack of a virilisation effect would greatly enhance their therapeutic potential, particularly in women (Gao and Dalton, 2007).

These properties of SARMs, high anabolic and low androgenic, have attracted the attention of some athletes. Consequently, WADA added the SARMs to the prohibited list in January 2008.

Tibolone

Tibolone has a steroidal structure related to norsteroids but it lacks androgenic effects. It is commonly used in hormone replacement therapy during menopause (Van Eenoo and Delbeke, 2006).

4.9   References

Aguilera, R., Becchi, M., Grenot, C. et al. (1996). Detection of testosterone misuse: Comparison of two chromatographic sample preparation methods for gas chromatographic-combustion/isotope ratio mass spectrometric analysis. *Journal of Chromatography B* **687**, 43–53.

Aguilera, R., Chapman, T.E. and Catlin, D.H. (2001). Performance characteristics of a carbon isotope ratio method for detecting doping with testosterone based on urine diols: Controls and athletes with elevated testosterone/epitestosterone ratios. *Clinical Chemistry* **47**, 292–300.

Alén, M. and Rahkila, P. (1988). Anabolic-androgenic steroid effects on endocrinology and lipid metabolism in athletes. *Sports Medicine* **6**, 327–332.

Archer, J. (1991). The influence of testosterone on human aggression. *British Journal of Psychology* **82**, 1–28.

Ayotte, C. (2006). Significance of 19-noradrosterone in athletes' urine samples. *British Journal of Sports Medicine* **40**, i25–i29.

Bahrke, M.S. (2000). Psychological effects of endogenous testosterone and anabolic-androgenic steroids. In *Anabolic steroids in sport and exercise*, ed. C. Yesalis, Human Kinetics Publishers, Champaign, Illinois. 94–106.

Baume, N., Schumacher, Y.O., Sottas, P.E. *et al.* (2006). Effects of multiple oral doses of androgenic anabolic steroids on endurance performance and serum indices of physical stress in healthy male subjects. *European Journal of Applied Physiology* **98(4)**, 329–340.

Bhasin, S., Calof, O.M., Storer, T.W. *et al.* (2006). Drug insight: Testosterone as selective androgen receptor modulators as anabolic therapies for chronic illness and ageing. *Nature Clinical Practice Endocrinology and Metabolism* **2**, 146–159.

Bhasin, S., Woodhouse, L. and Storer, T.W. (2001). Proof of the effect of testosterone on skeletal muscle. *Journal of Endocrinology* **170**, 27–38.

Blazevich, A.J. and Giorgi, A. (2001). Effect of testosterone administration and weight-training on muscle architecture. *Medicine and Science in Sport and Exercise* **33**, 1688–1693.

Catlin, D.H., Ahrens, B.D. and Kucherova, Y. (2002). Detection of norbolethone an anabolic steroid never market in athletes urine. *Rapid Communications in Mass Spectrometry* **16**, 1273–1275.

Catlin, D.H., Fitch, K.D. and Ljungqvist, A. (2008). Medicine and science in the fight against doping in sport. *Journal of Internal Medicine* **264**, 99–114.

Catlin, D.H., Kammerer, R.C., Hatton, C.K. *et al.* (1987). Analytical chemistry at the Games of the XXIII Olympiad in Los Angeles, 1984. *Clinical Chemistry* **33**, 319–327.

Catlin, D., Wright, J., Pope, H. *et al.* (1993). Assessing the threat of anabolic steroids. *Physical and Sports Medicine* **21**, 37–44.

Catlin, D.H., Leder, B.S., Ahrens, B. *et al.* (2000). Trace contamination of over-the-counter andiostenedino and positive urine tests results for a nandrolone metabolite. *Journal of the American Medical Association* **284**, 2618–2621.

Catlin, D.H., Sekera, M.H., Ahrens, B.D. *et al.* (2004). Tetrahydrogestrinone: Discovery, synthesis and detection in urine. *Rapid Communications in Mass Spectrometry* **18**, 1245–1249.

Choi, P.Y.L. (1998). Illicit anabolic androgenic steroid use in women: A case of pseudo-hermaphroditism. *Journal of Performance Enhancing Drugs* **2**, 24–26.

Choo, J-J., Horon, M.A., Little, R.A. *et al.* (1992). Clenbuterol and skeletal muscle are mediated by β2 adrenoceptor activation. *American Journal of Physiology* **263**, 50–56.

Costill, D.L., Pearson, D.R. and Fink, W.J. (1984). Anabolic steroid use among athletes. Changes in HDC-C levels. *Physician and Sports Medicine* **12**, 113–117.

Dehennin, L., Bonnaire, Y. and Plou, P. (1999). Urinary excretion of 19-norandrosterone of endogenous origin in man: Quantitative analysis by gas chromatography mass spectrometry. *Journal of Chromatography B* **721**, 301–307.

Dugal, R., Dupuis, C. and Bertrand, M.J. (1977). Radioimmunoassay of anabolic steroids: An evaluation of three antisera for the detection of anabolic steroids in biological fluids. *British Journal of Sports Medicine* **11**, 162–169.

Elashoff, J.D., Jacknow, A.D., Shain, S.G. *et al.* (1991). Effects of anabolic-androgenic steroids on muscular strength. *Annals of Internal Medicine* **115**, 387–393.

Elliot, D.I. and Goldberg, I. (2000). Women and anabolic steroids. In *Anabolic steroids in sport and exercise*, ed. C. Yesalis, Human Kinetics Publishers, Champaign, Illinois. 225–240.

Evans, N.A. (1997). Gym and tonic: A profile of 100 male steroid users. *British Journal of Sports Medicine* **31**, 54–58.

Ferstle, J. (1999a). The nandrolone story. *Athletics Weekly*, 15 September 1999, 16.

Ferstle, J. (1999b). Nandrolone part 2. *Athletics Weekly*, 22 September 1999, 26–27.

Franke, W.N. and Berendonk, B. (1997). Hormonal doping and androgenisation of athletes: A secret program of the German Democratic Republic government. *Clinical Chemistry* **43**, 1262–1297.

Friedl, K.E. and Yesalis, C.E. (1989). Self-treatment of gynaecomastia in body builders who use anabolic steroids. *Physician and Sports Medicine* **17**, 67–79.

Gao, W.Q. and Dalton, J.T. (2007). Expanding the therapeutic use of androgens via selective androgen receptor modulators (SARMs). *Drug Discovery Today* **12**, 241–248.

Goldman, B. (1984). *Death in the locker room: Steroids and sports*. Century Publishing, London.

Graham, M.R., Davies, B., Grace, F.M. *et al.* (2008). Anabolic steroid use. Patterns of use and detection of doping. *Sports Medicine* **38**, 505–525.

Green, G.A., Uryasz, F.D., Petr, T.A. *et al.* (2001). NCAA study of substance use and abuse habits of college student-athletes. *Clinical Journal of Sports Medicine* **11**, 51–56.

Greenblatt, R.B., Chaddha, J.S., Teran, A.Z. *et al.* (1985). Aphrodisiacs. In *Psychopharmacology: Recent advances and future prospects*, ed. S.D. Iverson, British Association for Psychopharmacology Monograph No. 6, Oxford University Press, Oxford. 290–302.

Hartgens, F. and Kuipers, H. (2004). Effects of androgenic anabolic steroids in athletes. *Sports Medicine* **34**, 513–554.

Haupt, H.A. and Rovere, G.D. (1984). Anabolic steroids: A review of the literature. *American Journal of Sports Medicine* **12**, 469–484.

Herbst, K.I. and Bhasin, S. (2004). Testosterone action on skeletal muscle. *Current Opinions on Nutrition and Metabolic Care* **7**, 271–277.

Hobbs, C.J., Jones, R.E. and Plymate, S.R. (1996). Nandrolone, a 19-nortestosterone, enhances insulin dependent glucose uptake in normal men. *Journal of Endocrinology and Metabolism* **81**, 1582–1585.

Holma, P.K. (1979). Effects of an anabolic steroid (methandienone) on spermatogenesis. *Contraception* **15**, 151–162.

Johnson, R. (1999). Abnormal testosterone: Epitestosterone ratio dehydroepiandrostenedrine supplements. *Clinical Chemistry* **45**, 163–164.

Kadi, F. (2008). Cellular and molecular mechanisms responsible for the action of testosterone on human skeletal muscle. A basis for illegal performance enhancement. *British Journal of Pharmacology* **154**, 522–528.

Karila, T.A., Hovatta, O. and Seppälä, T. (2004). Concomitant abuse of anabolic androgenic steroids and human chorionic gonadotrophin impairs spermatogenesis in power athletes. *International Journal of Sports Medicine* **25(4)**, 257–263.

Karila, T.A., Karjalainen, J.E., Mantysaari, M.J. *et al.* (2003). Anabolic androgenic steroids produce dose-dependent increase in left ventricular mass in power athletes and this effect is potentiated by concomitant use of growth hormone. *International Journal of Sports Medicine* **24**, 337–343.

Kashkin, K.B. and Kleber, H.D. (1989). Hooked on hormones? An anabolic steroid addiction hypothesis. *Journal of the American Medical Association* **262**, 3166–3170.

Kennedy, M.C. and Lawrence, C. (1993). Anabolic steroid abuse and cardiac death. *Medical Journal of Australia* **158**, 346–348.

Kicman, A.T. (2008). Pharmacology of anabolic steroids. *British Journal of Pharmacology* **154**, 502–521.

Kinze, P., Cirimele, V. and Ludes, B. (1999). Noradrosterone et noretiocholanone: Les métaboltes révélateurs. *Acta Clinica Belgica* **S1999–1**, 68–73.

Korkia, P., Leneham, P. and McVenigh, J. (1996). Medical use of androgens among women. *Journal of Performance Enhancing Drugs* **1**, 71–76.

Kuipers, H., Wijnen, J.A.G., Hartgens, F. *et al.* (1991). Influence of anabolic steroids on body composition, blood pressure, lipid profile and liver functions in body builders. *International Journal of Sports Medicine* **12**, 413–418.

Laseter, J.T. and Russell, J.A. (1991). Anabolic steroid–induced tendon pathology: A review of the literature. *Medicine and Science in Sports and Exercise* **23**, 1–3.

Le Bizec, B., Bryand, F., Gausin, I. *et al.* (2002). Endogenous nandrolone metabolites in human urine: Preliminary results to discriminate between endogenous and exogenous origin. *Steroids* **67**, 105–110.

Le Bizec, B., Monteau, F., Gaudin, I. and Andre, F. (1999). Evidence for the presence of endogenous 19-norandrostenedione in human urine. *Journal of Chromatography B* **723**, 157–172.

Lombardo, J.A., Hickson, P.C. and Lamb, D.R. (1991). Anabolic/androgenic steroids and growth hormone. In *Perspectives in exercise science and sports medicine, vol. 4: Ergogenics—Enhancement of performance in exercise and sport*, ed. D.R. Lamb and M.H. Williams, Brown and Benchmark. 249–278.

Lukas, S.E. (1993). Current perspectives on anabolic-androgenic steroid abuse. *Trends in Pharmacological Sciences* **14**, 61–68.

Maganaris, C.N., Collins, D., and Sharp, M. (2000). Expectancy effects and strength training: Do steroids make a difference? *Sports Psychologist* **14**, 272–278.

Mareck, U., Geyer, H., Opfermann, G. *et al.* (2008). Factors influencing the steroid profile in doping control analysis. *Journal of Mass Spectrometry* **43**, 877–891.

Mareck-Engelke, U., Schultz, G., Geyer, H. *et al.* (2002). The appearance of 19-noradrosterone during pregnancy. *European Journal of Sports Science* **2**, 1–7.

Mark, P.B., Watkins, S. and Dargie, H.J. (2005). Cardiomyopathy induced by performance enhancing drugs in a competitive body builder. *Heart* **91**, 888.

Middleman, A.B., and DuRant, P.H. (1996). Anabolic steroid use and associated health risk behaviours. *Sports Medicine* **21**, 251–255.

Millar, A.P. (1994). Licit steroid use—hope for the future. *British Journal of Sports Medicine* **28**, 79–83.

Mottram, D.R. and George, A.J. (2000). Anabolic steroids. *Clinical Endocrinology and Metabolism* **14**, 55–69.

Nieminen, M.S., Ramo, M.P., Viitasalo, M. *et al.* (1996). Serious cardiovascular side effects of large doses of anabolic steroids in weight lifters. *European Heart Journal* **17**, 1576–1583.

Pagonis, T.A., Angelopoulos, N.V., Koukoulis, G.N. *et al.* (2006). Psychiatric side effects induced by supraphysiological doses of combinations of anabolic steroids correlate to the severity of abuse. *European Psychiatry* **21**, 551–562.

Pärssinen, M., Kinjala, U., Vartiainen, E. *et al.* (2000). Increased premature mortality of competitive powerlifters suspected to have used anabolic agents. *International Journal of Sports Medicine* **21**, 225–227.

Pärssinen, M. and Seppälä, T. (2002). Steroid use and long-term health risks in former athletes. *Sports Medicine* **32**, 83–94.

Perry, H.M., Wright, D. and Littlepage, B.N.C. (1992). Dying to be big: A review of anabolic steroid use. *British Journal of Sports Medicine* **26**, 259–261.

Pope, H.G., Gruber, A.J., Choi, P. *et al.* (1997). Muscle dysmorphia. *Psychosomatics* **38**, 548–557.

Pope, H.G. and Katz, D.L. (1988). Affective and psychotic symptoms associated with anabolic steroid use. *American Journal of Psychiatry* **145**, 487–490.

Prendergast, H.M., Bannen, T., Erickson, T.B. *et al.* (2003). The toxic torch of the modern Olympic Games. *Veterans Human Toxicology* **45**, 97–102.

Reznik, U., Dehennin, L., Coffin, C. *et al.* (2001). Urinary nandrolone metabolites of endogenous origin in man: A confirmation by output regulation under human chorionic gonadotropin stimulation. *Journal of Clinical Endocrinology and Metabolism* **86**, 145–150.

Rockhold, R.W. (1993). Cardiovascular toxicity of anabolic steroids. *Annual Review of Pharmacology and Toxicology* **33**, 497–520.

Rogol, A.D. and Yesalis, C.E. (1992). Anabolic-androgenic steroids and athletes: What are the issues? *Journal of Endocrinology and Metabolism* **74**, 465–469.

Ryan, A.J. (1981). Anabolic steroids are fool's gold. *Federation Proceedings* **40**, 2682–2688.

Saudan, C., Baume, N., Robinson, N. *et al.* (2006). Testosterone and doping control. *British Journal of Sports Medicine* **40**, i21–i24.

Schänzer, W. (2002). Analysis of non-hormonal nutritional supplements for anabolic-androgenic steroids—An international study. Available at www.olympic.org (accessed May 2002).

Sekera, M.H., Ahren, B.D., Chang, Y.-C. *et al.* (2005). Another designer steroid: Discovery, synthesis and detection of "madol" in urine. *Rapid Communications in Mass Spectrometry* **19**, 781–784.

Sinha-Hikim, I., Artaza, J., Woodhouse, I. *et al.* (2002). Testosterone-induced increase in muscle size in healthy young men in association with muscle fibre hypertrophy. *American Journal of Physiology, Endocrinology and Metabolism* **283**, E154–E164.

Sjöqvist, F., Garle, M. and Rane, A. (2008). Use of doping agents, particularly anabolic steroids, in sports and society. *Lancet* **371**, 1872–1882.

Sklarek, H.M., Mantovani, R.P., Erens, E. *et al.* (1984). A.I.D.S. in a body builder using anabolic steroids. *New England Journal of Medicine* **311**, 861–862.

Spann, C. and Winter, M.E. (1995). Effects of clenbuterol on athletic performance. *Annals Pharmacotherapy* **29**, 75–77.

Street, C., Antonio, J. and Cudlipp, D. (1996). Androgen use by athletes: A re-evaluation of the health risks. *Canadian Journal of Applied Physiology* **21**, 421–440.

Thiblin, I., Lindquist, O. and Rajs, J. (2000). Cause and manner of death among abusers of anabolic androgenic steroids. *Journal of Forensic Science* **45**, 16–23.

Thiblin, I. and Petersson, A. (2005). Pharmacoepidemiology of anabolic androgenic steroids: A review. *Fundamentals of Clinical Pharmacology* **19**, 27–44.

Tokish, J.M., Kocher, M.S. and Hawkins, R.J. (2004). Ergogenic aids: A review of basic science, performance, side effects and status in sports. *American Journal of Sports Medicine* **32**, 1543–1553.

Ueki, M. and Okano, M. (1999). Doping with naturally occurring steroids. *Journal of Toxicology—Toxin Reviews* **18**, 177–195.

Van Eenoo, P. and Delbeke, F.T. (2006). Metabolism and excretion of anabolic steroids in doping control—New steroids and new insights. *Journal of Steroids Biochemistry and Molecular Biology* **101**, 161–178.

Wagner, J.C. (1991). Enhancement of athletic performance with drugs. *Sports Medicine* **12**, 250–265.

Walker, C.J., Cowan, D.A., James, V.H.T. *et al.* (2009). Doping in sport-1. Excretion of 19-norandrosterone by healthy women, including those using contraceptives containing norethisterone. *Steroids* **74(3)**, 329–334.

Wallace, M.B., Lim, J., Cutler, A. *et al.* (1999). Effects of dhydro epiandrosterone vs. androsteredine supplementation in men. *Medicine and Science in Sports and Exercise* **31**, 1788–1792.

Warren, M.P. and Shantha, S. (2000). The female athlete. *Clinical Endocrinology and Metabolism* **14**, 37–54.

Williamson, P.J. and Young, A.H. (1992). Psychiatric effects of androgenic and anabolic-androgenic steroid abuse in men: A brief review of the literature. *Journal of Psychopharmacology* **6**, 20–26.

Wilson, J.D. (1988). Androgen abuse by athletes. *Endocrinological Reviews* **9**, 181–199.

Wright, F., Bricout, V., Doukani, A. *et al.* (2000). Nandrolone et norsteroids: Substances endogenes ou xenobitiques? *Science & Sports* **15**, 111–124.

Wright, J.E. (1980). Anabolic steroids and athletics. *Exercise and Sport Science Reviews* **8**, 149–202.

Wu, F.C.W. (1997). Endocrine agents of anabolic steroids. *Clinical Chemistry* **43**, 1289–1292.

Yang, Y.T. and McElliott, M.A. (1989). Multiple actions of β-adrenergic agonists on skeletal muscle and adipose tissue. *Biochemistry Journal* **261**, 1–10.

Yates, W.R., Perry, P.J., MacIndoe, J. *et al.* (1999). Psychosexual effects of 3 doses of testosterone cycling in normal men. *Biological Psychiatrist* **45**, 254–260.

Yesalis, C.E. and Bahrke, M.S. (2000). Doping among adolescent athletes. *Clinical Endocrinology and Metabolism* **14**, 25–35.

Yesalis, C.E., Herrick, R.T., Buckley, W.E. *et al.* (1988). Self-reported use of anabolic androgenic steroids by elite power lifters. *Physician and Sports Medicine* **16**, 91–100.

Chapter 5

Peptide hormones and related substances

Alan J. George and David R. Mottram

5.1 Introduction

The World Anti-Doping Agency prohibits the use of a number of peptide hormones and related substances (Table 5.1), most of which occur naturally in the body.

5.2 Erythropoiesis-stimulating agents

This group of agents includes the endogenous peptide erythropoietin (EPO), which is commercially available as recombinant-EPO and the synthetically produced darbepoetin (dEPO) and methoxy polyethylene glycol-epoetin beta (CERA). The modes of action and use of these agents is reviewed in Chapter 9 of this book.

5.3 Human growth hormone (hGH)

Introduction

Human growth hormone (hGH) is one of the major hormones influencing growth and development in humans. The period of human growth extends from birth to the age of 20 years. A large number of hormones influence this period, producing many complex interactions. Besides hGH, testosterone, oestradiol, cortisol, thyroxine and insulin have important roles at different stages of growth and development. The exact role of hGH is difficult to evaluate, because of the many different developmental and metabolic processes that hGH can influence. A review of hGH and its abuse in sport has been published by Holt and Sonksen (2008). The regulation of muscle mass by hGH and growth factors has been reviewed by Velloso (2008).

Release of human growth hormone

The anterior pituitary, a small endocrine gland at the base of, but not part of, the brain, contains somatotroph cells, which secrete growth hormone. Release of

Table 5.1 The list of peptide hormones, growth factors and related substances on the WADA prohibited list (January 2010)

1. Erythropoiesis-stimulating agents (e.g. erythropoietin [EPO], darbepoetin [dEPO], methoxy polyethylene glycol-epoetin beta [CERA], hematide)
2. Chorionic gonadotropin (CG) and luteinizing hormone (LH) in males
3. Insulins
4. Corticotropins
5. Growth hormone (GH), insulin-like growth factor-1 (IGF-1), mechano growth factors (MGFs), platelet-derived growth factors (PDGF), vascular-endothelial growth factor (VEGF) and hepatocycte growth factor (HGF) as well as any other growth factor affecting muscle, tendon or ligament protein synthesis/degradation, vascularisation, energy utilization, regenerative capacity or fibre type twitching
6. Platelet-derived preparations (e.g. platelet-rich plasma, "blood spinning") administered by intramuscular route. Other routes of administration require a declaration of use in accordance with the International Standard for Therapeutic Use Exemptions.

And other substances with similar chemical structure or similar biological effect(s).

hGH is under the control of two hypothalamic hormones: somatostatin, which inhibits secretion, and somatocrinin, which stimulates secretion. Oestradiol also stimulates hGH secretion while testosterone has very little effect. Various brain neurotransmitter systems also influence hGH secretion. This is thought to occur via a controlling influence on the hypothalamic production of somatostatin and somatocrinin, but direct effects on the somatotroph cells cannot be ruled out. Drugs such as clonidine, which stimulate α_2 adrenergic receptors, cause increases in hGH secretion while drugs that stimulate β_2-receptors, such as salbutamol, decrease hGH secretion. The factors influencing hGH secretion have been reviewed in detail by Macintyre (1987) and Muller (1987).

Daily hGH secretion is episodic: the highest levels (0.5–3.0 mg.l^{-1}) occur 60–90 minutes after the onset of sleep. Human GH is metabolised in the liver; the plasma half-life is only 12–45 minutes. The physiological regulation of hGH release is complex. Systemic factors stimulating hGH secretion include hypoglycaemia, a rise in blood amino acid concentration, and stress and exercise, while conversely hGH secretion is inhibited by hyperglycaemia. Both endurance exercise and resistance training have been shown to cause an increase in hGH secretion in female athletes (Consitt et al., 2002).

Human growth hormone action

The most obvious action of hGH is that it stimulates somatic growth in pre-adolescents but it also has metabolic effects. The importance of these metabolic actions in homeostatic regulation of fuel usage and storage is unclear as is the overall role of hGH in the adult; this is discussed in detail by Macintyre (1987). Receptors for hGH are present on the surface of every cell in the body (Holt, 2004).

Discussion of the actions of hGH is further complicated by the involvement of the plasma growth factors or somatomedins in the action of hGH. hGH stimulates the release mainly from the liver of two hormonal polypeptides, somatomedin C (or insulin-like growth factor I) and somatomedin A (insulin-like growth factor II) and a full account of this is provided by Macintyre (1987) and Kicman and Cowan (1992). The somatomedin hypothesis suggests that growth hormone exerts its anabolic actions through the generation of IGF-I (Le Roith *et al.*, 2001).

In this chapter somatomedin C will be known as IGF-I and somatomedin A as IGF-II. IGF-I is the most important of these growth factors but there is still doubt whether many, if any, of the important metabolic effects of hGH are mediated via IGFs (Sonksen, 2001).

In addition, the liver produces three binding proteins with affinity for insulin-like growth factors. These are called IGFBP 1,2,3, of which IGFBP-3 seems to be the most important (Sonksen, 2001). IGFs are carried in the plasma in two different forms: as ternary complexes and simpler low molecular weight complexes (Boisclair *et al.*, 2001). The ternary complexes that contain the IGF in combination with IGFBP-3 and a protein called ALS (acid-labile sub unit) render the IGF biologically inactive, unable to enter tissue spaces and resistant to metabolism. The simple complexes, however, allow the IGFs to enter tissue spaces from the blood capillaries (Boisclair *et al.*, 2001). Very little IGF remains free in the blood.

Effects on muscle

hGH seems to have some effects on muscle growth but the effect of IGF-I is greater. This action *appears* similar to that of insulin in that it promotes amino acid uptake and stimulates protein synthesis, resulting, in children, in an increase in the length and diameter of muscle fibres, while only the growth of the latter occurs in adults. This stimulation of muscle protein synthesis and growth is qualitatively different to that induced by work, since insulin is required for hGH-stimulated muscle growth but not for that induced by work (Macintyre, 1987). However, the action of insulin is more likely to be an anti-catabolic effect on muscle protein rather than a direct stimulatory effect on muscle protein synthesis (Sonksen, 2001).

Effects on bone

hGH stimulates both directly and via the IGFs the elongation of bone in pre-adolescents. This is achieved by a stimulation of cartilage proliferation in the epiphyseal plates situated at each end of each long bone. Cartilage cells possess receptors for hGH and IGFs.

Effects on metabolism

The actions of hGH on metabolism are complex at both the cellular and organ level and appear to be biphasic. In the first or acute phase, which seems to involve the action of hGH alone, amino acid uptake into muscle (via mobilisation of muscle membrane amino acid transporters) and liver is stimulated, and there is increased glucose uptake into muscle and adipose tissue together with reduced fat metabolism (Smith and Perry, 1992). During the second, chronic phase, mediated by the IGFs, there is increased lipolysis (triglyceride breakdown) in adipose tissue resulting in a rise in the plasma concentration of fatty acids and increased fatty acid utilisation, thus sparing glucose.

Effects on adipose tissue

Treatment of GH-deficient adults has shown that GH can increase lean body mass by several kilograms and decrease fat mass, especially visceral fat, by an equivalent amount (Marcus and Hoffman, 1998). Whether the same effect would be achieved in someone with normal GH secretion is unknown.

Treatment with hGH causes a rise in blood free fatty acid levels or rise in the blood glucose level and a reduction in the triglyceride content of adipose tissue, which contributes to a decrease in adipose tissue mass and an increase in fat-free weight (Kicman and Cowan, 1992).

Effects of exercise on hGH

Within 20 minutes of beginning exercise to 75–90 per cent VO_2max, hGH levels rise. The intensity of the response depends on age, level of fitness and body composition. The type of exercise undertaken also produces varying hGH responses. Intermittent intense exercise is claimed to result in the highest hGH levels (Macintyre, 1987).

Administration and supply of hGH

hGH is a peptide and must be injected. Human GH is produced synthetically. Therapeutically, hGH administration is usually recommended as either three single injections, intramuscularly (i.m.) or subcutaneously (s.c.) or as daily s.c. injections in the evening.

Many hGH supplies are known to be illicitly obtained by theft from pharmaceutical company production lines and from retail pharmacies (Sonksen, 2001). The prevalence of hGH use by athletes is difficult to determine as much of the evidence arises through anecdotal reports (McHugh et al., 2005).

Growth hormone disorders

Inadequate secretion of hGH is one of the causes of the conditions known as dwarfism. This disorder is usually recognised in childhood when the rate of growth is below the ninetieth percentile for that child's age, race and sex. Further tests involve "challenges" to the pituitary in the form of arginine, clonidine or insulin. If these fail to evoke adequate hGH secretion then a diagnosis of dwarfism, due to inadequate hGH, can be made. The treatment is regular administration of synthetic hGH until the end of puberty. Treatment after adolescence is ineffective in stimulating growth in stature because by this time the epiphyseal plates in the long bones have fused, terminating any further bone growth. Overproduction of hGH as a result of a tumour may occur in puberty and adolescence when it gives rise to gigantism; the individual is well above average adult height for his or her age, sex and race, and the limbs and internal organs are also enlarged.

In late adulthood, a tumour of the anterior pituitary can cause increased hGH secretion; this is a condition known as acromegaly. The affected individual does not grow any taller because the epiphyses have fused but internal organs enlarge (especially the heart) and the fingers grow and the skin thickens. Metabolic disorders occur, which often precipitate Type II diabetes mellitus.

A deficiency in hGH secretion in adulthood has been recognised in elderly people, some of whom have responded favourably to hGH therapy (Marcus and Hoffman, 1998; Gotherstrom et al., 2005). The investigations of this syndrome, while providing interesting data on the effects of hGH, have not indicated a universal benefit of hGH treatment for the elderly.

It has been suggested by a number of geriatricians that hGH might be used to reverse some of the bodily changes occurring in old age. Normal ageing is associated with a reduction in lean body mass, an increase in fat mass and a reduction in skin thickness. Trials of hGH treatment in the elderly have shown that the hormone is able to reverse these changes (Jorgensen and Christiansen, 1993), but a review of world-wide clinical trials of hGH in the elderly was not favourable (Marcus and Hoffman, 1998).

5.4   The abuse of hGH in sport

There appear to be four major abuses of hGH in sport: (1) to increase muscle mass and strength, (2) to increase lean body mass, (3) to improve the "appearance of musculature", and (4) to increase final adult height. Scientific evidence from controlled trials that hGH increases muscle strength is controversial. There is some evidence to support the claim that hGH administration may increase lean body mass. Lombardo et al. (1991) describe experiments where hGH administration has caused significant reductions in "fat weight", and increases in fat-free weight compared to placebo.

As early as 1988, Cowart reviewed anecdotal reports by body builders of increases in strength following hGH administration. There are also several positive findings of increased muscle growth, strength and protein synthesis in hGH-deficient adults treated with human growth hormone (Marcus and Hoffman, 1998). When Taaffe et al. (1996) examined the effects of growth hormone treatment on muscle strength and lean body mass in elderly men they found no increases in strength but an increase in lean body mass and a decrease in fat mass. Similarly when Yarasheski et al. (1993) examined resistance training schedules before and during hGH administration in elderly men they found hGH did not further enhance muscle strength improvements induced by exercise regimes. In younger adult men there is a similar picture. Sixteen healthy men, 21–34 years old, who had not previously trained were given hGH (0.56 IU/kg/12 weeks) or placebo during 12 weeks of heavy resistance training. At the end of the study, lean body mass and total body water increased in the hGH group compared to placebo, but there was no difference in muscle strength or limb circumference (Yarasheski *et al.*, 1992). Negative results have also been obtained with seven weightlifters who were given hGH 0.56 IU/Kg week during a 14-day heavy session. Muscle protein synthesis did not increase and there was no change in whole body protein breakdown. When slightly higher doses, 0.631U/Kg/week, were administered to 22 male power athletes ages 20–28 for six weeks, no increases in biceps or quadriceps maximal strength occurred in the hGH group compared to placebo (Deyssig *et al.*, 1993).

The above evidence conflicts with positive anecdotal reports (Cowart, 1988) and the continuing popularity of hGH abuse suggested by surveys (Bidlingmaier *et al.*, 2000). The potential performance-enhancing effects of hGH is still debated amongst users (Saugy *et al.*, 2006). Effects may be attributed to other substances used in combination with hGH.

Ehrnborg *et al.* (2000) reviewed previous experiments on hGH use and concluded that possibly the studies are "too short and included too few subjects". As with early studies on anabolic steroids the doses used may have been too low and some of the hGH abusers may also have been concurrently abusing anabolic steroids (Schnirring, 2000). Yarasheski *et al.* (1993) concluded that increases in lean body mass can occur without increases in strength if it is non-contractile protein that is produced.

It is claimed that hGH administration improves the appearance of the body builder, making his/her muscles more salient or "sculpted" and improving their photogenicity. There is no way this effect can be measured directly or objectively but it appears to be a logical development associated with loss of fat tissue.

The desire to produce tall offspring either for cosmetic reasons, athletic potential or so that they can qualify for a vocation where there is a minimum height limit has prompted hGH abuse amongst children in the USA. In addition to the ethical problems that it presents, the child may later resent its tallness particularly if later it fails to qualify as a professional sportsperson. An apparent relentless drive for "bigness" and "tallness" in sport and society by selective and drug-induced means is discussed in a review by Norton and Olds (2001).

Overall, there continues to be debate as to whether the adverse effects of hGH outweigh the potential performance-enhancing effects (Rennie, 2003).

Side effects associated with hGH abuse in sport

The long-term risks of hGH in athletes are not well known since epidemiological data derived from users in sport are not available (Saugy *et al.*, 2006).

The potential risk of hGH therapy in children is clear. In the UK, the recommended standard replacement dose of hGH is about 0.6 IU/kg body weight per week. It is widely assumed that athletes who abuse the drug are taking ten times this dose (Smith and Perry, 1992). Major side effects include skeletal changes, enlargement of the fingers and toes, growth of the orbit and lengthening of the jaw. The internal organs enlarge and the cardiomegaly that is produced is often one of the causes of death associated with hGH abuse. Although the skeletal muscles increase in size, there are often complaints of muscle weakness. Adverse biochemical changes include impaired glucose regulation (usually hyperglycaemia), hyperlipidaemia and insulin resistance. The changes described above contribute to the prevalence of diabetes in hGH abusers. Arthritis and impotence often occur after chronic hGH abuse (Kicman and Cowan, 1992).

A consequence of the increased protein synthesis during hGH abuse is changes to the skin. This includes thickening and coarsening—the "elephant epidermis" that has been known to make the skin almost impenetrable by standard gauge syringe needles (Taylor, 1988). Other skin effects include activation of naevocytes and an increase in dermal viscosity (Ehrnborg et al. 2000). This combination of side effects, particularly the cardiomegaly, hyperlipidaemia and hyperglycaemia, almost certainly contributes to the shortened life spans seen in those suffering from overproduction of hGH (Smith and Perry, 1992). The effect of hGH on blood lipids seems equivocal: whereas long periods of abuse may cause elevation of blood lipids, abuse for up to six weeks may decrease plasma cholesterol and apolipoproteins (Zuliani et al., 1989).

It is believed that many athletes use doses of hGH 10 times or so higher that those used therapeutically and it is reasonable to expect that many side effects may develop (Holt and Sonksen, 2008). It is likely that the longer-term effect of hGH administration would also occur with IGF-I (Holt and Sonksen, 2008), as described in clinical trials for mecasermin rinfabate (Kemp, 2007).

Who abuses growth hormone and why?

The reasons for hGH abuse appear to be based on some false premises: that it is as effective as anabolic steroids, with fewer side effects and is less easily detected. Abusers believe hGH may protect the athlete who has abused anabolic steroids and who wishes to stop "muscle meltdown" when anabolic steroids are withdrawn.

There are few scientific studies available on the prevalence of hGH abuse in sport. Macintyre (1987) identified American football players and body builders as the most likely abusers based on lab reports from accredited testing agencies. An early UK investigation by Perry et al. (1992) revealed no hGH abuse. However, by 1997, Korkia and Stimson reported that 2.7 per cent of the anabolic steroid abusers in their UK survey were also abusing hGH while Evans (1997) found concordant abuse of anabolic steroids and hGH in 12.7 per cent of abusers in his gymnasia survey.

Five per cent of adolescents in a survey (Rickert *et al.*, 1992) admitted using hGH and 24.5 per cent claimed to know of someone who was abusing it. Fifty per cent of the abusers could not name one side effect of hGH. Those who abused hGH were most likely to be involved in wrestling or American football and to have obtained their information about hGH from another person such as a coach. There was also some evidence of co-abuse of anabolic steroids and hGH in the same adolescent sample.

Because a validated test for hGH has not been available, reports of hGH abuse have been mostly anecdotal or as observations by anti-doping agencies (Stow *et al.*, 2009). On a number of occasions, athletes have confessed to using hGH, having tested positive for other substances. This was the case with Ben Johnson after the 1988 Seoul Olympics and for a number of high-profile athletes after the BALCO affair in 2003. A review of the use of hGH by athletes can be found in Holt *et al.* (2009).

Detection of hGH abuse

Human GH is a peptide that has a very short half-life in the blood and appears in very low concentrations in the urine. Furthermore, secretions of naturally occurring hGH from the pituitary gland are pulsatile. Therefore, blood levels fluctuate significantly. Since hGH secretion is affected by factors such as emotion, stress, sleep and nutritional status, there is a high variability within individuals and between individuals (Saugy *et al.*, 2006). In addition, exercise can influence hGH secretion (Wallace *et al.*, 2001). Therefore, traditional methods for the detection of performance-enhancing substances in athletes are ineffective. There is no urine test for hGH currently available.

Up to the 2004 Athens Olympic Games a validated method to detect hGH was not in use, despite significant attempts to develop such a method. After the 1996 Atlanta Games, a research project entitled GH-2000 was set up, comprising a consortium of endocrinologists with expertise in growth hormone research from four European countries, with collaboration from two leading pharmaceutical companies (Holt *et al.*, 2009). The project team reported their results in 1999 (GH-2000, 1999), with a proposal for a test based on the measurement of two markers for hGH, IGF-1 and type III pro-collagen (P-III-P) (Powrie *et al.*, 2007). Despite significant support for the proposed test, it was recommended that further research was required to ensure the test would work within ethnic groups other than Caucasians and that the test was not affected by injury. Unfortunately, funding for the extension of the research was not forthcoming from the IOC, the main sponsor of GH-2000 (Holt *et al.*, 2009).

However, following the foundation of WADA in 1999, a second phase of research into hGH testing was set up, entitled GH-2004, with significant financial support from the US Anti-Doping Agency. GH-2004 directed its efforts towards the "markers" approach to hGH testing. At the same time, WADA focused its funding on an "isoform" approach to testing (Barroso *et al.*, 2009).

The indirect "markers" approach to hGH doping detection

The indirect approach does not aim to detect hGH itself but to build up a database of the normal range of a number of markers for hGH, such as IGF-I, P-III-P, IGFBPs or markers for bone turnover. Having established cut-off levels for these markers, individuals who exceed these levels could be construed as having used exogenous hGH (Wallace *et al.*, 1999). It has been suggested that this approach would not stand up in a court as an absolute proof of doping (Saugy *et al.*, 2006). However, the results of the GH-2000 and GH-2004 studies supported the choice of IGF-I and P-III-P as markers to detect hGH in samples for several days after recombinant hGH administration (Erotokritou-Mulligan *et al.*, 2007).

The direct "isoform" approach to hGH doping detection

This approach involves immunoassays to quantify different types of hGH isoforms that differentiate between naturally secreted hGH and recombinant hGH that has been injected by the athlete.

This test was used, experimentally, at the Athens Olympic Games in 2004 and at the Torino Winter Olympic Games in 2006 (Saugy *et al.*, 2006). To fulfil WADA requirements, two double tests were applied to serum samples. The first test quantified the 22kDa isoform that is derived from recombinant hGH. The second test measured the other isoforms derived from naturally occurring hGH. When recombinant hGH is administered, endogenous growth hormone secretion is inhibited; therefore, the ratio of 22kDa to total GH increases. The ratio between these isoforms is calculated. A second double sample test was used for confirmatory purposes (Bidlingmaier *et al.*, 2000).

The direct test was also used at the 2008 Beijing Olympic Games. However, as in Athens and Torino, no positive test results were detected. It has been suggested that this is unsurprising as this method has a relatively short (less than 24 hour) window of opportunity. Therefore, any athlete who discontinues use of hGH on the day before the test would not be detected (Holt *et al.*, 2009).

National anti-doping organisations, such as UK Sport, are continuing research into improving the direct and indirect approaches for the detection of hGH (Stow *et al.*, 2009). Ultimately, the aim is a combined approach using both the differential isoform immunoassay and the markers detection both in and out of competition (Barroso *et al.*, 2009).

Another approach being adopted by international federations is longitudinal studies on athletes' biological profiles. By regularly monitoring these haematological profiles, any abnormalities would reveal potential doping activity.

Other approaches to hGH detection are being investigated by research groups around the world, including urine-based tests (Barroso *et al.*, 2009).

5.5   Human chorionic gonadotropin (hCG)

Human chorionic gonadotropin (hCG) is produced by placental trophoblast cells during pregnancy and also by a number of different types of tumour cells.

Its major physiological role is stimulating the corpus luteum in pregnant females, maintaining synthesis and secreting the hormone progesterone during pregnancy. However, when injected into males, hCG also stimulates the Leydig cells of the testes to produce testosterone and epitestosterone, and so it can mimic the natural stimulation of testicular hormone produced by luteinizing hormone (LH). Administration of hCG stimulates secretion of testosterone and epitestosterone in a normal ratio.

The Leydig cells of the testes possess receptors that, when stimulated by LH or hCG, activate testosterone synthesis. This increase in synthesis is rapid, a 50 per cent increase in plasma testosterone concentration has been measured two hours after i.m. injection of 6000 IU of hCG (Kicman et al., 1991). Injection of hCG also stimulates production of nandrolone (19 nortestosterone) metabolites and this may indicate that it can stimulate production of endogenous nandrolone itself (Reznik et al., 2001).

An excellent review of hCG has been published by Stenman et al. (2008).

Therapeutic use

hCG is used to stimulate ovulation in conjunction with FSH in infertile women. Occasionally, hCG is used to stimulate testicular hormone production when puberty is delayed.

hCG abuse in sport

Human CG has been used because it stimulates the secretion from the testes of both testosterone and epitestosterone. This led to the banning of hCG by the IOC in 1987.

A standard doping regime for hCG has been described (Brooks et al., 1989) in which the abuser first injects testosterone. Apart from any gains in strength or competitiveness the testosterone inhibits LH secretion from the pituitary. When testosterone is withdrawn before competition (to avoid detection) the athlete would be at a disadvantage with lower than normal plasma testosterone levels. However, administration of hCG stimulates testicular testosterone secretion and also that of epitestosterone. In a small, elegant experiment, Kicman et al. (1991) reproduced this situation in three normal men and showed that hCG can stimulate the testosterone substitution claimed by abusers and retain the testosterone/ epitestosterone ratio within WADA limits. In all three cases, the hCG could be detected in the urine by radioimmunoassay as long as plasma testosterone levels were raised. Brower (2000) described three separate regimes to restore endogenous testosterone secretion to normal following its suppression due to administration of testosterone or anabolic steroids. He has recorded descriptions of hCG 50 IU/Kg producing a doubling of endogenous testosterone secretion within three to four days of administration.

A review by Hendelsman (2006) concluded that whilst hCG produces marked increases in blood testosterone levels in men, the effects are negligible in women and therefore prohibition and testing for hCG should be restricted to men.

Hendelsman *et al.* (2009) showed a prominent dose-dependent and sustained effect on blood and urine hCG, LH and testosterone levels after administration of recombinant CG. They further concluded that testosterone:LH ratio measurements may be a sensitive test to detect hCG administration for at least one week after injection.

Side effects of hCG in sport

The side effects of hCG will be similar to those for anabolic steroids. However, the incidence of gynaecomastia may be greater as hCG also stimulates oestradiol production by the Leydig cells. The increase of oestradiol may be linked to nandrolone metabolite production in the process of aromatisation (Reznik *et al.*, 2001).

Prevalence of hCG abuse

Though hCG abuse is mentioned in the survey by Yesalis and Bahrke (2000), it is not quantified. In two UK surveys the prevalence of hCG abuse was 22.7 per cent (Korkia and Stimson, 1997) and 49 per cent (Evans, 1997). In an earlier UK survey, Perry *et al.* (1992) did not record any hCG abuse, suggesting that in the UK its abuse has occurred or been detected only in recent years. WADA statistics from 2003 to 2008 show a variable rate of abuse (see Chapter 25) with 46 cases identified as adverse analytical findings in 2008.

5.6   Luteinizing hormone (LH) and its use in sport

Luteinizing hormone is produced by the gonadotroph cells of the anterior pituitary in both males and females. In males, LH stimulates testicular sperm production and the synthesis and secretion of testosterone, while in females it stimulates ovulation and the production of progesterone. There are structural similarities between LH and hCG and a detailed comparison is made by Kicman and Cowan (1992). LH secretion is subject to negative feedback control by testosterone; therefore, as plasma testosterone levels rise, LH secretion is reduced. A recent study on the effects of single doses of recombinant LH, up to 750 IU, found that it had no influence on serum or urine LH or testosterone (Hendelsman *et al.*, 2009).

LH abuse is limited by its scarcity and its high costs and because its plasma half-life is 50 per cent less than hCG (Kicman and Cowan, 1992). "Designer" synthesis of LH, a dual chain peptide, is difficult owing to the complexity of its structure. Problems associated with the detection of LH are reviewed at length by Stenman *et al.* (2008).

It is much more likely that the LH-releasing hormone, the substance regulating LH release, will become a drug of abuse. It could be used to stimulate endogenous LH release, which will in turn stimulate the testes to secrete testosterone in males withdrawing from anabolic steroid abuse. Brower (2000) has described several LH treatment regimes, which could be used to restore testosterone secretion in males suffering anabolic steroid withdrawal syndromes or in those who need to restore normal testosterone before an event or test.

WADA statistics from 2003 to 2008 show low rates of detection for LH (see Chapter 25) with just one case reported in 2008. This is possibly due to the unreliable methods of detection for LH (Hendelsman *et al.*, 2009).

5.7   Insulin and its use in sport

An innocent enquiry by a Russian medical official at the Nagano Winter Olympics in 1998 led to the investigation of insulin by sports authorities and insulin's subsequent prohibition in non-diabetic athletes.

Insulin has powerful effects on carbohydrate, fat and protein biochemistry and simultaneously has a co-operative effect on these processes with other hormones, particularly hGH and IGF-I.

Insulin enhances glucose uptake into muscle and aids the formation and storage of muscle glycogen. It inhibits glucose output from the liver, encouraging liver glycogen storage. In adipose tissue, insulin encourages triglyceride formation and thus the formation of fat. The action of insulin on muscle and muscle protein is more complex. There has always been weak evidence that insulin increases muscle protein synthesis, but it now seems that in normal physiology, hGH and IGF-I are more important than insulin in stimulating this process. Insulin's role now seems to be inhibition of protein catabolism, an action it may share with supra-physiological doses of anabolic steroids. So what is the basis for the use of insulin? This can be briefly summarised as follows:

1   increasing muscle glycogen stores;
2   enhancing muscle glycogen storage during training schedules to increase stamina;
3   as a co-operative muscle-building stimulant with hGH.

In example 3, insulin would enhance the effects of hGH while the latter would oppose the insulin-stimulated deposition of triglycerides in adipose tissue. A full account of the physiology of insulin as a doping agent is provided by Sonksen (2001).

It has been suggested that around 25 per cent of body builders using anabolic steroids take them in combination with insulin in order to improve their effects (Evans and Lynch, 2003).

Because insulin is a naturally occurring peptide hormone, whose plasma and urinary levels vary considerably throughout the day, detecting insulin abuse is difficult (Holt and Sonksen, 2008). Research on the identification of analogue insulin, which is distinguishable from human insulin, has been undertaken (Thomas *et al.*, 2007).

5.8   Corticotropins

The peptide hormone adrenocorticotropic hormone (ACTH) is produced and secreted by the corticotroph cells of the anterior pituitary. It is a polypeptide consisting of 39 amino acids, of which only the 24 N-terminal amino acids are necessary for its biological activity. ACTH stimulates the reticularis and fasciculata cells of the adrenal cortex to synthesise and secrete corticosteroids such as cortisol and corticosterone.

Administration of ACTH

ACTH itself is never used for treatment or abuse; instead a synthetic derivative, the peptide tetracosactrin consisting of the first 24 N-terminal amino acids of ACTH, is administered by injection. Tetracosactrin administration stimulates a rise in blood cortisol and corticosterone concentration within two hours.

Abuse of ACTH

ACTH abuse is limited to short-term boosting of plasma cortisol and corticosterone in an attempt to reduce lethargy and produce "positive" effects on mood during training and competition. It is for this reason that it is banned by WADA along with corticosteroids. ACTH and corticosteroids are unsuitable for chronic use because they decrease muscle protein synthesis, leading to skeletal muscle wasting.

Detection of ACTH

Tetracosactrin abuse and endogenous ACTH are difficult to detect in urine samples. In the blood a rise in ACTH levels and therefore of corticosteroids occurs naturally during exercise. Kicman and Cowan (1992) investigated blood analysis for tetracosactrin, which should enable abuse to be detected.

5.9   References

Barroso, O., Schamasch, P. and Rabin, O. (2009). Detection of GH abuse in sport: Past, present and future. *Growth Hormone and IGF Research* **19**, 369–374.

Bidlingmaier, M., Wu, Z. and Strasburger, C.J. (2000). Test method: GH. *Best Clinical Endocrinology and Metabolism* **14**, 99–109.

Boisclair, Y.R., Rhoads, R.P., Ueki, I. *et al.* (2001). The acid labile subunits (ALS) of the 150 KDq IGF-binding protein complex: An important but forgotten component of the circulating IGF system. *Journal of Endocrinology* **170**, 3–70.

Brooks, R.V., Collyer, S.P., Kicman, A.T. *et al.* (1989). HCG doping in sport and methods for its detection. In *Official proceedings of second IAF world symposium on doping in sport*, ed. P. Bellot, G. Benzi and A. Ljungavist , London. 37–45.

Brower, K.J. (2000). Assessment and treatment of anabolic steroid abuse, dependence and withdrawal. In *Anabolic steroids in sport and exercise*, 2nd ed., ed. C. Yesalis, Human Kinetics, Champaign, Illinois. 305–332.

Consitt, L.A., Copeland, J.L. and Tremblay, M.S. (2002). Hormonal responses to exercise in women. *Sports Medicine* **32,** 1–22.

Cowart, V. (1988). Human growth hormone: The latest ergogenic aid? *Physician and Sport Medicine* **16,** 175–175.

Deyssig, R., Firsch, H., Blum, W.F. *et al.* (1993). Effect of growth hormone treatment and hormonal parameters, body composition and strength in athletes. *Acta Endocrinologica (Copenhagen)* **128,** 313–318.

Ehrnborg, C., Bengtsson, B.A. and Rosen, T. (2000). Growth hormone abuse. *Best Clinical Endocrinology and Metabolism* **14,** 71–77.

Erotokritou-Mulligan, I., Bassett, E.E. and Kniess, A. (2007). Validation of the growth hormone (GH)-dependent marker method of detecting GH abuse in sport through the use of independent data sets. *Growth Hormone and IGF Research* **17,** 416–423.

Evans, N.A. (1997). Gym and tonic: A profile of 100 anabolic steroid users. *British Journal of Sports Medicine* **31,** 54–58.

Evans, P.J. and Lynch R.M. (2003). Insulin as a drug of abuse in body building. *British Journal of Sports Medicine* **37,** 356–357.

GH-2000. (1999). GH-2000 group. Final report to the International Olympic Committee and European Union, 1999. Available at http://www.gh2004.soton.ac.uk (accessed 8 November 2009).

Gotherstrom, G., Bengtsson, B.-A., Sunnerhagen, K.S. *et al.* (2005). The effect of five-year growth hormone replacement therapy on muscle strength in elderly hypopituitary patients. *Clinical Endocrinology* **62,** 105–113.

Hendelsman, D.J. (2006). The rationale for banning human chorionic gonadotrophin and estrogen blockers in sport. *Journal of Clinical Endocrinology and Metabolism* **91,** 1646–1653.

Hendelsman, D.J., Goebel, C., Idan, A. *et al.* (2009). Effects of recombinant human LH and hCG on serum and urine LH and androgens in man. *Clinical Endocrinology* **71,** 417–428.

Holt, R.I.G. (2004). The metabolic effects of growth hormone. *CME Bulletin of Endocrinological Diabetes* **5,** 11–17.

Holt, R.I.G., Erotokritou-Mulligan, I. and Sonksen, P.H. (2009). The history of doping and growth hormone abuse in sport. *Growth Hormone and IGF Research*, **19,** 320–326.

Holt, R.I.G. and Sonksen, P.H. (2008). Growth hormone, IGF-1 and insulin and their abuse in sport. *British Journal of Pharmacology*, **154,** 542–556.

Jorgensen, J.O.L. and Christiansen, J.S. (1993). Brave new senescence, hGH in adults. *Lancet* **341,** 1247–1248.

Kemp, S.F. (2007). Mecasermin rinfabate. *Drugs Today* **43,** 149–155.

Kicman, A.T., Brooks, R.V. and Cowan, D.A. (1991). Human chorionic gonadotrophin and sport. *British Journal of Sports Medicine* **25,** 73–80.

Kicman, A.T. and Cowan, D.A. (1992). Peptide hormones and sport: Misuse and detection. *British Medical Buletin* **48,** 496–517.

Korkia, P. and Stimson, G.V. (1997). Indications and prevalence, practice and effects of anabolic steroid use in Great Britain. *International Journal of Sports Medicine* **18**, 557–562.

Le Roith, D., Bondy, C., Yakar, S. *et al.* (2001). The somatomedin hypothesis. *Endocrinological Review* **22**, 53–74.

Lombardo, J.A., Hickson, P.C. and Lamb, D.R. (1991). Anabolic/androgenic steroids and growth hormone. In *Perspectives in exercise science and sports medicine, vol. 4: Ergogenics—Enhancement of performance in exercise and sport*, ed. D.R. Lamb and M.H. Williams, Brown and Benchmark, New York. 249–278.

Macintyre, J.G. (1987). Growth hormone and athletes. *Sports Medicine* **4**, 129–142.

Marcus, R. and Hoffman, A.R. (1998). Growth hormone as therapy for older men and women. *Annual Review of Pharmacology and Toxicology* **38**, 45–61.

McHugh, C.M., Park, R.T., Sonksen, P.H. *et al.* (2005). Challenges in detecting the abuse of growth hormone in sport. *Clinical Chemistry* **51**, 1587–1593.

Muller, E.E. (1987). Neural control of somatotropic function. *Physiological Review* **3**, 962–1053.

Norton, K. and Olds, T. (2001). Morphological evolution of athletes over the 20th century. *Sports Medicine* **31**, 763–783.

Perry, M.H., Wright, D. and Littlepage, B.N.C. (1992). Dying to be big: A review of anabolic steroid use. *British Journal of Sports Medicine* **26**, 259–261.

Powrie, J.K., Bassett, E.E., Rosen, T. *et al.* (2007). Detection of growth hormone abuse in sport. *Growth Hormone and IGF Research* **17**, 220–226.

Rennie, M.J. (2003). Claims for the anabolic effects of growth hormone: A case of the emperor's new clothes? *British Journal of Sports Medicine* **37**, 100–105.

Reznik, Y., Dehennin, L., Coffin, C. *et al.* (2001). Urinary nandrolone metabolites of endogenous origin in man: A confirmation by output regulation under human chronic gonadotrophin stimulation. *Journal of Clinical Endocrinology and Metabolism* **86**, 146–150.

Rickert, V.I., Pawlak-Morello, C., Sheppard, V. *et al.* (1992). Human growth hormone: A new substance of abuse among adolescents? *Clinical Paediatrics* **31**, 723–726.

Saugy, M., Robinson, M., Saudan, C. *et al.* (2006). Human growth hormone doping in sport. *British Journal of Sports Medicine* **40**, i35–i39.

Schnirring, L. (2000). Growth hormone doping: The search for a test. *Physician and Sports Medicine* **28**, 1–6.

Smith, D.A. and Perry, P.J. (1992). The efficacy of ergogenic agents in athletic competition. Part II. Other performance enhancing agents. *Annals of Pharmacotherapy* **26**, 653–659.

Sonksen, P. (2001). Insulin growth hormone and sport. *Journal of Endocrinology* **170**, 13–15.

Stenman, U.-H., Hotakainen, K. and Alfthan, H. (2008). Gonadotrophins in doping: Pharmacological basis and detection of illicit use. *British Journal of Pharmacology* **154**, 569–583.

Stow, M.R., Wojek, N. and Marshall, J. (2009). The UK sport perspective on detecting growth hormone abuse. *Growth Hormone and IGF Research* **19**, 375–377.

Taaffe, D.R., Jin, I.H., Vu, T.H. *et al.* (1996). Lack of effect of recombinant human growth hormone (GH) on muscle morphology and GH-insulin-like growth factor expression in resistance trained elderly men. *Journal of Clinical Endocrinology & Metabolism* **81**, 421–425.

Taylor, W.N. (1988). Synthetic human growth hormone. A call for federal control. *Physician and Sports Medicine* **16**, 189–192.

Thomas, A., Thevis, M., Delahaut, P. *et al.* (2007). Mass spectrometric identification of degradation products of insulin and its long-acting analogues in human urine for doping control purposes. *Analytical Chemistry* **79**, 2518–2524.

Velloso, C.P. (2008). Regulation of muscle mass by growth hormone and IGF-1. *British Journal of Pharmacology* **154**, 557–568.

Wallace, J.D., Cuneo, R.C., Baxter, R. *et al.* (1999). Responses of the growth hormone (GH) and insulin-like growth facts axis to exercise, GH administration, and GH withdrawal in trained adult males: A potential test for GH abuse in sport. *Journal of Clinical Endocrinology and Metabolism* **84**, 3591–3601.

Wallace, J.D., Cuneo, R.C., Bidlingmaier, M. *et al.* (2001). The response of molecular isoforms of growth hormone to acute exercise in trained adult males. *Journal of Clinical Endocrinology and Metabolism* **86**, 200–206.

Yarasheski, K.E., Campbell, J.A., Smith, K. *et al.* (1992). Effect of growth hormone and resistance exercise on muscle growth in young men. *American Journal of Physiology* **262**, 261–267.

Yarasheski, K.E., Zachweija, J.J., Angelopoulis, T.J. *et al.* (1993). Short-term growth hormone treatment does not increase muscle protein synthesis in experienced weightlifters. *Journal of Applied Physiology* **74**, 3073–3076.

Yesalis, C.E. and Bahrke, M.S. (2000). Doping among adolescent athletes. *Best Clinical Endocrinology and Metabolism* **14**, 25–35.

Zuliani, U., Bernardini, B., Catapano, A. *et al.* (1989). Effects of anabolic steroids, testosterone and HGH on blood lipids and echocardiographic parameters in body builders. *International Journal of Sports Medicine* **10**, 62–66.

Chapter 6

Beta-2 agonists

David J. Armstrong and David R. Mottram

6.1 Introduction

Maximum performance in aerobic events, at whatever level of competition, is only achievable if respiratory function is optimal. Participants will always be concerned about respiratory problems whether they are from a major disease (e.g. asthma) or a minor ailment (e.g. the common cold). Their recourse to medications either to control or to alleviate symptoms of these conditions has brought many sportspersons into conflict with their national federations and Olympic committees.

In the case of asthma, the best classes of drugs to treat this condition are beta-2 agonists (β_2-agonists). These drugs produce their therapeutic effect through bronchodilation. Clearly, such an effect has the potential to enhance athletic performance by improving oxygen uptake. β_2-agonists are therefore on the World Anti-Doping Agency (WADA) prohibited list. As first-line drugs for the treatment of asthma and other conditions involving bronchoconstriction, β_2-agonists are necessary in the treatment regimes for such patients. A Therapeutic Use Exemption (TUE) is therefore required for asthmatic athletes in order to allow them to compete on equal terms with fellow competitors.

This chapter will review the condition of asthma, the types of drugs used in its treatment, with particular emphasis on β_2-agonists, the misuse of these drugs in sport and the systems in place for prohibiting β_2-agonists as performance-enhancing agents whilst permitting TUE, where appropriate.

6.2 Asthma and its treatment

Definition

Asthma is a chronic inflammatory disorder of the airways. In susceptible individuals this inflammation causes recurrent episodes of coughing, wheezing, chest tightness, and difficult breathing. Inflammation makes the airways sensitive to stimuli such as allergens, chemical irritants, tobacco smoke, cold air or exercise. When exposed to these stimuli, the airways may become swollen, constricted, filled with mucus and hyper-responsive to stimuli. The resulting airflow limitation is reversible (but not completely so in some patients), either spontaneously or with treatment. When asthma therapy is adequate, inflammation can be reduced over the long term, symptoms can usually be controlled and most asthma-related problems prevented (Global Initiative for Asthma, 2008).

Epidemiology

Asthma is one of the most common chronic conditions. It affects children more than adults. It is estimated that 1 in 7 children (ages 2–15) and 1 in 25 adults (ages 16 and older) in the UK have asthma symptoms currently requiring treatment. That is equivalent to 1.5 million children and 1.9 million adults (National Asthma Audit, 1999/2000). The global incidence of asthma is estimated to be over 100 million (Global Initiative for Asthma, 2008).

Pathophysiology

An asthma attack always consists of an early phase and frequently a late phase. The early phase occurs within minutes of exposure to a trigger factor, reaches a maximum within 15 to 20 minutes and normally resolves within an hour. The early phase is caused by bronchoconstriction. The late phase occurs 2 to 4 hours after exposure to the trigger factor and reaches a maximum after 6 to 8 hours. The late phase is caused by inflammation of the airways.

Historically, it was thought that airway obstruction and hence difficulty of breathing in asthma were caused by contraction of airway smooth muscle, i.e. bronchoconstriction. However, postmortem findings in asthma have revealed the cardinal features of inflammation. There is disruption of the airway epithelium (desquamation) and exposure of sub-epithelial tissue. The sub-epithelium demonstrates increased blood flow (hyperaemia), oedema (caused by increased vascular permeability), hypertrophy of airway smooth muscle and accumulations of pro-inflammatory cells (particularly eosinophils and mononuclear cells). The molecular mechanisms of the inflammation are extremely complex and not fully understood. The putative mediators of asthma parallel the chronology of the discovery of inflammatory mediators. Thus they have changed from histamine to the cyclo-oxygenase-mediated metabolites of arachidonic acid, to platelet-activating factor and currently to the lipoxygenase-mediated metabolites of arachidonic acid (namely the leukotrienes). It is unlikely that the inflammatory processes in asthma can be attributed to either a single mediator or a family of mediators. Nevertheless, appreciation of the change of emphasis from bronchoconstriction to inflammation as the cause of airway obstruction has underpinned the change in approach to the management of asthma.

Trigger factors

There are numerous factors that can trigger an asthma attack. The commonest are allergens. These can be either inhaled, e.g. pollens and/or animal danders (hairs and feathers), or ingested, e.g. dairy produce or strawberries. Viral, but not bacterial, infection of the upper respiratory tract can trigger asthma. Indeed, the initial presenting feature of asthma may be a persistent wheeze after a self-limiting, viral infection of the upper respiratory tract. Occupational pollution can cause asthma. Asthma attacks can be precipitated by emotional factors. This should not be misinterpreted as an indication that asthma is psychosomatic. Rather it is a reflection of neuroendocrine changes that, as yet, are poorly understood. Certain drugs may precipitate an asthma attack. Beta blockers and non-steroidal anti-inflammatory drugs (NSAIDs), particularly aspirin, can evoke a potentially fatal asthmatic attack. Beta blockers cause bronchoconstriction by blocking the bronchodilating β_2-receptors on airway smooth muscle. They should not be administered to asthmatics. The mechanism by which NSAIDs evoke bronchospasm is hypothetical but may involve a shift in balance between bronchodilating and bronchoconstricting metabolites of arachidonic acid. Approximately 10 per cent of asthmatics are aspirin-sensitive and will bronchoconstrict if given the drug. Finally, and most importantly in the context of sport, exercise can cause bronchoconstriction in which case either exercise-induced asthma (EIA) or exercise-induced bronchoconstriction (EIB) is diagnosed (WADA, 2009). An asthmatic may be sensitive to a variety of trigger factors or to just one.

6.3   Exercise and asthma

Exercise is the most common trigger of bronchospasm in those who are known to be asthmatic, and 50–90 per cent of all individuals with asthma have airways that are hyper-reactive to exercise (Parsons and Mastronarde, 2005). Furthermore, EIB also occurs in up to 10 per cent of subjects who are not known to be atopic or asthmatic. Asthma presents a twofold problem to elite sportspersons. First, it can impair performance if not treated correctly. However, many athletes compete successfully at the highest level despite having asthma. Second and perhaps of greater concern, treatment can expose the sportsperson to drugs that are on the WADA lists of prohibited classes of substances.

Prevalence of asthma in athletes

Asthma is reported to be more common in elite athletes than in the general population. A review of previous studies, by Parsons and Mastronarde (2005), revealed that prevalence rates for brochospasm related to exercise ranged from 11 to 50 per cent. Furthermore, up to 90 per cent of subjects with asthma will have exercise-induced asthma (EIA). The highest prevalence of EIA has been noted in athletes competing in the winter season, due to exposure to cold, dry air (Weiler and Ryan, 2000). The high prevalence of asthma in swimmers and other athletes training in indoor pools can be explained by exposure to chlorine and its derivatives (Langdeau and Boulet, 2001). Pedersen et al. (2008) believe that elite swimmers do not have particularly susceptible airways when they take up competitive swimming when young but that they develop respiratory symptoms, airway inflammation and airway hyper-responsiveness later on during their swimming careers. Similarly, Fitch (2006) reported that of the 193 athletes who met the IOC's criteria for the use of β_2-agonists at the 2006 Winter Olympics, only 32.1 per cent had childhood asthma and 48.7 per cent of athletes reported onset at age 20 years or older. This led the authors to speculate that years of intense endurance training may be a causative factor in bronchial hyper-reactivity.

The higher prevalence of airway hyper-responsiveness measured in athletes coupled with the use of subjective methods to diagnose asthma may mean that the prevalence of respiratory problems in athletes is underdiagnosed (Langdeau and Boulet, 2003). A recent review by Carlsen et al. (2008a) confirms the view that the prevalence of asthma and bronchial hyper-responsiveness is markedly increased in athletes, especially within endurance sports and that environmental factors often contribute to this increase. These authors also provide recommendations for the diagnosis of asthma in athletes.

Pathogenesis of exercise-induced asthma (EIA)

Exercise may be one of a number of trigger factors for an individual's asthma or it may be the only trigger factor. This led to the concept of EIA as a syndrome discrete from asthma. Thus, EIA has been defined in terms of the trigger factor, i.e. as reversible airway obstruction that occurs during or after exertion. The initial response to exercise in both non-asthmatics and asthmatics is bronchodilation. However, in the asthmatic, initial bronchodilation is not sustained and bronchoconstriction develops, most dramatically once the exercise has been terminated. The maximum decrease in peak expiratory flow rate (PEFR) and forced expiratory volume in the first second (FEV_1) normally occur between 3 to 15 minutes after the exercise has been completed (Rupp, 1996). The ventilatory changes in EIA are identical to those observed during a spontaneous asthma attack, i.e. decreased V_t, (tidal volume), PEFR, FEV_1, forced vital capacity (FVC) and increased residual volume (RV) leading to hyperventilation and dyspnoea. The symptoms include coughing, wheezing, excessive sputum production, dyspnoea and/or chest tightness (Lacroix, 1999). All of these changes are observed in asthma induced by factors other than exercise. In the laboratory, the exercise needs to be six to eight minutes in duration at greater than 80 per cent of predicted maximal heart rate (Lacroix, 1999). Although in their sport the early phase may take longer to develop, the maximum decrease in lung function occurs after 15 minutes and returns towards normal function after approximately one hour. This is known as the early phase of EIA. EIA may consist of just an early phase or, in approximately 30 per cent of EIA patients, may also develop a late phase after six to eight hours (Lacroix, 1999). In 50 per cent of individuals affected by EIA, a second period of exercise within two hours of the initial period evokes a weaker bronchoconstrictor response (less than 50 per cent of the original response). This period during which the response is reduced is referred to as the refractory period. Advantage can be taken of the refractory period for both training and competition. EIA occurs in up to 90 per cent of people with chronic asthma and 40 per cent of people with allergic rhinitis (Rupp, 1996; Lacroix, 1999). Random testing of asymptomatic children found that 7 per cent had EIA (Nastasi *et al.*, 1995).

The pathophysiology of EIA is only partially understood and is likely to be multifactorial (Parsons and Mastronarde, 2005). It is accepted that the severity of EIA is dependent upon the level of ventilation and the temperature and humidity of the inspired air. Cold, dry air is more asthmogenic than warm, humid air. This challenges the homeostatic regulation of airway temperature and water loss. Water loss from the airway epithelial cells decreases the cell volume and increases the viscosity of mucus. The latter can obstruct airflow and stimulate the cough reflex. After the challenge has subsided, the airways must be re-warmed and the intracellular fluid that was lost must be replaced. This can cause reactive hyperaemia (increased blood flow to the airway wall) and rebound increase in cell volume. This may be the key event that causes release of mediators and triggers bronchoconstriction and inflammatory changes in the airway wall. It may also explain the time course of the changes in lung function. Moreover, cycling may be the most asthmogenic sport because both training and competition involve longer periods of challenge to the respiratory tract. Typical cycling road races can last in excess of four hours whereas marathons last two and a half hours and football matches last one and a half hours. Finally, the environment in which the exercise takes place is important. Thus cross-country skiing, which is conducted in cold, dry air environments, has one of the highest incidences of reported EIA (Larsson *et al.*, 1993).

6.4   Management of asthma

Non-drug treatment of asthma involves avoidance of known trigger factors. Drug treatment of asthma is now directed at arresting and reversing the inflammatory process. The emphasis has shifted from the excessive and inappropriate use of β_2-agonist bronchodilator therapy towards the early use of anti-inflammatory drugs. β_2-Agonists merely relieve the symptoms of asthma without addressing the underlying inflammation. This has been likened to "painting over rust". Guidelines for treatment of chronic asthma have been prepared in several countries. They constitute a systematic approach to the treatment of increasing severity of symptoms. It must be remembered that the treatment of asthma can also be stepped down if the severity of the symptoms declines. The following are guidelines published by the British Thoracic Society in 2008.

- **Step 1. Mild intermittent asthma**
  - ○   Inhaled short-acting β_2-agonists should be used as required.

- **Step 2. Regular preventer therapy**
  - Inhaled short-acting β_2-agonists should be used as required;
  - *Add*;
  - Inhaled steroid, 200–800 mcg/day.

- **Step 3. Initial add-on therapy**
  - Inhaled short-acting β_2-agonists should be used as required;
  - Inhaled steroid, 200–800 mcg/day;
  - *Add*;
  - Inhaled long-acting β_2-agonist (LABA);
  - Assess control of asthma;
  - Good response to LABA—continue LABA;
  - Benefit from LABA but control still inadequate—continue LABA and increase inhaled steroid dose to 800 mcg/day (if not already on this dose);
  - No response to LABA—stop LABA and increase inhaled steroid dose to 800 mcg/day. If control still inadequate, institute trial of other therapies, leukotriene receptor antagonist or slow-release theophylline.

- **Step 4. Persistent poor control**
  - Consider trials of:
  - Increasing inhaled steroid up to 2000 mcg/day;
  - Addition of a fourth drug, e.g. leukotriene receptor antagonist, slow-release theophylline or β_2-agonist tablet.

- **Step 5. Continuous or frequent use of oral steroids**
  - Use daily steroid tablets in lowest dose, providing adequate control.
  - Maintain high dose of inhaled steroid at 2000 mcg/day.
  - Consider other treatments to minimise the use of steroid tablets.
  - Refer patient to specialist care.

Stepping down

Regular review of patients as treatment is stepped down is important. When deciding which drug to step down first and at what rate, the severity of asthma, the side effects of the treatment, the time on concurrent doses, the beneficial effects achieved and the patient's preference should all be taken into account.

6.5 Management of exercise-induced asthma (EIA)

The management of EIA consists of both non-drug and drug interventions and is directed at two goals:

1   optimal control of base-line symptoms;
2   prevention of an asthmatic attack following exercise.

Relief of symptoms of EIA should be considered as an indication that the first two goals have not been achieved satisfactorily.

Non-drug treatment

A   Aerobic fitness. Fitness does not prevent EIA as indicated by the number of Olympians who suffer from the syndrome. However, aerobic fitness does improve lung function, retards deterioration in lung function with age (in non-asthmatics) and enables asthmatics to exercise with less EIA. It also facilitates social interactions and improves self-esteem of asthmatics. There is no evidence to suggest that aerobic training is deleterious to asthmatics, provided that their treatment is optimal and that they have a satisfactory management plan that includes access to appropriate bronchodilator therapy, if required. The only contra-indication for strenuous aerobic activity in asthmatics would be if they demonstrated significant arterial desaturation upon exercise-testing during laboratory investigations.

B   Minimise cooling and drying of the airways. This can be achieved in several ways. First, if possible, select a physical activity such as walking and swimming, which are less likely to evoke bronchoconstriction. Second, utilise nasal breathing whenever possible. Third, seek to avoid exercising in a cold, dry environment. If this is unavoidable, then a face mask may reduce cooling and drying of the airways.

C   Warm up. This can help to maximise the benefit of the training session and, if possible, should take account of the refractory period that many asthmatics experience after an initial episode of EIA. The warm-up should be 15 minutes long. It is debatable whether this should involve high-intensity bursts to increase ventilation rapidly or moderate sustained activity. It is also advisable to cool down gradually after the exercise to minimise rebound warming of the airways.

D   Monitoring of PEFR. This will provide objective assessment of the current status of base-line control of asthma. Inadequate base-line control requires revision of maintenance therapy. Concurrent conditions, e.g. hay fever and allergic rhinitis, should also be satisfactorily controlled. If possible, training and participation should not be undertaken on days when symptoms are poorly controlled.

Drug treatment with β_2-agonists

These drugs are the most effective prophylactic treatment of EIA. Short-acting β_2-agonists (i.e. salbutamol or terbutaline) should be administered 15 (Rupp, 1996) to 30 minutes (Lacroix, 1999) before commencing exercise. They induce bronchodilation within five minutes and afford protection against EIA for approximately three to six hours (Rupp, 1996; Lacroix, 1999). They prevent asthma symptoms in 90 per cent of patients (Lacriox, 1999). β_2-Agonists should be available to the athlete for rapid relief of symptoms should they develop despite pre-exercise treatment. Salmeterol, a long-acting β_2-agonist, should be taken 30 minutes before exercise and is effective for up to nine hours (Nelson *et al.*, 1998). Its long duration of action makes it suitable for children who require prophylaxis against EIA throughout the school day. Because of its slower onset of action, salmeterol should not be used as a rescue medication to relieve symptoms of an asthma attack. Salbutamol or terbutaline should be used instead. There is controversy about the relative merits of the long-term prophylactic use of short- and long-acting β_2-agonists. Tachyphylaxis to salmeterol has been shown to develop after four weeks of regular use (Nelson *et al.*, 1998). Alternatives to regular use of salmeterol are either short-acting β_2-agonists before exercise and "on-demand" for relief of symptoms or leukotriene antagonists before exercise.

A recent review (Carlsen *et al.*, 2008a) of the treatment of EIA concluded that EIA should be treated in athletes along the same principles as for non-athletes. They concluded that there is a very high level of evidence for the lack of improvement in athletic performance by inhaled β_2-agonists.

6.6   Pharmacology of β_2-agonists

Bronchodilation

The first β-agonist to be used in the treatment of asthma was isoprenaline. The increase in asthma mortality, which paralleled the introduction of isoprenaline, prompted the development of a new generation of selective for use as bronchodilators. There are currently seven selective β_2-agonists licensed in the UK for the treatment of asthma (Table 6.1).

All the selective β_2-agonists are potent bronchodilators. They differ in their time to onset and duration of action. Salbutamol and terbutaline are short-acting and the most frequently used β_2-agonists in the UK. There are many formulations of salbutamol and terbutaline, including tablets, slow-release tablets, elixirs, aerosols and dry powder and solutions for injection and inhalation from a nebuliser. Inhalation is the route of choice because it is the most rapidly effective (one to two minutes) and is associated with the fewest side effects. Tremor is the only common side effect after inhalation. However, other side effects of

Table 6.1 Selective β_2-adrenoceptor agonists

Salbutamol (Ventolin™)
Terbutaline (Bricanyl™)
Bambuterol (Bambec™)
Fenoterol (Berotec™)
Formoterol/Eformoterol (Foradil™ /Oxis™)
Salmeterol (Serevent™)
Tulobuterol (Respacal™)

β_2-agonists are common (Cockcroft, 2006). This led Backer *et al.* (2007) to conclude that anti-asthmatic treatment is necessary for asthmatics but should not be used by non-asthmatic elite athletes due to possible systemic effects and side effects.

The side effects after oral administration include fine tremor (usually of the hands), nervous tension and headache. Tachycardia, peripheral vasodilation and hypokalaemia may occur after oral dosing but are more common after intravenous injection. Tachycardia is most uncommon after nebulisation. The duration of action of salbutamol and terbutaline after aerosol administration is approximately four hours. Formoterol (eformoterol) and salmeterol are the most frequently prescribed long-acting β_2-agonists with a duration of approximately 12 hours.

The properties of different β_2-agonists determine their use in the treatment of asthma. Rapid onset, short-acting β_2-agonists are used to give immediate and/or emergency relief from symptoms. There are differences between the time to onset of action for formoterol and salmeterol. The former begins to take effect within 1 to 3 minutes whilst the latter takes 10 to 20 minutes. Nevertheless, long-acting β_2-agonists should not be used for immediate relief of symptoms. Instead, they should be used in addition to inhaled corticosteroids to treat troublesome nocturnal symptoms and to prevent EIA when their longer duration of action confers a definite advantage. It was thought that short-acting β_2-agonists should be used a maximum of four times a day. However, this provides no clear clinical benefit when compared with their use "as required". Indeed, a clinical trial has shown greater efficacy of formoterol compared with terbutaline when used "as required" in terms of improved lung function, symptoms and quality of life (Tattersfield *et al.*, 2001).

Anabolic effects of β_2-agonists

β_2-Agonists possess anabolic activity, although the extent of this activity varies between drugs. Anabolic effects of oral β_2-agonists in animals has been clearly demonstrated (Ryall *et al.*, 2006). Clenbuterol is a long-acting β_2-agonist that is licensed for the treatment of asthma in several countries, including Germany, Italy and Spain. It is not licensed for human use in either the UK or the USA. It is licensed for veterinary use (Ventopulmin®, Boehringer Ingelheim) in horses for the treatment of bronchoconstriction caused by several equine respiratory diseases.

The therapeutic dose of clenbuterol for the treatment of asthma is 20–30 µg per day. It is misused in humans as an anabolic agent when doses of 100–140 µg per day are commonly employed. β_2-Agonists can promote normal skeletal muscle growth and experiments with clenbuterol show that it can increase muscle weight in rats by 10–12 per cent after two weeks of treatment (Yang and McElliott, 1989). It has been shown that clenbuterol can reverse experimentally induced muscle fibre atrophy by increasing muscle protein synthesis as well as inhibiting amino acid loss. In contrast salbutamol has no significant effect on muscle protein though this difference may be related to the short half-life of salbutamol, since continuous infusion of salbutamol causes anabolic effects similar to that of clenbuterol.

Clenbuterol does not produce its anabolic effects by interacting with testosterone, growth hormone or insulin (Choo *et al.*, 1992) but via β_2-receptor stimulation. Similarly the fat-mobilising action of clenbuterol is also mediated via β_2-receptors.

The molecular mechanism of the anabolic effect is complex. Colloquially, clenbuterol is described as either a "fat burner" or a "repartitioning agent". In the high doses at which the drug is abused, it is reported to increase non-shivering thermogenesis by increasing metabolism in brown fat. A one-degree increase of body temperature will increase basal calorific utilization by 5 per cent. The evidence for the anabolic effect of clenbuterol in animals is considerable. It increases muscle mass by causing hypertrophy but not hyperplasia. It inhibits muscle protein catabolism, which is why it is reported to be abused in humans after discontinuation of steroids to reduce the catabolic phase (Prather *et al.*, 1995). The combination of an increase in lipolysis and an increase in muscle mass results in an increase in lean body mass, hence the description of "a repartitioning agent".

As with any drug, clenbuterol has side effects. One advantage of clenbuterol is that it is not a steroid and therefore does not cause steroid-related side effects. However, it is a β_2-agonist and has side effects that are typical of this group of drugs (i.e. tremor, restlessness, agitation, headache, increased blood pressure and palpitations). These side effects are dose-related and purported to decrease after 8 to 10 days. This is due to a decrease or down-regulation of β_2-receptors. A consequence of this is also a decrease in the anabolic effect of the drug. Other adverse, dose-dependent effects include tissue desensitization and cell necrosis in heart and slow-twitch soleus muscle (Burniston *et al.*, 2005).

Zilpaterol, like clenbuterol, was introduced as a growth promoter in cattle. It has a similar pharmacological profile to clenbuterol (Davies *et al.*, 2008). It has a reputation as an anabolic agent with body builders, despite little published work on its efficacy in this respect.

6.7 β_2-agonists and the WADA prohibited list

Up to January 2010, all β_2-agonists were prohibited. This includes both their D- and L-isomers. However, since this class of drugs has several important applications in clinical therapy, WADA regulations permitted the use of selected members of this class subject to TUE regulations. Therefore, formoterol, salbutamol, salmeterol and terbutaline, when administered by inhalation, also required a TUE in accordance with the relevant section of the International Standard for TUE.

However, in January 2010, WADA changed the rules with respect to the β_2-agonists salbutamol and salmeterol. This decision was made to "allow anti-doping organizations to manage a number of substances and methods in a significantly more administrative and cost-effective way". WADA's rationale was that over the past few years almost all cases where salbutamol has been detected were covered by a TUE. Therefore from January 2010 the therapeutic use of inhaled salbutamol or salmeterol will not require a TUE. For monitoring purposes, athletes using inhaled salbutamol will be required to declare their use on the Doping Control Form when they are tested.

The WADA regulations still stipulate that salbutamol will be prohibited for urinary concentrations in excess of 1000 ng/ml. In such circumstances, there will be a presumption that the substance was not taken by inhalation and the athlete will have to prove through a controlled pharmacokinetic study that the level found in his or her urine was the result of therapeutic inhaled use. It is specified that the maximum dose for the controlled pharmacokinetic study cannot exceed the maximum therapeutic dose for inhaled salbutamol, 1600 µg/day.

β_2-Agonists such as clenbuterol, zeranol and zilpaterol appear on the WADA prohibited list under anabolic agents (subsection of other anabolic agents), reflecting their potential anabolic properties.

Therapeutic Use Exemption regulations with respect to β_2-agonists

At the 2000 Sydney Olympic Games, 607 competing athletes (5.5 per cent) notified the IOC Medical Commission that they wished to use β_2-agonists for the treatment of asthma. This was a significant increase from the Atlanta Games in 1996 (3.6 per cent) (Holzer et al., 2002). The IOC raised concerns over the accuracy of diagnosis of asthma in elite athletes. It was concluded that respiratory symptoms alone cannot be relied on to make a diagnosis of asthma. For this reason, in 2001, the IOC introduced criteria that required athletes to demonstrate, objectively, current asthma, EIA, EIB or airway hyper-responsiveness (Fitch et al., 2008). These criteria were used at the 2002 Winter Olympics in Salt Lake City. The criteria to demonstrate asthma included bronchial provocation challenge tests to enable correct asthma diagnosis. These provocation tests include methacholine, eucapnic voluntary hyperpnoea (EVH) and osmotic challenge with mannitol (Holzer et al., 2002).

By the 2004 Athens Olympic Games, the need to provide objective testing evidence for asthma resulted in a statistically significant reduction in the number of athletes seeking approval to use β_2-agonists to 445 (4.6 per cent of competitors), of whom 45 were rejected (Anderson et al., 2006). Anderson et al. suggested that objective evidence had provided information for the athletes' doctors that was likely to improve the health of the athletes because many appeared to be undertreated at the time of the testing.

Following a review in 2008, the IOC reaffirmed that athletes should continue to be required to demonstrate the presence of asthma, EIB or airway hyper-responsiveness to be approved to inhale β_2-agonists at the Olympic Games (Fitch et al., 2008).

WADA has drawn up a set of International Standards for TUE, which specify minimum requirements that must be adopted during the medical examination for the granting of a TUE. These are outlined in Table 6.2.

Guidance is provided on these requirements.

Medical history. Physicians should consider history of asthma; age of onset; respiratory symptoms that suggest asthma; triggering factors such as environment and season; alternative causes of symptoms; past history of acute episodes of asthma.

Clinical examination. Clinical examination of the respiratory system with baseline measurement of resting spirometry including forced expiratory volume (FEV_1) and forced vital capacity (FVC).

Bronchodilator reversibility challenge. A bronchodilator test is deemed positive if FEV_1 increases by more than 12 per cent from baseline value following short-acting β_2-agonist administration.

Bronchoprovocation challenge. The challenge may be with exercise, EVH or mannitol. A positive diagnosis is made if a fall in FEV_1 greater than 10 per cent following an exercise or EVH challenge, or greater than 15 per cent following a mannitol challenge.

The application for a TUE is considered by a TUE committee (TUEC), which is composed of at least three physicians with experience in the care and treatment of athletes and a sound knowledge of clinical, sports and exercise medicine. In order to ensure independence of decisions, the majority of the members of any TUEC should be free of conflicts of interest or political responsibility in the anti-doping organisation to which the athlete belongs.

Some researchers, who investigated the criteria for applying the rules for TUE to athletes concluded that up to a third of asthmatic athletes would be denied the

Table 6.2 WADA minimal requirements for the medical file to be used for the TUE process in the case of asthma and its clinical variants

The file must reflect current best medical practice to include:

1) a complete medical history;
2) a comprehensive report of the clinical examination with specific focus on the respiratory system;
3) a report of spirometry with the measure of the forced expiratory volume in one second (FEV_1);
4) if airway obstruction is present, the spirometry will be repeated after inhalation of a short-acting β_2-agonist to demonstrate the reversibility of bronchoconstriction;
5) in the absence of reversible airway obstruction, a bronchial provocation test to establish the presence of airway hyper-responsiveness;
6) exact name, speciality, address (including telephone, e-mail, fax) of examining physician.

Available at http://www.wada-ama.org.

use of β_2-agonists during competition (Naranjo Orellana *et al.*, 2006). Haahtela *et al.* (2008) examined 69 potential Olympic athletes from Finland who had symptoms suggesting asthma. All had respiratory symptoms; 20 per cent had a history of asthma dating back to childhood but the majority had developed symptoms during their sports careers. These two distinct phenotypes exhibited differing responsiveness to the set of criteria set by the IOC for approval of use of β_2-agonists. The authors concluded that there is a significant problem for both under- and over-diagnosing asthma in athletes and re-confirmed the need for robust objective testing for the approval of TUE.

6.8   The use of β_2-agonists in sport

Prevalence of β_2-agonists in sport

β_2-Agonists have been a target for athletes for many years. They have appeared in large numbers on the IOC/WADA annual statistics for adverse analytical findings. From 1997 to 2002, around 400 cases a year were recorded (Mottram, 2005). This trend has continued since 2003 (Table 6.3).

These annual figures for positive test results for β_2-agonists do include cases where athletes have received permission to use the drugs for therapeutic purposes. However, it has been acknowledged that there has been a marked increase by athletes in the application to use short-acting β_2-agonists (Fitch *et al.*, 2008). Figures for the percentage of all athletes applying to inhale β_2-agonists at summer Olympic Games show 3.6% at Atlanta in 1996, 5.7% at Sydney in 2000 and 4.6% at Athens in 2004 (Carlsen *et al.*, 2008a). The equivalent figures for winter Olympic Games were higher, with 5.6% at Nagano in 1998, 6.3% at Salt Lake City in 2002 and 8.3% at Torino in 2006 (Carlsen *et al.*, 2008a), perhaps reflecting the higher incidence of EIA in cold conditions.

Table 6.3 WADA statistics for the number of positive results for substances classed as β_2-agonists (2003–2008)

	2003	2004	2005	2006	2007	2008
Salbutamol	189	251	357	391	60	56
Terbutaline	76	78	171	175	182	163
Formoterol	–	4	18	42	107	91
Salmeterol	–	1	4	16	37	30
Fenoterol		–	3	5	11	10
Reproterol	–	1	4	2	2	–
Orciprenaline	1	–	–	–	–	–
Clenbuterol[+]	31	46	52	53	53	73
Total	297	381	609	684	452	423

Results on β_2-agonists include adverse findings for which the athlete may have been granted the Therapeutic Use Exemption under WADA regulations.
[+] Recorded under anabolic agents from 2006.

Cases involving β₂-agonists

Barcelona Olympics, 1992

The 1992 Olympics in Barcelona turned the spotlight on a new controversy surrounding selective β_2-agonists, namely the putative anabolic effects of β_2-agonists in general, and clenbuterol in particular. Two British weightlifters were withdrawn from the Olympic Games when they tested positive for clenbuterol. A US competitor and a German athlete also tested positive and were banned for using clenbuterol.

The "Festina Affair", 1998

Clenbuterol was one of the frequently used drugs cited by Willy Voet in his account of the notorious "Festina Affair" in the 1998 Tour de France cycle race (Voet, 2001).

Jessica Hardy, 2008

Jessica Hardy was dropped from the US Olympic team one month before the 2008 Beijing Olympic Games because she tested positive for clenbuterol. She claimed that she had accidentally ingested the banned substance when taking a nutritional supplement. The Arbitration Panel for Sport accepted her claim and reduced her suspension from two years to one year.

Do β₂-agonists enhance performance?

Several studies have investigated the effects of inhaled β_2-agonists, in both asthmatic and healthy athletes. Few studies have reported an increase in exercise performance following inhaled treatment (Signorile *et al.*, 1992; van Baak *et al.*, 2004). The majority of studies failed to show an ergogenic effect (Morton and Fitch, 1992; Norris *et al.*, 1996; Larsson *et al.*, 2005; Carlsen *et al.*, 2008b). Inhaled salbutamol, even in high doses, did not have a significant effect on endurance performance in non-asthmatic, highly trained cyclists (Goubault *et al.*, 2001). These authors did note that salbutamol had a slight but significant bronchodilator effect, which may be sufficient to improve respiratory adaptation at the beginning of exercise. However, they further concluded that it is unlikely that the widespread use of salbutamol by athletes is driven by the weak effects of the inhaled drug. Within a recent review in which 20 randomised, placebo-controlled studies were evaluated, only three studies reported a performance-enhancing effect from inhaled β_2-agonists (Kindermann and Meyer, 2006), although methodological shortcomings were cited as being factors in the findings. These authors concluded that there is no ergogenic potential of inhaled β_2-agonists in non-asthmatic athletes and questioned the inclusion of inhaled β_2-agonists on the list of WADA-prohibited substances.

In cold environments, where athletes with EIA are more likely to experience symptoms of the condition, inhaled formoterol did not improve endurance performance in healthy, well-trained male athletes (Tjørhom *et al.*, 2007). The authors therefore concluded that formoterol can be used in competitive sports without fear of a possible performance-enhancing effect.

With respect to the anabolic effects of β_2-agonists, these depend on the receptor density of muscles (Beerman, 2002). Since chronic administration of β_2-agonists produces down-regulation of receptors (Johnson, 2006), this may limit the effectiveness and therefore the value of β_2-agonists as anabolic agents (Davies *et al.*, 2008).

6.9   References

Anderson, S.D., Sue-Chu, M., Perry, C.P. *et al.* (2006). Bronchial challenges in athletes applying to inhale a β_2-agonist at the 2004 Summer Olympics. *Journal of Allergy and Clinical Immunology* **117**, 767–773.

Backer, V., Lund, T. and Pedersen, L. (2007). Pharmaceutical treatment of asthma symptoms in elite athletes—Doping or therapy? *Scandinavian Journal of Medicine and Science in Sports* **17**, 615–622.

Beerman, D.H. (2002). β-Adrenergic receptor agonist modulation of skeletal muscle growth. *Journal of Animal Science* **80E (Suppl. 1)**, E18–E23.

British Thoracic Society. (2008). The British guidelines on asthma management. Available at http://www.brit-thoracic.org.uk/ClinicalInformation/Asthma/Asthma Guidelines/tabid/83/Default.aspx (accessed 9 January 2009).

Burniston, J.G., Chester, N., Clark, W.A. *et al.* (2005). Dose-dependent apoptotic and necrotic myocyte death induced by the β_2-adrenergic receptor agonist, clenbuterol. *Muscle Nerve* **32**, 767–774.

Carlsen, K.H., Anderson, S.D., Bjermer, L. *et al.* (2008a). Exercise induced asthma, respiratory and allergic disorders in elite athletes: Part I of the report from the Joint Task Force of European Respiratory Society (ERS) and European Academy of Allergy and Clinical Immunology (EAACI) in cooperation with GA²LEN. *Allergy* **63**, 387–403.

Carlsen, K.H., Anderson, S.D., Bjermer, L. *et al.* (2008b). Treatment of exercise induced asthma, respiratory and allergic disorders in sports and the relationship to doping: Part II of the report from the Joint Task Force of European Respiratory Society (ERS) and European Academy of Allergy and Clinical Immunology (EAACI) in cooperation with GA²LEN. *Allergy* **63**, 492–505.

Choo, J-J., Horon, M.A., Little, R.A. *et al.* (1992). Clenbuterol and skeletal muscle are mediated by β2 adrenoceptor activation. *American Journal of Physiology* **263**, 50–56.

Cockcroft, D.W. (2006). Clinical concerns with β_2-agonists: Adult asthma. *Clinical Reviews in Allergy and Immunology* **31(2–3)**, 197–207.

Davies, E., Loiacono, R. and Summers, R.J. (2008). The rush to adrenaline: Drugs in sport acting on the β-adrenergic system. *British Journal of Pharmacology* **154**, 584–597.

Fitch, K. (2006). β_2-Agonists at the Olympic Games. *Clinical Reviews in Allergy and Immunology* **31(2–3)**, 259–268.

Fitch, K., Sue-Chu, M., Anderson, S. *et al.* (2008). Asthma and the elite athlete: Summary of the International Olympic Committee's Consensus Conference, Lausanne,

Switzerland, January 22–24, 2008. *Journal of Allergy and Clinical Immunology* **122**, 254–260.

Global Initiative for Asthma. (2008). Available at http://www.ginasthma.com (accessed 9 January 2009).

Goubault, C., Perault, M.C., Leleu, E. *et al.* (2001). Effects of inhaled salbutamol in exercising non-asthmatic athletes. *Thorax* **56**, 675–679.

Haahtela, T., Malmberg, P. and Moreira, A. (2008). Mechanisms of asthma in Olympic athletes—Practical implications. *Allergy* **63**, 685–694.

Holzer, K., Anderson, S.D. and Douglass, J. (2002). Exercise in elite summer athletes: Challenges for diagnosis. *Journal of Allergy and Clinical Immunology* **110**, 374–380.

Johnson, M. (2006). Molecular mechanisms of β_2-adrenergic receptor function, response and regulation. *Journal of Allergy and Clinical Immunology* **117**, 18–24.

Kindermann, W. and Meyer, T. (2006). Inhaled β_2 agonists and performance in competitive athletes. *British Journal of Sports Medicine* **40(Suppl. 1)**, i43–i47.

Lacroix, V.J. (1999). Exercise-induced asthma. *The Physician and Sports Medicine* **27 (12)**, 75–92.

Langdeau, J.B. and Boulet, L.P. (2001). Prevalence and mechanisms of development of asthma and airway hyperresponsiveness in athletes. *Sports Medicine* **31(8)**, 601–616.

Langdeau, J.B. and Boulet, L.P. (2003). Is asthma over- or under-diagnosed in athletes? *Respiratory Medicine* **97**, 109–114.

Larsson, K., Carlsen, K.H. and Bonini, S. (2005). Anti-asthmatic drugs: Treatment of athletes and exercise-induced bronchoconstriction. *European Respiratory Monthly* **33**, 73–88.

Larsson, K., Ohlsen, P., Larsson, L. *et al.* (1993). High prevalence of asthma in cross-country skiers. *British Medical Journal* **307**, 1326–1329.

Morton, A.R. and Fitch, K.D. (1992). Asthmatic drugs and competitive sport. An update. *Sports Medicine* **14**, 228–242.

Mottram, D.R. (2005). Prevalence of drug misuse in sport. In *Drugs in Sport*, 4th ed., ed. D.R. Mottram, Routledge, London. 357–380.

Naranjo Orellana, J.N., Prada, R.A.C. and Marquez, M.D.C. (2006). Use of β_2 agonists in sport: Are the present criteria right? *British Journal of Sports Medicine* **40**, 363–366.

Nastasi, K.J., Heinly, T.L. and Blaiss, M.S. (1995). Exercise-induced asthma and the athlete. *Journal of Asthma* **32(4)**, 249–257.

National Asthma Audit. (1999/2000). Available at http://www.asthma.org.uk/infofa18.html (accessed 13 March 2001).

Nelson, J.A., Strauss, L., Skowronski, M. *et al.* (1998). Effect of long-term salmeterol treatment on exercise-induced asthma. *New England Journal of Medicine* **339**, 141–146.

Norris, S.R., Petersen, S.R. and Jones, R.L. (1996). The effects of salbutamol on performance in endurance cyclists. *European Journal of Applied Physiology and Occupational Physiology* **73**, 364–368.

Parsons, J.P. and Mastronarde, J.G. (2005). Exercise-induced bronchoconstriction in athletes. *Chest* **128**, 3966–3974.

Pedersen, L., Lund, T.K., Barnes, P.J. *et al.* (2008). Airway responsiveness and inflammation in adolescent elite swimmers. *Journal of Allergy and Clinical Immunology* **122**, 322–327.

Prather, I.D., Brown, D.E., North, P. *et al.* (1995). Clenbuterol: A substitute for anabolic steroids? *Medicine and Science in Sports and Exercise* **27**, 1118–1121.

Rupp, N.T. (1996). Diagnosis and management of exercise-induced asthma. *The Physician and Sports Medicine* **24 (1)**, 77–87.

Ryall, J.G., Sillence, M.N. and Lynch, G.S. (2006). Systemic administration of β_2-adrenoceptor agonists, formoterol and salmeterol, elicit skeletal muscle hypertrophy in rats at micromolar doses. *British Journal of Pharmacology* **147**, 587–595.

Signorile, J.F., Kaplan, T.A., Applegate, B. *et al.* (1992). Effects of acute inhalation of the bronchodilator, albuterol, on power output. *Medicine and Science in Sports and Exercise* **24**, 638–642.

Tattersfield, A.E., Lofdahl, C.G., Postma, D.S. *et al.* (2001). Comparison of formoterol and terbutaline for as-needed treatment of asthma. *The Lancet* **357**, 257–261.

Tjørhom, A., Riiser, A. and Carlsen, K.H. (2007). Effects of formoterol on endurance performance in athletes at an ambient temperature of –20°C. *Scandinavian Journal of Medicine and Science in Sports* **17**, 628–635.

Van Baak, M.A., de Hon, O.M., Hartgens, F. *et al.* (2004). Inhaled salbutamol and endurance cycling performance in non-asthmatic athletes. *International Journal of Sports Medicine* **25**, 533–538.

Voet, W. (2001). *Breaking the chain*. Yellow Jersey Press, London.

Weiler, J.M. and Ryan, E.J. III (2000). Asthma in United States Olympic athletes who participated in the 1998 Olympic Winter Games. *Journal of Allergy and Clinical Immunology* **106**, 267–271.

World Anti-Doping Agency (WADA). (2009). Medical information to support the decisions of TUECs: Asthma. Available at http://www.wada-ama.org/rtecontent/document/Asthma_en.pdf (accessed 6 November 2009).

Yang, Y.T. and McElliott, M.A. (1989). Multiple actions of β-adrenergic agonists on skeletal muscle and adipose tissue. *Biochemical Journal* **261**, 1–10.

Chapter 7

Hormone antagonists and modulators

David R. Mottram

7.1 Introduction

Androgenic anabolic steroids were one of the first major classes of drugs to be used by athletes in modern times (see Chapter 2). They have maintained their pre-eminent position as the most widely used class of drugs, as evidenced by the annual statistics from IOC/WADA-accredited laboratories (see Chapter 25). However, sophisticated and sensitive testing procedures for anabolic steroids have deterred many of those athletes who have sought to gain an unfair advantage by using such drugs to enhance muscle mass and strength. Some of these athletes have turned to strategies that have involved indirect methods to increase levels of the endogenous anabolic steroid, testosterone. This has included the use of certain hormone antagonists and modulators.

7.2 Hormone antagonists and modulators and the WADA prohibited list

The WADA 2010 prohibited list categorises hormone antagonists and modulators as substances and methods inhibited at all times, both within competition and out of competition. Within the class of hormone antagonists and modulators, there are four subclasses:

1   *Aromatase inhibitors* including, but not limited to, anastrozole, letrozole, aminoglutethamide, exemestane, formestane, testolactone, androsta-1,4,6-triene-3,17-dione (androstatriene) and 4-androstene-3,6,17 trione (6-oxo);
2   *Selective oestrogen receptor modulators (SERMs)* including, but not limited to, raloxifene, tomoxifen, toremifene;
3   *Other anti-oestrogenic substances* including, but not limited to, clomiphene, cyclofenil, fulvestrant;
4   *Agents modifying myostatin function(s)* including, but not limited to, myostatin inhibitors.

The annual number of positive test results within this class has remained low, ranging from 6 to 30 per year between 2003 and 2007, during which period the

Table 7.1 WADA statistics for the number of positive results for substances classed as agents with anti-oestrogenic activity (2003–2008)

	2003	2004	2005	2006	2007	2008
Tamoxifen	5	8	11	11	6	12
Aminoglutethamide	1	−	2	1	−	2
Clomiphene	−	−	7	4	5	1
Anastrazole	−	−	1	4	−	4
Formestane	−	−	−	5	2	−
6-oxo-androstenedione	−	−	−	1	−	2
Androst-1,4,6-triene-3,17-dione	−	−	−	1	2	3
Cyclofenil	−	−	−	1	−	−
Exemestane	−	−	−	1	−	−
Letrozole	−	−	−	1	1	5
6-Alpha-methylandrostendione	−	−	−	−	2	−
Total	6	8	21	30	18	29

class was entitled "agents with anti-estrogenic activity", and 29 in 2008 when the class became "hormone antagonists and modulators" (see Table 7.1).

Currently, this class of drugs is prohibited for use in all athletes. However, there is justification for suggesting that prohibition of some of the subclasses should be restricted to men (Handelsman, 2006).

All subclasses of hormone antagonists and modulators are used clinically for therapeutic purposes, except agents modifying myostatin function, which are still under clinical investigation.

7.3   Clinical use of hormone antagonists and modulators

Aromatase inhibitors

Aromatase inhibitors have been used in the treatment of breast tumours, particularly in post-menopausal women. Since oestrogens have been implicated in the development and progression of such tumours, the objective of treatment is to deprive the tumour of oestrogens. This can be accomplished by inhibiting aromatase, the enzyme that catalyses the final step in the biosynthesis of oestrogen (Njar and Brodie, 1999). Post-menopausal women tend to have tumours that are positive for oestrogen receptors and are therefore more responsive to treatment involving hormone antagonism.

Aromatase inhibitors include both steroidal and non-steroidal mechanism-based inhibitors. The steroidal agents are mostly analogs of androstenedione and include testolactone, formestane, exemestane and atamestane, whilst the non-steroidal analogues include fadrozole, letrozole, anastrozole, vorozole and finrazole (Handelsman, 2006).

Selective oestrogen receptor modulators (SERMs)

The first drugs to be used clinically as blockers of oestrogen receptors were non-steroidal drugs such as clomiphene and tamoxifen. Newer anti-oestrogens such as raloxifene, toremifene, droloxifene and lasoxifene have been developed. These drugs also possess partial agonist activity and are now described as selective oestrogen receptor modulators (SERMs). Tamoxifen and other SERMs have been the most widely used anti-oestrogens in the management of hormone-receptor positive breast cancer in post-menopausal women. Tamoxifen has both an antagonist and a partial agonist effect on oestrogen receptors. As a result, long-term use has been associated with an increased risk of endometrial cancer (Bundred and Howell, 2002). The partial agonist effect of tamoxifen has also been associated with the development of "tamoxifen resistence", where the drug ceases to inhibit tumour growth and appears to promote it (Bundred and Howell, 2002).

Other anti-oestrogenic substances

This subclass of drugs is also used primarily for the treatment of breast cancer in post-menopausal women. Fulvestrant is an oestrogen receptor antagonist that competitively binds to the receptors with an affinity similar to that of oestradiol but higher than that of tamoxifen (McKeage *et al.*, 2004). The binding of fulvestrant to the oestrogen receptor sets off a series of changes to down-regulate receptor function. Unlike tamoxifen, fulvestrant has no partial oestrogen receptor agonist activity and therefore has fewer side effects.

Agents modifying myostatin function(s)

Myostatin is a growth factor that contributes both to developing muscles during growth and to negatively regulating muscle growth in adulthood. Studies in animals and humans have demonstrated that decreasing the levels of this growth factor or inhibiting its function can dramatically increase muscle size (Fedoruk and Rupert, 2008). Myostatin is a member of the transforming growth factor-β group of proteins that regulates muscle growth during embryogenesis (Matsakas and Diel, 2005). The clinical applications for the development of myostatin-based medicines include muscular dystrophy, cachexia (muscular atrophy associated with AIDS and other chronic diseases), myopathies resulting from inflammation and sarcopenia and the loss of muscle associated with increasing age (Wagner, 2005). Strategies for inhibiting myostatin function are under clinical investigation and several of these are reviewed by Fedoruk and Rupert (2008). However, drugs that manipulate myostatin signalling are also being considered as lifestyle drugs in anti-aging therapies and for their potential to enhance physical performance in athletes (Matsakas and Diel, 2005).

7.4   The use of hormone antagonists and modulators in sport

The natural androgens, testosterone and androstenedione, are the precursors of the principal oestrogen, estradiol. The conversion of the androgens to estradiol is achieved in the body by the enzyme aromatase. Clearly, the inhibition of aromatase will elevate levels of testosterone and androstenedione, thereby increasing anabolic effects. Another natural androgen, dihydrotestosterone, the most potent natural androgen, cannot be aromatized and cannot therefore be converted to an oestrogen (Handelsman, 2008).

Aromatase inhibitors have also been used by anabolic steroid abusers in an attempt to treat breast enlargement (gynaecomastia), a common side effect associated with androgen use in men, although the clinical efficacy for this is debatable (Handelsman, 2008).

Athletes use synthetic anabolic steroids primarily for their anabolic effects. However, most anabolic steroids have some androgenic effects that inhibit the release of gonadotropin-releasing hormone from the hypothalamus and follicle-stimulating hormone and leutinizing hormone from the anterior pituitary gland. With prolonged use, the resulting hypogonadotropic state results in testicular atrophy. This decreases serum testosterone levels, causing impotence and decreased libido. Clomiphene has been reported to be used to treat these conditions by an anti-oestrogen effect on the hypothalamus, resulting in increased gonadotropin-releasing hormone release and oestrogen-like effects on the pituitary, increasing the sensitivity to gonadotropin-releasing hormone (Bickelman et al., 1995).

In women, it has been argued that there is no convincing evidence that oestrogen blockers cause any consistent, biologically significant increase in blood testosterone concentrations (Handelsman, 2008). Furthermore, Handelsman suggests that oestrogen blockade poses no unusual medical risks to female athletes and there is therefore no basis to ban oestrogen blockade in female athletes.

The use of hormone antagonists is not confined to competitive sport. In one study on recreational gym users it was found that 22 per cent of members surveyed used tamoxifen, described by the authors as an enormous increase in use compared with previous studies (Baker et al., 2006). The increase in use appeared to be predominantly for cosmetic reasons.

Hormone antagonists and modulators are easily detected through the standard testing regimes operated by WADA-accredited laboratories (Mareck et al., 2005, 2006; Parr et al., 2009; Thevis et al., 2009).

In humans, resistance or endurance training has been shown to suppress myostatin expression (Raue et al., 2006). This allows muscle to grow in size. It is not surprising, therefore, that suppression of myostatin function is deemed to be a potential method for increasing growth response to training or even to stimulate muscle growth independently of training. This is why WADA introduced agents modifying myostatin function(s) to the prohibited list in January 2008. While data suggest myostatin blockade is likely to increase muscle mass in humans, to date there is no robust evidence to show that this would translate into improved athletic performance.

While a number of strategies to inhibit myostatin function are under clinical review (Fedoruk and Rupert, 2008), there are no therapeutic agents available at present. There is, however, an herbal preparation, albeit of questionable efficacy, available on the market. This product is derived from the sea weed *Cystoseira canariensis*, the active principles of which are sulphated polysaccharides that have been shown to bind to myostatin (Ramazanov *et al.*, 2003). The effectiveness of this product is open to debate. However, despite the lack of evidence, the prospect of an agent that may increase muscle growth and possibly enhance performance is sure to be attractive to some athletes.

Manipulation of myostatin function using gene therapy for clinical application is not being actively pursued at present (Fedoruk and Rupert, 2008). However, the prospect of gene doping is a reality and is discussed in Chapter 11 of this book. It has been suggested that manipulation of myostatin gene expression may be one of the first types of gene doping attempted (Baoutina *et al.*, 2007).

7.5 References

Baker, J.S., Graham, M.R. and Davies, B. (2006). Steroid and prescription medicine abuse in the health and fitness community. A regional study. *European Journal of Internal Medicine* 17(7), 479–484.

Baoutina, A., Alexander, T.E., Rasko, J.E. *et al.* (2007). Potential use of gene transfer to athletic performance enhancement. *Molecular Therapy* 15, 1751–1766.

Bickelman, C., Ferries, L. and Eaton, R.P. (1995). Impotence related to anabolic steroid use in a body builder. Response to clomiphene citrate. *Western Journal of Medicine* 162, 158–160.

Bundred, N. and Howell, A. (2002). Fulvestrant (Faslodex): Current status in the therapy of breast cancer. *Expert Review in Anticancer Therapy* 2(2), 151–160.

Fedoruk, M.N. and Rupert, J.L. (2008). Myostatin inhibition: A potential performance enhancement strategy. *Scandinavian Journal of Medicine and Science in Sports* 18, 123–131.

Handelsman, D.J. (2006). The rationale for banning human chorionic gonadotropin and estrogen blockers in sport. *Journal of Clinical Endocrinology and Metabolism* 91, 1648–1653.

Handelsman, D.J. (2008). Indirect androgen doping by oestrogen blockade in sports. *British Journal of Pharmacology* 154, 598–605.

Mareck, U., Geyer, H., Guddat, S. *et al.* (2006). Identification of the aromatase inhibitors anastrozole and exemestane in human urine using liquid chromatography/tandem mass spectrometry. *Rapid Communications in Mass Spectrometry* 20(12), 1954–1962.

Mareck, U., Sigmund, G., Opfermann, G. *et al.* (2005). Identification of the aromatase inhibitor letrozole in urine by gas chromatography/mass spectrometry. *Rapid Communications in Mass Spectrometry* 19(24), 3689–3693.

Matsakas, A. and Diel, P. (2005). The growth factor myostatin, a key regulator in skeletal muscle growth and homeostasis. *International Journal of Sports Medicine* **26(2)**, 83–89.

McKeage, K., Curran, M.P. and Plosker, G.L. (2004). Fulvestrant. A review of its use in hormone receptor-positive metastatic breast cancer in postmenopausal women with disease progression following antiestrogen therapy. *Drugs* **64(6)**, 633–648.

Njar, V.C.O. and Brodie, A.M.H. (1999). Comprehensive pharmacology and clinical efficacy of aromatase inhibitors. *Drugs* **58(2)**, 233–256.

Parr, M.K., Fußhöller, G., Schlörer, N. *et al.* (2009). Metabolism of androsta-1, 4, 6-triene-3, 17-dione and detection by gas chromatography/mass spectrometry in doping control. *Rapid Communications in Mass Spectrometry* **23**, 207–218.

Ramazanov, Z., Jimenez del Rio, M. and Ziegenfuss, T. (2003). Sulfated polysaccharides of brown seaweed *Cystoseira canariensis* bind to serum myostatin protein. *Acta Physiologica et Pharmacologica Bulgarica* **27**, 101–106.

Raue, U., Slivka, D., Jemiolo, B. *et al.* (2006). Myogenic gene expression at rest and after a bout of resistance exercise in young (18–30 yr) and old (80–89 yr) women. *Journal of Applied Physiology* **101**, 53–59.

Thevis, M., Kuuranne, T., Geyer, H. *et al.* (2009). Annual banned substance review: The prohibited list 2008—Analytical approaches in human sports drug testing. *Drug Testing and Analysis* **1**, 4–13.

Wagner, K.R. (2005). Muscle regeneration through myostatin inhibition. *Current Opinions in Rheumatology* **17**, 720–724.

Chapter 8

Diuretics and other masking agents

David R. Mottram

8.1 History of diuretics and other masking agents in sport

Masking agents are drugs that do not possess performance-enhancing properties but are taken in an attempt to disguise the fact that other prohibited substances are being used. Athletes quickly realised the potential for this type of subterfuge; therefore these drugs have been used for as long as athletes have been subject to drug testing.

Diuretics were first added to the IOC prohibited list, as a class of doping substances, in 1985. Two years later, probenecid and other masking agents were added under doping methods as part of the class referred to as pharmacological chemical and physical manipulation.

Over the years both the IOC and WADA classified and re-classified diuretics and other masking agents. From 1985 to 2003 diuretics were listed as a class of drugs alongside other major classes of drugs, such as anabolic agents and stimulants. In 2004 they were re-classified under substances prohibited in certain sports. The following year they were combined with other masking agents under the section of substances and methods prohibited at all times (in and out of competition), where they have remained to the current (2010) list. In 2003, masking agents were identified as a discrete class of substances, where they remained until 2005 when they were combined with diuretics, as described above.

The principal reason for the variation in classification described in the previous paragraphs lies in the fact that diuretics have been used over the years not only as masking agents but also as drugs to produce short-term weight loss in sports where weight categories apply. These sports include boxing, wrestling and horse racing where jockeys are required to attain specific weight levels.

The extent to which diuretics and other masking agents have been used in sport can be gauged by looking at Table 8.1.

It can be seen that there has been a steady increase in the numbers of adverse findings for most of the types of substances within this class. The rate of increase is greater than that seen prior to 2003 (Mottram, 2005).

The statistics in Table 8.1 include alpha reductase inhibitors and epitestosterone; however, it should be noted that WADA removed both of these groups of

Table 8.1 WADA statistics for the number of positive results for substances classed as diuretics and other masking agents (2003–2008)

	2003	2004	2005	2006	2007	2008
Diuretics						
Furosemide	48	62	91	90	111	104
Hydrochlorothiazide	42	44	67	88	103	137
Canrenone	14	9	14	8	15	15
Triamterene	10	7	9	7	15	7
Amiloride	6	4	10	10	10	6
Bumetanide	1	1	1	5	7	11
Chlorothiazide	–	1	3	1	7	27
Chlortalidone	3	4	1	8	6	4
Indapamide	1	2	4	5	4	12
Acetazolamide	3	4	6	2	4	6
Bendroflumethazide	1	7	5	2	3	–
Althiazide	–	–	–	1	2	3
Spironolactone	–	1	1	–	1	4
Trimethylchlorothiazide	–	–	–	–	1	–
Diclofenamide	–	–	–	1	–	–
Epitizide	–	–	–	1	–	–
Piretanide	–	–	1	–	–	1
Clopamide	1	1	–	–	–	–
Torasemide	1	1	–	–	–	2
Bemithizide	–	–	–	–	–	1
Thiazide	–	–	–	–	–	1
Alpha reductase inhibitors						
Finasteride	1	–	28	44	53	84
Epitestosterone	10	6	5	15	14	8
Probenecid	–	2	–	2	3	3
Hydroxyethyl starch	–	1	–	–	–	–
Total	142	157	246	290	359	436

drugs from the class of diuretics and masking agents in 2009. Alpha reductase inhibitors were removed completely from the prohibited list, whilst epitestosterone was re-classified under anabolic agents. The rationale for this is described in section 8.4 of this chapter.

There have been a number of high-profile cases involving this class of substances.

Case studies involving masking agents

Pedro Delgardo, 1988

In 1988, the professional road race cyclist Pedro Delgardo tested positive for the masking agent probenecid, whilst leading in the twelfth stage of the Tour de France.

Probenecid was included on the IOC prohibited list at that time. However, the governing body for cycling, the Union Cycliste International (UCI), did not prohibit the drug. Pedro Delgardo was therefore allowed to continue the race, which he eventually won. Remarkably little comment ensued, despite the fact that probenecid possesses no performance-enhancing properties itself but had been used solely as a masking agent. This should have raised the question as to what the cyclist was trying to mask. This case was a classic example of the lack of harmonization that existed in international doping control at that time, a position that would not be rectified until the establishment of WADA more than 10 years later.

8th Swimming World Championships, Australia, 1998

These championships were marred by a number of doping-related events surrounding the Chinese swimming team. In addition to the discovery of vials of human growth hormone by Australian customs officials prior to the Games, out-of-competition pre-testing at the Games resulted in adverse analytical findings for the diuretic triamterene in four members of the Chinese squad.

World Nordic Skiing Championships, Finland, 2001

At the time, before a validated test for EPO had been widely adopted by laboratories, the International Ski Federation had reduced the acceptable "safe" haemoglobin limit in blood to 17.5 mg/dl for men in an attempt to control the use of erythropoietin (EPO). Some athletes realised that by combining EPO with plasma volume expanders they could elevate haemoglobin and total blood volume while holding haemoglobin below the legal limit. At the World Nordic Skiing Championships in 2001, six Finnish skiers tested positive for hydroxyl ethyl starch (HES), having not realised that the WADA laboratories had devised a detection method for HES but had not generally announced this fact (Seiler, 2001). In this case, it was further revealed that the use of EPO along with the intravenous administration of HES had been undertaken systematically with the collusion of the head coach and two national team doctors. It served to remind that such personnel can be implicated as accessories to athlete doping.

Zach Lund, 2006

In February 2006, the skeleton sled racer Zach Lund was banned from competition for one year, having tested positive for finasteride (a constituent in his hair growth stimulant) on the eve of the Winter Olympic Games in Torino, Italy. The one-year ban was a reduction from the two-year ban recommended by WADA since the Court of Arbitration for Sport had determined that Lund "bears no significant fault or negligence". Finasteride was removed from the WADA prohibited list in January 2009.

8.2   Action and use of diuretics in sport

Clinical uses of diuretics

The main function of the kidneys is to maintain a constant interior environment to the body by regulating the volume, electrolyte content and pH of extracellular fluid in response to variations in diet and fluctuations in external environmental conditions. The kidneys are also responsible for eliminating waste and noxious products from the body. Within the kidneys, fluid salts and low-molecular weight constituents of the plasma are extracted from the blood and mostly re-absorbed, leaving excess water, ions and "foreign" chemicals to be excreted within the urine so produced.

Diuretics act on the kidneys to increase the excretion of ions, particularly sodium (Na^+), and water. There are different types of diuretics classified according to their mode of action (Table 8.2). Diuretics can also be classified according to their chemical structure, which is diverse. This does not pose a problem with

Table 8.2 Classification of diuretics and their major clinical uses

Class of diuretic	Examples	Major clinical uses
Loop diuretics	Furosemide Bumetanide Torasemide	Chronic heart failure Renal failure
Thiazide diuretics	Bendroflumethazide Hydrochlorothiazide Chlortalidone Indapamide Metolazone Chlorothiazide Cyclopenthiazide Xipamide	Hypertension Oedema
Potassium sparing diuretics	Amiloride Triamterene	In conjunction with loop or thiazide diuretics to maintain potassium balance
Aldosterone antagonists (also potassium sparing)	Spironolactone Eplerenone Canrenone	Primary hyperaldosteronism Cirrhosis of the liver
Carbonic anhydrase inhibitors	Acetazolamide Dorzolamide Brinzolamide	Rarely used except orally (Acetazolamide) or topically to treat glaucoma
Osmotic diuretics	Mannitol	Cerebral oedema

respect to doping analysis (Deventer *et al.*, 2002; Morra *et al.*, 2006). Major clinical uses of diuretics are also presented in Table 8.2.

Diuretics as masking agents

One of the principal reasons for athletes' use of diuretics is for their masking effect through the production of copious volumes of urine. This attempt at disguising other drugs being excreted is highly unlikely to succeed, considering the levels of sensitivity and accuracy exhibited by modern analytical testing regimes.

Diuretics in sports requiring weight limitation or categorisation

A number of sports require weight categorisation in order to ensure some degree of equivalence between competitors. Most of these sports involve physical contact, such as boxing, judo and wrestling, or compare the ability to lift weights. Such sports require a weigh-in prior to competition. Clearly, athletes must ensure that they meet the limits of their respective weight category and often need to resort to weight-lowering strategies in order to achieve that objective. These strategies have sometimes included the use of diuretics.

Another sport in which weight is of prime importance is professional horse racing, where jockeys are required to maintain very low body weight and precise weight control. All jockeys routinely adopt practices of restricting food intake and sauna-induced sweating. However, a study in which professional jockeys in Australia were questioned on their weight management revealed that 22 per cent of subjects frequently resorted to diuretics for rapid weight loss (Moore *et al.*, 2002). This practice is widespread and reports date back many years (Price, 1973).

Sports federations within which weight control is a factor reserve the right to administer dope control testing at the time of the weigh-in as well as at the time of competing, since the weigh-in may take place some period of time before the competition.

Diuretic use with other prohibited substances

Diuretics have been shown to have a widespread appeal as part of the culture of polydrug use in activities such as body building (Delbeke *et al.*, 1995). In this context, the principal function of diuretics is to counter the fluid-retentive properties of anabolic steroids. In the case of body builders this is an essential property in order to attain the required "cut" look. A similar result was found in gym users, where polypharmacy was practiced by more than 80 per cent of steroid users, with 22 per cent using diuretics as part of their regime (Evans, 1997).

Other uses of diuretics associated with sport

Acetazolamide is a weak diuretic but has been used for prophylaxis against mountain sickness, an indication for which it is not licensed. However, it is not suitable for altitude acclimatisation. A study into the effect of acetazolamide on exercise performance and muscle mass at high altitude concluded that the subjects taking acetazolamide had few symptoms of acute mountain sickness than controls, although the difference was not statistically significant (Bradwell *et al.*, 1986). The authors also showed that weight loss, including muscle mass, was greater in controls and this correlated with a fall in exercise performance, leading to the conclusion that acetazolamide is useful for climbers and trekkers who are acclimatised to high altitudes and that the drug could be most useful at extreme altitudes. There is no published evidence for benefits of acetazolamide at altitudes where most sports are undertaken.

Diuretics have been used in sports for weight loss other than in sports where weight categories apply. In a study by Martin *et al.* (1998), the use of diuretics by female basketball, softball and volleyball players was investigated. Volleyball players (23.6 per cent), in particular, used diuretics for weight loss purposes but in 79.6 per cent of cases this was specifically for appearance enhancement.

8.3   Action and uses of other masking agents in sport

Probenecid

Probenecid is an inhibitor of renal tubular transport mechanisms. Because it inhibits the resorption of uric acid it increases the elimination of urate through the kidneys. This therefore reduces plasma uric acid and the likelihood of this substance crystallising out in joints and soft tissue, the effects of which lead to the painful symptoms of gout.

Probenecid has an opposite effect on the elimination of other substances, such as penicillins, where it inhibits urinary excretion leading to increased plasma concentrations. This has been used to therapeutic advantage in the case of penicillins, which are otherwise rapidly and effectively excreted, leading to the necessity for frequent dosing in order to maintain therapeutically effective plasma levels of the drug.

Probenecid has also been shown to inhibit the urinary excretion of other drugs, including anabolic steroids and their metabolites, and has therefore been used as a masking agent. However, the urinary excretion of anabolic steroids and their metabolites is not completely inhibited by probenecid, therefore athletes would still record an adverse analytical finding during drug testing. It is therefore not surprising to find that probenecid has, in recent years, infrequently appeared in WADA's laboratory statistics (see Table 8.1).

Plasma expanders

Plasma expanders contain large molecules that, when administered by intravenous infusion, do not readily leave the blood vessels. Within blood vessels they exert osmotic pressure and hold extra fluid in the blood, thereby elevating plasma volume and total blood volume. This can disguise elevated red blood cell levels. This property of plasma expanders was exploited by athletes using erythropoietin (EPO) prior to the validated test for EPO that was introduced in 2000. Before the introduction of this test, evidence for EPO use relied on blood tests showing elevated haematocrit levels.

Albumin is an endogenous plasma protein. Its concentration in the plasma can be increased through intravenous infusion of albumin solution, derived by extraction from whole blood that has had most other constituents removed. Albumin also has the potential to bind drugs, thereby delaying their excretion via the urine. There are a number of side effects associated with albumin infusion, the most serious of which is the risk of hypersensitivity reactions leading to anaphylaxis.

Other plasma expanders include dextran, gelatin and hydroxyethyl starch (HES), which are plasma substitutes. They expand and maintain increased blood volume and are only slowly metabolised. They also expose the user to the risk of hypersensitivity reactions. HES was added to the prohibited list in 2000 after reports of its use by athletes. This led to the search for a validated method to identify this substance in urine (Thevis et al., 2000). Rapid screening techniques for HES and dextran are now available (Guddat et al., 2008a).

Epitestosterone

Testosterone is an endogenous anabolic steroid and has been taken by athletes for decades to promote anabolic effects. Testing for the use of testosterone is problematic as it is difficult to determine what constitutes a normal level within the body. A number of direct and indirect methods for detecting testosterone abuse are available (Saudan et al., 2006). One method for detecting testosterone use relies on the measurement of relative concentrations of testosterone and its isomer epitestosterone, which is produced by the body along with testosterone. The concentration of epitestosterone is not increased by exogenous administration of testosterone (Stárka, 2003). This fact provides the basis for identifying testosterone abuse. WADA regulations require further investigations if the ratio of testosterone/epitestosterone (T/E) is greater than 4:1, a level that has recently been questioned (Sottas et al., 2008). The further investigations include isotope ratio mass spectrometry (IRMS) analysis for the determination of the $^{13}C/^{12}C$ ratio, since pharmaceutically synthesised testosterone contains less ^{13}C than endogenous testosterone (Aguilera et al., 2001). Unsurprisingly, athletes have resorted to taking epitestosterone in order to mask the use of testosterone.

For reasons outlined in Section 8.4 of this chapter, WADA, in 2009, transferred epitestosterone from the class of diuretics and other masking agents to anabolic agents. Despite this transfer, epitestosterone remains on the prohibited list as a masking agent because it does not possess anabolic effects.

Alpha reductase inhibitors

Alpha reductase inhibitors, such as finasteride and dutasteride are used clinically to treat benign prostatic hyperplasia, a non-malignant increase in the size of the male prostate gland. They decrease the activity of the enzyme 5-α-reductase. These drugs are also sometimes used to treat male baldness. Alpha reductase inhibitors influence the metabolic pathways of endogenous and exogenously administered steroids. These effects can complicate the evaluation of steroid profiles in drug testing (Thevis *et al.*, 2007). Despite this, in 2009 WADA considered that systems based on athlete passports and steroid profiling were sufficiently robust to render alpha reductase inhibitors ineffective as masking agents and therefore removed them from the prohibited list (see Section 8.4).

8.4   Current WADA classification of diuretics and masking agents

A number of significant changes were made to the section on diuretics and other masking agents within the 2009 WADA anti-doping code and prohibited list. The 2009 list included modifications in relation to the status of "specified substances". This meant that where athletes can clearly establish how a specified substance entered their body or came into their possession, and that such a substance was not intended to enhance sport performance, the sanction could be reduced as low as a reprimand and no period of ineligibility. The prohibited list clearly identified which classes of substances and methods would not be considered as specified substances and would not therefore be considered for more flexible sanctions. Diuretics and other masking agents were all classed as specified substances. Consequently, epitestosterone was moved from diuretics and other masking agents to the class of anabolic agents since it is an isomer of testosterone, and within the class of anabolic agents it would maintain its status as a non-specified substance for the purposes of sanctions.

A second major change in 2009 was the removal of alpha reductase inhibitors from the list. They were no longer prohibited as they had been rendered ineffective as masking agents by closer consideration of steroid profiles within WADA laboratories. Steroid profiling of urine samples was introduced as part of the standard doping control process for WADA-accredited laboratories. Steroid profiles are a major component of "athlete passports". The objective of this was to monitor an athlete's biological parameters over time in order to detect abnormal variations that could indicate potential doping. Steroid profiling has been described as one of the most versatile and informative screening tools for the detection of steroid abuse in sport (Mareck *et al.*, 2008). The urinary steroid profile contains concentrations and ratios of endogenously produced steroidal hormones, their precursors and their metabolites. Using athlete passports to routinely record these data, an alteration of the concentration of one or more of these parameters raises suspicion of doping malpractice. The steroid profile is highly sensitive to administrations of endogenous as well as synthetic anabolic steroids, masking agents and bacterial activity (Mareck *et al.*, 2008). On the other hand, the majority of parameters are not influenced by exercise, severe physical endurance, menstrual cycle, circadian rhythms or annual rhythms.

The final major change to the 2009 list was that the words "intravenous administration" preceded the examples of plasma expanders to reflect that these substances are only prohibited when administered by this route. Mannitol was also added as an example, although mannitol, by inhalation, is permitted when used, for example, to perform bronchial provocation testing in asthma. The difficulty for drug testers is to distinguish between mannitol taken by the prohibited method of intravenous infusion rather than by permitted routes (Guddat *et al.*, 2008b).

Following these changes, the revised section on diuretics and other masking agents in the 2010 WADA prohibited list is shown in Table 8.3.

The WADA prohibited list cites three diuretics that are not prohibited. Drospirenone is an analogue of spironolactone, an aldosterone antagonist diuretic, and has weak diuretic effects. However, its principal pharmacological effect lies in the fact that it is a progestin, a synthetic version of the hormone progestogen. As such, it is used clinically in combined oral contraceptive pills. The diuretic effect of drospirenone is therefore deemed insufficient, by WADA, to warrant its prohibition as a masking agent. Similarly, WADA does not prohibit the carbonic anhydrase inhibitors dorzolamide and brinzolamide in topical eyedrop preparations for the treatment of glaucoma, as they will not be absorbed into the systemic circulation in sufficient quantities to act as masking agents.

Table 8.3 List of substances included under diuretics and other masking agents in the WADA prohibited list, 2010

Masking agents are prohibited. They include:
Diuretics, probenecid, plasma expanders (e.g. glycerol; intravenous administration of albumin, dextran, hydroxyethyl starch and mannitol) and other substances with similar biological effect(s)

Diuretics include:
Acetazolamide, amiloride, bumetanide, canrenone, chlorthalidone, etacrynic acid, furosemide, indapamide, metolazone, spironolactone, thiazides, triamterine and other substances with a similar chemical structure or similar biological effect(s) (except drosperinone, pamabrom and topical dorzolamine and brinzolamide, which are not prohibited)

A Therapeutic Use Exemption for diuretics and masking agents is not valid if an athlete's urine contains such substances in association with threshold or sub-threshold levels of an exogenous Prohibited Substance(s).

Finally, it is worth noting that diuretics have a number of important clinical uses (see Table 8.2) and therefore athletes may apply for a Therapeutic Use Exemption (TUE), where appropriate. However, the footnote to the WADA prohibited list for this class of drugs renders a TUE invalid if another exogenous substance from the list is found within an athlete's urine sample.

8.5 References

Aguilera, R., Chapman, T.E., Starcevic, B. *et al.* (2001). Performance characteristics of a carbon isotope ratio method for detecting doping with testosterone based on urine diols: Controls and athletes with elevated testosterone/epitestosterone ratios. *Clinical Chemistry* **47**, 292–300.

Bradwell, A.R., Coote, J.H., Milles, J.J. *et al.* (1986). Effect of acetazolamine on exercise performance and muscle mass at high altitude. *Lancet* **327**, 1001–1005.

Delbeke, F.T., Desmet, N. and Debackere, M. (1995). The abuse of doping agents in competing body builders in Flanders (1988–1993). *International Journal of Sports Medicine* **16(1)**, 66–70.

Deventer, K., Delbeke, F.T., Roels, K. *et al.* (2002). Screening for 18 diuretics and probenecid in doping analysis by liquid chromatography-tandem mass spectrometry. *Biomedical Chromatography* **16**, 529–535.

Evans, N.A. (1997). Gym and tonic: A profile of 100 male steroid users. *British Journal of Sports Medicine* **31**, 54–58.

Guddat, S., Thevis, M., Thomas, A. *et al.* (2008a). Rapid screening of polysaccharide-based plasma volume expanders dextran and hydroxyethyl starch in human urine by liquid chromatography-tandem mass spectrometry. *Biomedical Chromatography* **22**, 695–701.

Guddat, S., Thevis, M. and Schänzer, W. (2008b). Identification and quantification of the osmodiuretic mannitol in urine for sports drug testing using gas chromatography-mass spectrometry. *European Journal of Mass Spectrometry*, **14(3)**, 127–133.

Mareck, U., Geyer, H., Opfermann, G. *et al.* (2008). Factors influencing the steroid profile in doping control analysis. *Journal of Mass Spectrometry* **43**, 877–891.

Martin, M., Schlaback, G. and Shibinski, K. (1998). The use of non-prescription weight loss products among female basketball, softball and volleyball athletes from NCAA Division 1 institutions: Issues and concerns. *Journal of Athletic Training* **33(1)**, 41–44.

Moore, J.M., Timperio, A.F., Crawford, D.A. *et al.* (2002). Weight management and weight loss strategies of professional jockeys. *International Journal of Sports Nutrition* **12(1)**, 1–13.

Morra, V., Davit, P., Capra, P. *et al.* (2006). Fast gas chromatographic/mass spectrometric determination of diuretics and masking agents in human urine. Development and validation of a productive screening protocol for antidoping analysis. *Journal of Chromatography A* **1135**, 219–229.

Mottram, D.R. (2005). Prevalence of drug misuse in sport. In *Drugs in Sport*, 4th ed., ed. D.R. Mottram, Routledge, London. 357–380.

Price, D. (1973). Abuse of diuretics by jockeys. *British Medical Journal* **1(5856)**, 804.

Saudan, C., Baume, N., Robinson, N. *et al.* (2006). Testosterone and doping control. *British Journal of Sports Medicine* **40 Supp. 1**, i21–i24.

Seiler, S. (2001). Doping disaster for Finnish ski team: A turning point for drug testing? *Sportscience* **5(1)**, 1–3.

Sottas, P.-E., Saudan, C., Schweizer, C. *et al.* (2008). From population- to subject-based limits of T/E ratio to detect testosterone abuse in elite sports. *Forensic Science International* **174**, 166–172.

Stárka, L. (2003). Epitestosterone. *Journal of Steroid Biochemistry and Molecular Biology* **87**, 27–34.

Thevis, M., Geyer, H., Mareck, U. *et al.* (2007). Doping control analysis of the 5 alpha-reductase inhibitor finasteride: Determination of its influence on urinary steroid profiles and detection of its major urinary metabolite. *Therapeutic Drug Monitoring* **29(2)**, 236–247.

Thevis, M., Opfermann, G. and Schänzer, W. (2000). Detection of plasma volume expander hydroxyethyl starch in human urine. *Journal of Chromatography B – Analytical Technologies in the Biomedical and Life Sciences* **744(2)**, 345–350.

Chapter 9

Enhanced oxygen transfer

David J. Armstrong

9.1 Introduction

In sports events or strenuous exercise lasting more than one minute, the predominant mode of energy production is aerobic. This means that performance is limited by the oxygen that is delivered to and utilized by the active muscles. The level of performance is determined by the nature of training, which can affect both central and peripheral physiological factors. When the muscles are well trained, as in the case of elite endurance athletes, the limiting factors in determining the maximal oxygen uptake are the cardiac output and the oxygen-carrying capacity of the blood. The maximal cardiac output is also highly important when exercise is conducted in the heat because it then subserves two functions: the distribution of blood to the skin for thermoregulatory purposes and the supply of oxygen to the active muscles for energy metabolism.

The oxygen-carrying capacity of the blood is determined by the haemoglobin content, which helps bind oxygen within the red blood cells. It is the total body haemoglobin rather than its relative concentration that is correlated with the maximal oxygen uptake. When the total haemoglobin level falls, exercise performance is impaired. Athletes and their mentors are cognisant of this relationship and many performers regularly take iron supplements to prevent anaemia. Often this practice of supplementation is unnecessary as haemoglobin levels are normal and iron stores are adequate. It is also well recognised by sports practitioners that "blood boosting" can enhance endurance performance. Consequently, various ways have been devised of augmenting the oxygen-carrying capacity of the blood of athletes. These methods include the procedures of "blood doping".

The WADA prohibited list differentiates between the substances used to enhance oxygen transport (erythropoiesis-stimulating agents, ESAs) and the methods that are subclassified into blood doping and that artificially enhance the uptake, transport and delivery of oxygen. The scientific background, methods of detection and examples of abuse for blood doping will be discussed according to that WADA classification.

9.2   Physiology

Erythropoiesis

Erythropoiesis, the production of the red blood cells, takes place in haemopoietically active bone marrow. Nearly all bones contain haemopoietically active "red" marrow for the first two to three years of life. In a normal adult the only sites of haemopoietically active marrow are to be found in the skull, bony thorax, vertebrae, iliac crests and the upper ends of the femur and humerus. The majority of bone marrow consists of fatty or "yellow" marrow, which is haemopoietically inactive. It can become active once more in times of pathologically elevated demand for production of red blood cells.

Although erythropoiesis takes place within the bone marrow (i.e. medullary) it is extravascular—that is, it occurs outside the blood vessels that supply and drain the bone marrow. The most primitive stem cells, which are found in the endothelial lining of the medullary sinusoids, are pluripotential haematopoietic stem cells (PHSC), which are self-regenerating and can develop into any type of blood cell, red cell or white cell, either lymphoid or non-lymphoid. The PHSCs give rise to pluripotential myeloid stem cells or colony-forming units-spleen (CFU-S). These in turn are stimulated to mature into unipotential, committed precursor cells (e.g. burst-forming units erythroid [BFU-E]) by a number of growth factors (including stem cell factor [SCF]; interleukin-3 [IL-3], granulocyte-macrophage colony-stimulating factor [GM-CSF] and IGF-1) that function synergistically with erythropoietin cytokines including interleukin-1 (IL-1), interleukin-6 (IL-6) and granulocyte-colony stimulating factor (G-CSF). BFU-E cells then give rise to discrete colony-forming unit-erythrocyte (CFU-E) cells that, in turn, generate discrete colonies of developing erythrocytes. The CFU-E is the first red cell precursor to possess receptors for erythropoietin (Bick et al., 1993).

The BFU-E compartment contains thousands of erythroblasts. The cells reach a maximum size by 14 days and produce 3–6 CFU-E. Each CFU-E forms clusters of erythrocytes (approximately 20–25) within seven days. The BFU-E cells develop as islands of erythroblasts centred about a single histiocyte or macrophage. This cell, which has processes extending between the developing erythroblasts, is responsible for engulfing the extruded nuclei of the late normoblasts as they mature into reticulocytes (Bick et al., 1993).

The first recognizable precursor of an erythrocyte is a pronormoblast. This cell is 15–20 μm in diameter, with a nucleus containing 1–2 nucleoli, mitochondria but no haemoglobin. It divides mitotically three times, giving three generations of normoblasts: early or basophilic, intermediate or neutrophilic, and late or eosinophilic. The terms baso-, neutro- and eosinophilic refer to the affinity for histological stains. As the normoblasts develop they synthesize haemoglobin, which stains with eosin and confers a pink tinge upon the cytoplasm. The development of normoblasts is also characterized by a decrease in cell diameter and condensation of nuclear material, such that the cytoplasm:nucleus ratio increases from early to intermediate to late normoblast. The late normoblast is approximately 10–12 μm in diameter, has a dense pyknotic nucleus and is almost fully haemoglobinized. It is incapable of mitotic division and further development occurs by maturation. Intramedullary development from pronormoblast to late normoblast takes approximately three days.

Development to this stage has been intramedullary but extravascular. The developing erythrocyte must now enter the circulation. The late normoblast loses its nucleus by extrusion. The residue of the cell passes between the junctions of the medullary capillaries by diapedesis (amoeboid-like movement) and enters the circulation as a reticulocyte. This cell is slightly smaller than a late normoblast (8–10 μm diameter) and lacks a nucleus. It contains residual ribosomal material and mitochondria that have an affinity for haematoxylin, and which confer a blue reticular appearance upon the cytoplasm, hence the name of the cell. Reticulocytes normally constitute less than 1 per cent of the circulating red cell count. An increased reticulocyte count is indicative of increased erythropoiesis. Final maturation to the mature erythrocyte involves completion of haemoglobinization and loss of reticular material. This occurs either during sequestration in the spleen or in the circulation and takes 24–48 hours.

The mature red blood cell is a biconcave disc, diameter 6.7–7.7 μm, volume 85 ± 8 fl containing an average of 29.5 ± 2.5 pg of haemoglobin. Mature erythrocytes do not have a nucleus, RNA or mitochondria. They are unable to synthesize enzymes or to produce adenosine triphosphate (ATP) aerobically. They metabolize glucose by glycolysis, to produce ATP for maintenance of cationic pumps, and by the hexose monophosphate pathway for generation of reduced NAD^+P for maintenance of haemoglobin in the reduced state (Bick *et al.*, 1993). They have a finite lifespan of 120 days. After that time, they are removed by the reticuloendothelial system, principally the spleen. If anaemia is not to develop, the rate of production of new erythrocytes must equal the rate of destruction. Consequently, 0.83 per cent of the circulating red cell mass must be replaced each day. Since the total red cell mass, the erythron, is approximately 3×10^{13} cells, that means that some 2.5×10^{11} erythrocytes must be produced and released each day, i.e. some 3×10^6/s. The total body haemoglobin contained in 3×10^{13} cells is approximately 900 g.

Oxygen transport

The solubility of oxygen in plasma is low such that at a PO_2 of 100 mmHg only 0.3 ml dissolves in 100 ml of whole blood. Because the basal oxygen requirement is 250 ml/min, this would require a resting cardiac output of approximately 80 l/min. The normal resting cardiac output of 5 l/min would therefore not be sufficient to meet the body's needs. Hence the need for haemoglobin.

Haemoglobin is a tetramer with each subunit consisting of a polypeptide chain (two α and two β chains) and a prosthetic group, haem. Each haem group contains one molecule of iron in the ferrous (Fe^{++}) state. Each ferrous ion combines with one molecule of oxygen so that each molecule of haemoglobin combines with four molecules of oxygen. Each gram of haemoglobin combines with 1.34 ml of oxygen under standard conditions. Since the average male haemoglobin concentration is approximately 15 g/dl, each decilitre of blood contains approximately 20 ml of oxygen. Therefore, the oxygen-carrying capacity of whole blood has been referred to as 20 per cent (i.e. 20ml of oxygen/100 ml of blood). Because the resting cardiac output is 5 l/min, this means that approximately 1000 ml of oxygen are transported around the body per minute.

The amount of oxygen bound to haemoglobin (i.e. the percentage saturation of a solution of haemoglobin) depends upon the partial pressure of oxygen. However, the relationship is not linear but sigmoidal (Figure 9.1) because of the subunit interactions. Reference to the oxyheamoglobin dissociation curve shows that at the partial pressure of oxygen in the lungs (100 mm Hg), Hb is almost 100 per cent saturated. By contrast, at the partial pressure of oxygen in the tissues (40 mmHg), Hb is only 75 per cent saturated. Therefore, 25 per cent of the

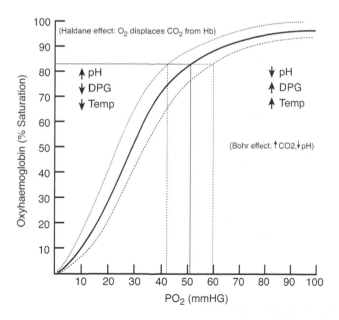

Figure 9.1 The oxyheamoglobin dissociation curve.

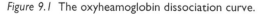

Reproduced from http://commons.wikimedia.org/wiki/File:Oxyhaemoglobin_dissociation_curve.png

oxygen that combined with Hb at the higher partial pressure in the lungs will be released at the lower partial pressure in the tissues. Thus, if Hb combines with 20 ml of oxygen/100ml of blood in the lungs, it will release 5 ml/100 ml in the tissues. This will equate to 50 ml/l and 250 ml/5l, which is the resting oxygen requirement.

An elite endurance athlete would be expected to have a maximum oxygen consumption in absolute terms of >6 l/min or, in relative terms, 6000ml/70 kg/min, which is approximately 80 ml/kg/min. Because the cardiac output of an elite endurance athlete can rise as high as 30 l/min, this could result in a sixfold increase in oxygen delivery from 250 ml/min to 1500 ml/min, or 1500/70 = 21.4 ml/kg/min. Thus an increase in cardiac output alone is insufficient to achieve the required VO_2 max of the elite athlete.

As can be seen from Figure 9.1, the affinity of Hb for oxygen depends on pH, CO_2, temperature and 2,3 DPG. If pH decreases and either CO_2, temperature or 2,3 DPG increase, the Hb dissociation curve will be shifted to the right, which constitutes a decreased oxygen affinity. Thus, whilst Hb will still become saturated with O_2 in the lungs, it will release more oxygen to the tissues. The maximum a-v O_2 (arterio-venous oxygen) difference is 17 ml/100ml. Therefore, if each 100 ml of blood can deliver 17 ml of oxygen and cardiac output reaches 30 l/min, total oxygen delivery can increase to 5100 ml/min and VO_{2max} could be increased to 5100/70 or 73 ml/kg/min.

This means that there are numerous prohibited substances and methods available to the unscrupulous athlete wishing to enhance oxygen transport. They are:

- to increase their haemoglobin concentration by

  o   stimulation of erythropoiesis using erythropoiesis-stimulating agents;
  o   transfusion of red blood cells (i.e. blood doping);
  o   infusion of haemoglobin-based oxygen carriers (HBOCs);

- to infuse a perfluorocarbon (PFC);
- to infuse an Hb modifier, which shifts the oxyhaemoglobin curve to the right.

Collectively, these substances and methods are described as blood doping. WADA defines blood doping as "the misuse of certain techniques and/or substances to increase one's red blood cell mass, which allows the body to transport more oxygen to muscles and therefore increase stamina and performance". These options will be discussed according to their classification on the prohibited list (WADA, 2010).

Regulation of erythropoiesis

Erythropoietin in health

The rate of production of red blood cells must be closely regulated because of the huge number of cells involved (3×10^6/s). Erythropoiesis is controlled by the circulating level of a glycoprotein hormone, *erythropoietin. Native erythropoietin* consists of 165 amino acids with a molecular weight of 30,400 daltons. It contains 14 sialic acid residues that determine the plasma half-life and *in vivo* biological activity of the hormone. In adults, *erythropoietin* is produced primarily in the endothelial cells of the peritubular capillaries within the cortex of the kidney (90 per cent) with a minor contribution from the liver (10 per cent). It has a half-life of six to nine hours and is cleared from plasma by the liver following desialylation. Normal serum concentration is 10–30 mU/ml (2–7 pmol/l) as determined by radioimmunoassay (Davison, 2004).

At the physiological level, the stimulus for the production of erythropoietin is reduced oxygen delivery to the kidney. This may happen as a result either of altitude-induced hypoxia (see Chapter 24), haemorrhage, cardiovascular disease, respiratory disease or anaemia. Anaemia is the most powerful stimulus for the production of EPO, which can increase 1000-fold in cases of severe anaemia. Production is decreased by hypophysectomy and starvation and increased by thyroxine. At the molecular level, EPO production is controlled by oxygen-dependent regulation of hypoxia-inducible factor (HIF-1_α). It has been postulated that the hypoxia-sensitive receptor contains a haem moiety. The deoxy form of the haem moiety stimulates, and the oxy form inhibits, the transcription of the erythropoietin gene to form erythropoietin mRNA (Barrett *et al.,* 2009). The system is extremely sensitive. A decrease in haematocrit below 20 per cent results in a hundredfold increase in erythropoietin.

9.3   Erythropoietin

Mode of action of erythropoietin

The effects of erythropoietin (EPO) are mediated by specific erythropoietin-sensitive receptors on the surface of the red cell progenitors. The EPO-receptor is a member of the JAK/STAT superfamily of cytokine receptors that lead to protein phosphorylation and transcription factor activation. The receptors are first expressed on the surface of BFU-Es but are present in greater numbers on the surface of CFU-Es (1000 per cell) and pronormoblasts. EPO works synergistically with other growth factors (SCF, GM-CSF, IL-3 and IGF-1) to cause maturation and proliferation of erythroid precursors. Ultimately, this increases their survival and prevents apoptosis (programmed cell death) (Fisher, 2003). The net effect is an increase in the number of erythrocytes that are produced and the rate at which they are released into the circulation.

Recombinant erythropoietin

The gene responsible for the synthesis of erythropoietin was cloned in 1985 and is located on chromosome 7 (band 7q21). Recombinant human erythropoietin (rHuEPO) was first patented by Amgen in 1989. There are currently three generations of rHuEPO in production: the prototype (erythropoietin), novel erythropoiesis-stimulating protein (NESP) and continuous erythropoietin receptor activator (CERA). Since the biological activity is determined by the sialylation of the protein moeity, the therapeutic target has been to prolong the half-life of the biopharmaceutical and hence to reduce the frequency of dosing. Second generation NESP (darbepoetin, Aranesp™) differs from EPO in having an additional eight sialic acid residue. Third-generation CERA differs in having a long polymer chain (methoxy polyethylene glycol) incorporated into the molecule. These genetically engineered modifications have increased the elimination half-lives from 8.5 to 25.3 to 142 hours, respectively. This has decreased the frequency of initial intravenous dosing from three times weekly to once weekly to once every two weeks, respectively. In addition to these innovator products, there are a number of biosimilars available on the market (e.g. Hemax™). Once the patent on the first-generation biopharmaceutical expired in 2004, the way was clear for other biotechnology companies to manufacture the equivalent of generic EPO. However, because these products were being manufactured in living cells (e.g. Chinese Hamster Ovary) and may have a different three-dimensional structure even though the chemical structure is identical, they are referred to as biosimilars. A biosimilar is defined as a biological medicinal product referring to an existing one and submitted to regulatory authorities for marketing authorization by an independent application after the time of the protection of the data has expired for the original product (Schellekens, 2009).

Detection of EPO

The first tests for EPO at the Olympic Games were introduced in Sydney in 2000. To be deemed culpable, the athlete had to test positive in both blood (Parisotto et al., 2001) and urine tests (Lasne and de Ceaurriz, 2000). Blood screening was done first and then urine analysis was performed to confirm a positive result. In 2003, WADA's executive committee accepted the results from an independent report that urine testing alone could be used to detect the presence of recombinant EPO. However, some international sporting federations still use a blood and urine analysis matrix for EPO detection. Blood screening has an advantage in that it is cheaper than urine screening. Recently, the method of screening urine was adapted for detecting newer erythropoiesis-stimulating agents in blood. In 2009, WADA published a Technical Document entitled "Harmonization of the method for the identification of recombinant erythropoietins (i.e. epoetins) and analogues (e.g. darbepoetin and methoxypolyethylene glycol-epoetin beta)", in which the methodology for detection was specified as were the results for the major commercially available epoetins (rEPO, Aranesp™ and Mircera™). Demonstration of the presence of an epoetin is based upon isoelectric focusing and chemiluminescence (Figure 9.2).

These techniques may be complemented with a further technique known as SDS-PAGE (sodium dodecyl sulfate polyacrylamide gel electrophoresis).

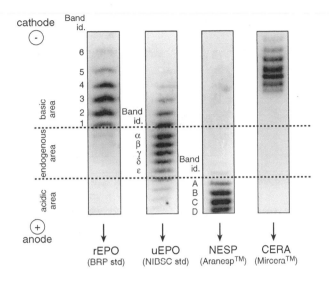

Figure 9.2 Results of epoietin detection obtained using isoelectric focusing and chemiluminescence.

Image courtesy of the World Anti-Doping Agency.

Note that the technique can identify not only r-HuEPO, NESP and CERA but also biosimilars (e.g. Hemax™ and Dynepo™) (Figure 9.3).

Abuse of EPO

The first clinical reports of EPO were published in 1987. Amagen received a licence for r-HuEPO in 1989. There were several newspaper articles during this time that linked the deaths of 18 Belgian and Dutch cyclists with rumours of EPO abuse in the peleton (Leith, 1992). In 1990, EPO was even implicated in the death of one such cyclist, Johannes Draaijer, by his widow. At that time, it was unlikely that the magnitude of the increase in red blood cell production was accurately controlled and the haematocrit (Hct) may have been raised to dangerously high levels. Values of 60 per cent were rumoured. Indeed, one cyclist, Marco Pantani, was found to have an Hct of 60.1 per cent when admitted to hospital after an accident in a 1995 race (Rendell, 2006). This concentration would cause significant increases in both systolic blood pressure and blood viscosity. In the short term there would be an increased risk of thrombosis and stroke. In the long term, chronically elevated Hct and blood viscosity could lead to left ventricular hypertrophy and, ultimately, to left ventricular failure and death.

In 1990, the IOC added EPO to the list of banned substances. There was much conjecture about abuse of EPO at this time. The former professional cyclist

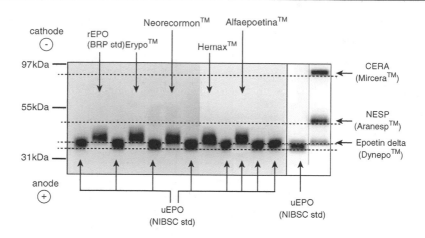

Figure 9.3 Results of epoietin detection obtained using SDS-PAGE.
Image courtesy of the World Anti-Doping Agency.

Paul Kimmage, referred in his book *Rough Ride* (1998) to such suspicions within the peleton. He also referred to the Donati dossier (1994), which was an account of EPO abuse involving elite Italian cyclists. The curriculum vitae of Sandro Donati is a fascinating insight into the politics of anti-doping in top level sport (Donati, 2001) as is the account of an interview with him conducted by Christopher Harrison (2003) and a report on the Ergogenics website (Donati, 2003). Proof of the extent of abuse of EPO did not exist until the 1998 Tour de France and what became known as the "Festina affair". Subsequent detention of the Festina team *soigneur*, Willy Voet, prompted Voet to publish a personal account of drug abuse within the peleton. He stated that provision and administration of EPO were formalised within the team and he provided evidence of drugs, doses and deductions from salaries according to drugs administered! It is difficult to imagine that other teams could compete with Festina without recourse to EPO, not least because there is undisputed evidence in sport-specific investigation of the ergogenic benefit derived from EPO (e.g. Ekblom and Berglund, 1991; Birkeland *et al.*, 2000). Thus the ergogenic effects of recombinant human EPO (r-HuEPO) were compared to those of transfusional polycythaemia by Ekblom and Berglund (1991). These authors reported that r-HuEPO increased Hb concentration from 152 g/l to 169 g/l and VO_{2max} from 4.52 to 4.88 l/min. These effects did not differ significantly from those evoked by re-infusion of 1350 ml of autologous blood. Significantly, systolic blood pressure was increased whilst cycling at 200 Watts from before to after r-HuEPO. In a later study, time to exhaustion was also increased from 493 ± 74 s to 567 ± 82 s following identical doses of r-HuEPO (Ekblom, 1997).

There have been many examples of positive tests (adverse analytical findings, or AAFs) for ESAs. Although by far the greatest number of AAFs have been for first-generation EPO, there have also been AAFs for second-generation ARANESP and third-generation CERA (WADA, 2008). Two commonly held misconceptions are (i) that EPO is mainly abused by cyclists and (ii) that it is used by athletes who are involved in endurance events (spectacularly so in the Tour de France). On the contrary, there have been many examples from a number of different sports of athletes who have abused EPO, including cross-country skiers, biathletes, swimmers, rowers, marathon runners, 5000 m runners, 400 m runners and 400 m hurdlers. A recent example is that of five Brazilian athletes who returned home prior to the 2009 World Championships in Berlin after testing positive for EPO in an out-of-competition test in Brazil. Amongst the five were two 400 m runners, an heptathlete, a 200 m runner and a 100 m runner. The latter confirmed that abuse of EPO is not restricted to participants in endurance events as demonstrated previously by USA sprinters (e.g. Marion Jones and Kelli White) who had also tested positive for EPO.

Given that there are well-defined methods for the detection of erythropoiesis-stimulating agents, why do athletes continue to abuse these drugs and risk sanctions? There are at least two possible explanations. First, the athletes believe they are abusing a drug for which there is no test available. This was possibly the case in the 2002 Winter Olympics in Salt Lake City when one former German skier (representing Spain) and two Russian skiers tested positive for the second-generation ESA, darbepoetin, and later in the 2008 Tour de France when two Italian cyclists and two Austrian cyclists tested positive for the third-generation ESA, CERA. On both occasions, the testers were one step ahead of the cheats rather than vice versa. Second, the athletes may believe they can somehow avoid detection, which is a strategy that has long been used by athletes. Various means of diluting red cell concentration have been employed in the past (e.g. the use of plasma volume expanders). Perhaps a more subtle and interesting strategy is to make combined use of the limitations of the test and the pharmacokinetics of the drug. One such strategy is to use a microdosing regime, which renders EPO undetectable within a short period of administration. In a study involving two well-trained male athletes, Ashenden et al. (2006) demonstrated that a three-week microdose regime could be utilised to maintain Hb concentrations at 164 g/l and 170 g/l (pre-EPO controls were 140 g/l and 148 g/l, respectively). Urine samples collected >24 hours after microdose injection typically had <80 per cent basic isoforms of EPO, which had been a criterion for an AAF. An approach such as this, whilst relatively simple to conduct within a laboratory setting, requires a degree of sophistication and support well beyond the compass of the athlete alone. In the past, this deception has been thought to involve the coaching and medical support staff. However, another possible level of collusion has come to light as the result of an ongoing investigation in Austria. Bernard Kohl, an Austrian cyclist, tested positive for CERA in the 2008 Tour de France and he subsequently confessed to blood doping and abuse of testosterone. His manager, Stefan Matschiner, was later questioned and arrested in connection with a doping network involving an unspecified number of top athletes in Europe. He reportedly had close ties with the Austrian skiing coach Walter Mayer, who had previously been banned from two Winter Olympics after his involvement in a blood doping scandal at the 2002 Winter Olympics. The investigations by the Austrian authorities led to a number of arrests including those of Walter Mayer and of a Vienna pharmacist and doctor. The latter two were connected to the supply of banned substances. Perhaps the most disturbing allegation to emerge from the affair was one made by Kohl, together with an admission from Matschiner, that the latter had bribed WADA employees at unspecified central European testing laboratories to provide information from tests on his athletes. These data were purportedly used to inform dosing regimes in order to avoid detection (http://uk.eurosport.yahoo.com/14082009/58/lab-staff-helped-kohl-cheat.html). Whilst this allegation remains unproven, it is not without precedent. In 1986, the IOC anti-doping laboratory in Rome was shown to have been complicit in providing athletes with data enabling them to avoid detection (Donati, 2003).

In addition to the risk to health posed by the more obvious increase in blood viscosity and the risk of thromboembolism, there is perhaps a more sinister and long-term potential side effect of abuse of ESAs. The risks of thromboembolism will decrease with time as the haematocrit falls. However, EPO-stimulated erythropoiesis vastly augments the demands of the sportsperson for ferrous iron for the synthesis of haemoglobin. Excess iron within the body is toxic. The body can protect itself to a certain extent from increased oral intake of iron by decreasing absorption from the gastrointestinal tract. Such are the requirements engendered by EPO administration: iron must be injected, thus bypassing the GIT regulation and leading to iron overload. There is evidence from both France and Italy that elite cyclists have ferritin levels indicative of severe iron overload. Thus recent investigations in Italy revealed that a large proportion of professional cyclists had elevated ferritin levels, often in excess of 1000 ng/ml (Cazzola, 2001). A study of elite riders in France revealed a mean ferritin level of 806 ng/ml with a range of 534–1997 ng/ml (Dine, 2001). These values are equivalent to those seen in congenital haemochromatosis. This condition is characterised by iron deposition in various tissues and organs, leading to multiple organ failure, including cirrhosis. It also increases the risk of hepatic carcinoma. A subsequent longitudinal follow-up study revealed that the situation had improved slightly from 1999 to 2002. In 1999, >45 per cent of riders had serum ferritin levels >300 ng/ml and 25 per cent exceeded 500 ng/ml. In 2002, the corresponding values were 27 per cent and 9 per cent, respectively (Zotter et al., 2004). The authors recommended that aggressive therapy should be initiated at or before the end of the careers of those riders with excessively elevated serum ferritin levels. Thus not only is EPO prohibited by WADA, but also it poses significant short- and long-term health problems to the abuser, inadvertent or not.

9.4   Blood doping

Blood transfusion

There are two forms of transfusional polycythaemia: autologous and homolo-gous. Autologous blood doping is the transfusion of one's own blood, which has been stored (refrigerated or frozen) until needed. Homologous blood doping is the transfusion of blood that has been taken from another person with the same blood type. The improved performance capability is achieved virtually overnight. Once the excess fluid is excreted, the athlete is left with a supranor-mally high red cell count, haemoglobin concentration, total body haemoglobin and hence oxygen-carrying capacity of the blood. This will ultimately increase the athlete's VO_2 max, conferring a positive ergogenic benefit in both training and competition.

The generally held opinion is that blood doping began after the 1968 Mexico Olympics when male athletes from Kenya, Tunisia and Ethiopia, who lived and trained at high altitudes, were notably successful in endurance athletic events. However, the first study of the ergogenic value of heterologous blood transfusion was in 1947 by Pace. The period from 1972 to 1984 marked the heyday of blood doping and there are numerous reports of allegations and admissions (e.g. Leigh-Smith, 2004; Eichner, 1987, 2007) that involved athletes from a variety of countries (including Finland, Italy, America, Russia and East Germany) partici-pating in a variety of different sports (e.g. long-distance running, cycling and skiing). The practice of blood doping was largely superseded in the late 1980s by abuse of EPO, which removed the risks associated with homologous transfusions and the inconvenience of autologous transfusions.

Methods of blood doping

The original method of autologous blood doping involved withdrawing one to four units of blood from an athlete. The blood was then centrifuged and separated into plasma, which was re-infused immediately, and packed RBCs that were stored at 4°C. The athlete then required 8–12 weeks to replenish the red cells that had been withdrawn. During that time, the ability to train and to compete would be reduced and the stored red cells would lyse at a rate of 1 per cent per day. In order to overcome these problems, the protocol was changed to removal of blood 16 weeks before the event, followed by re-infusion 8 weeks before the event. This enabled the athlete to benefit from a raised Hb and to resume maximum intensity of training prior to the event.

The advent of glycerol freezing of RBCs at –80°C, permitted storage for up to 10 years with only 10–15 per cent haemolysis. Of course, before re-infusion, the RBCs had to be thawed, washed and re-suspended in physiological saline. Detection of residual contaminants of the process has been proposed as a basis for testing for autologous transfusion.

At least two other techniques have been used to facilitate transfusional polycythaemia. Historically, athletes have been accompanied by their own heterologous blood donor in the form of a cross-matched family relative. More latterly, there were media reports that Operation Puerto had uncovered up to 100 plasma samples containing high levels of EPO. The assumption was that the plasma was spiked with EPO to augment the athletes' replenishment of their lost red cells.

Testing for blood doping

The history of testing for blood doping reflects concerns for both the ethics of sport and the health of participants. The International Olympic Committee (IOC) added blood doping to its banned procedures in 1985. In 1988 the Fédération Internationale de Ski (FIS) classified EPO as a doping substance. The FIS was the first federation to introduce blood sampling for detection of heterologous/ homologous erythrocyte infusions in 1989. Samples were analysed for blood groups, EPO and haemoglobin concentration. Erythropoietin was banned by the IOC in 1990. In 1997, the Union Cycliste Internationale (UCI) and the FIS accepted random blood testing before competition and fixed maximum haematocrit and haemoglobin levels. These tests were instigated, in part, for the benefit of the riders and skiers. Indeed, they were called health checks.

A test for blood doping using an homologous transfusion was introduced in the 2004 Summer Olympic Games in Athens. Detection is based upon a technique known as fluorescence-activated cell sorting (FACS) (Thevis et al., 2009). However, there is currently no method of detecting blood doping from the administration of an autologous transfusion (WADA, 2009). WADA is funding several scientific studies designed to address this shortcoming. Moreover, lack of a test for autologous transfusions is one of the reasons why WADA is supporting the development of the athlete/biological passport.

Abuse

The successful introduction of a test for EPO in 2000, the absence of a test for homologous transfusions until 2002 and the continuing lack of a test for autologous transfusions were probably three reasons for the re-emergence of blood doping in the new millennium. Just as the Festina affair in 1998 had highlighted the extent of EPO abuse in the Tour de France, so Operation Puerto highlighted the extent of blood doping within cycling and, indeed, other sports. Though the operation took place in 2006, its origins can be traced back to 2003 and a Spanish cyclist named Jesús Manzano. Manzano collapsed at stage 7 of the 2003 Tour de France. He later claimed that he had been given a 50 millilitre injection by the team doctor. In March of the following year, he gave an exclusive interview to the Spanish newspaper AS in which he detailed the practice of blood doping and use of performance-enhancing drugs within his team, Kelme. The accounts of systematic doping, funded by top-slicing of riders' salaries, were reminiscent of those published by Willy Voet after the Festina affair in 1998. At first, Manzano's allegations were dismissed as an act of revenge for his sacking. However, further revelations resulted in the withdrawal of Kelme's invitation to ride in the 2004 Tour de France. They later led directly to Operation Puerto and the arrest, in 2006, Eufemiano Fuentes (the Kelme team doctor in 2003) and Walter Virú (the former Kelme team doctor) amongst others. Police searches of a number of premises, including those of Dr. Fuentes, revealed thousands of doses of anabolic steroids, 100 packets of blood products and machines to manipulate and transfuse them. The ramifications of Operation Puerto were both short term and long term, individual and corporate. Allegedly, some 200 athletes were implicated in Operation Puerto. The Spanish Guardia Civil later named 34, all of whom were cyclists. None of the top five finishers in the 2005 Tour de France started the 2006 Tour. Numerous top cyclists were either suspended (Ivan Basso) or retired (most notably, Jan Ullrich). In August 2006, the main sponsor of the Kelme team, the Valencian Government, withdrew its sponsorship and the team folded. The following year, T-Mobile, who had sponsored a professional cycling team since 1991, withdrew its sponsorship. In 2009, Alejandro Valverde was prevented from competing in the Tour de France by the Italian Olympic Committee (CONI). CONI purportedly had DNA evidence that linked Valverde with Operation Puerto and imposed a two-year ban on his racing in Italy, commencing in May 2009. This effectively banned Valverde, because stage 16 of the 2009 Tour took the race in to Italy.

Although, at the time of Operation Puerto, athletes from other sports (including football and tennis) were allegedly linked to Dr. Fuentes, none were ever named. Dr. Fuentes is alleged to have been highly indignant that only cyclists were named and he said that he had worked with footballers and tennis players. In February 2009, following the tragic death of 21-year-old Belgian cyclist Frederiek Nolf, who died in his sleep, there were imputations that it was reminiscent of the deaths of Belgian and Dutch cyclists in the late 1980s. Sadly, however, cycling is not the only sport to be associated with sudden cardiac deaths in recent years. There have been a number of sudden deaths in football (including three Brazilians, one Portugese, one Cameroon, one Nigerian [*New Zealand Herald*, 2007] and two Spaniards, the latest of whom was the 26-year-old captain of Espanyol [*The Guardian*, 2009] and one in the rugby union [a Tongan playing for Perigueux; AFP/Expatica, 2009]). Such was the concern caused by the deaths of footballers that Union of European Football Associations (UEFA) introduced compulsory cardiac testing before EURO 2008. Whether or not this should be extended to all young athletes is contentious. However, analysis of 25 years of data from the USA revealed that one young competitive athlete died every three days from an unrecognised cardiovascular disorder (Maron *et al.*, 2006; cited in Drezner and Khan, 2008). The latter state that the existing evidence supports the use of a pre-participation screening that involves comprehensive recording of personal and family histories, a physical examination and a screening ECG.

9.5 Blood substitutes

The market in blood substitutes is potentially enormous. Over three million units of blood components are used each year in the UK. In Scotland some 300,000 units are used each year whilst the number of donations is approximately 240,000 (National Health Service, 2006). Because of problems with the availability of blood for transfusions and the associated risk of infections (e.g. Hepatitis C and variant Creutzfeldt-Jakob disease [vCJD]) from transfusions, there has been much research into blood substitutes and into drugs that can increase tissue oxygenation. There are two major types of blood substitutes: haemoglobin-based oxygen carriers (HBOCs) and perfluorocarbons (PFCs).

Haemoglobin-based oxygen carriers (HBOCs)

Free haemoglobin (Hb) is simple to prepare and purify but it is unstable, dysfunctional and ultimately toxic. Even autologous Hb, if infused, will dissociate into dimers that are dysfunctional and toxic. The dimers are filtered by the kidneys and cause renal tubule necrosis, chronic renal failure and death. Numerous techniques have been developed in order to overcome these problems. Haemoglobin has been polymerised, cross-linked, conjugated and even encapsulated in attempts to mimic the red cell. The first-generation HBOCs caused vasoconstriction because native Hb binds the endogenous vasodilator, nitric oxide (NO), the so-called NO-scavenging effect. Moreover, Hb is readily oxidised and causes a perturbation of the oxidant/anti-oxidant balance within the vasculature. Second-generation HBOCs incorporated antioxidants (e.g. catalase-superoxide dismutase) into the Hb molecule but again these were not protected by a red cell membrane mimic. Third-generation HBOCs have incorporated Hb and red cell enzymes into membranes, initially into liposomes and latterly into biodegradable polylactic acid nanoparticles.

It is not possible to test for HBOCs in urine because of their inherent design. However, they do impart a red colour to serum, which simplifies detection. Moreover, they can be detected by routine laboratory techniques including western immunoblotting or a combination of HPLC and mass spectrometry (Elliott, 2008). There has been one report of testing in humans performing exercise (Hughes et al., 1995). This study has been criticised on a number of points (Schumacher and Ashenden, 2004). It is of interest to note that the Hughes study pre-dates the concerns expressed by the then medical director of the IOC (Schamasch, 1998) about the rumours of abuse of blood substitutes. Concerns about the potential for abuse were echoed by Ashenden (2004).

There has been one case of a cyclist possessing an HBOC and another case of alleged administration of an HBOC. The 2001 Giro d'Italia was subjected to a raid upon team hotels in San Remo by 200 drug squad officers. An Italian cyclist, who was in second place overall at the time of the raid, withdrew from the race after it was revealed that banned substances (including Hemassist™) had been found in his hotel room (*The Guardian*, 2002). Hemassist is a synthetic haemo-globin, an HBOC, which was developed by Baxter Pharmaceutical Healthcare. However, a clinical trial was stopped after adverse results (Baxter Pharmaceuticals, 1998). Jesús Manzano claims that the drug that was administered to him on the morning of stage 7 of the 2003 Tour De France, during which he collapsed and was admitted to hospital, was Oxyglobin™. Oxyglobin is a first-generation HBOC that is licensed by the FDA but only for veterinary use (treatment of canine anaemia) in the USA since 1998.

Perfluorocarbons (PFCs)

The PFCs are synthetic, highly fluorinated, inert organic compounds that can dis-solve oxygen and other respiratory gases (Lowe, 2001). There is no chemical interaction between oxygen and the PFC. The amount of oxygen dissolved in the PFC particles is directly proportional to the partial pressure of oxygen. Thus, the PFC will dissolve oxygen in the lungs and then release it, in exchange for carbon dioxide, when it passes through the tissues. This process is repeated for the time that the PFC remains in the body. First-generation PFCs (e.g. perftoran) had a long half-life (65 days) but a low capacity to dissolve oxygen (5 ml/dl at a pO_2 of 500 mmHg). Second-generation PFCs (e.g. perflubron) have a shorter half-life (4–6 hrs) and a higher capacity to dissolve oxygen (16 ml/dl at a pO_2 of 500 mmHg). This is comparable to the oxygen-carrying capacity of whole blood. More significantly, because of the linear relationship between the partial pressure of oxygen and the amount of oxygen dissolved in the PFC, 12 ml/dl of oxygen will come out of solution in the tissues, which is greater than that released from whole blood under standard conditions of temperature and pressure (Gaudard *et al.*, 2003). The obvious drawback for the athlete wishing to abuse a PFC is that the latter functions best when the subject is inhaling oxygen at greater than ambient partial pressures.

PFCs, as inert organic chemicals, are immiscible in water and must be infused as an emulsion. The droplets are removed from circulation by phagocytosis by the cells of the reticulo-endothelial system (RES). They are not metabolised but gradually released back into the circulation and excreted in the expired air. They can be detected in both blood and expired air either by gas chromatography or by a combination of gas chromatography and mass spectrometry. Although these methods exist, they are not applied routinely and only under special circum-stances (e.g. when requested by the sporting federation) (Gaudard *et al.*, 2003).

There have been no published reports of studies of PFCs in humans perform-ing exercise. Neither have there been any confirmed reports of abuse of PFCs in sport. However, they are mentioned specifically in the 2010 WADA list of pro-hibited methods (under M1, enhancement of oxygen transport). There was one alleged incident in 1998 when a Swiss cyclist was withdrawn from a stage in the Tour of Romandie, Switzerland, and treated for a mysterious and near fatal ill-ness, which was initially diagnosed as an infection. The symptoms were difficulty in breathing, muscle pain, gastroenteritis and "intravascular coagulation". Doctors from a Lausanne hospital suspected that he had been given PFCs without his knowledge (Gains, 1998). The cyclist subsequently tried to sue the doctor who treated him and who subsequently made the allegations. However, the UCI did take the rumours sufficiently seriously to write a letter to all teams who were due to take part in the Giro d'Italia, just a few days later, warning them of the dangers of PFCs (Austen, 1999).

9.6   Haemoglobin modifiers

Another approach to increasing oxygen delivery to the tissues is to decrease the oxygen affinity of Hb, i.e. shifting the oxyhaemoglobin dissociation curve to the right. This is achieved physiologically by increases in $[H^+]$, pCO_2, temperature and 2,3 BPG. RSR13 is a drug that mimics the effects of 2,3 BPG and decreases the oxygen affinity of Hb by binding allosterically to the Hb tetramer. Unlike the naturally occurring 2,3, BPG, RSR13 binds to the α-subunits and not into the cleft between the β-subunits (Gaudard et al., 2003). Therefore, it has the potential to be used synergistically to augment the action of the endogenous allosteric inhibitor 2,3 BPG. One study demonstrated a dose-dependent shift in p50, which is the partial pressure of oxygen at which Hb is 50 per cent saturated. The peak pharmacological effect occurs immediately at the end of the infusion and lasts for three to six hours. The drug, which must be given by slow intravenous infusion, was in clinical trials in Canada and the USA as a radio-sensitizing agent in cancer therapy. However, it failed to meet a primary end-point in a phase 3 clinical trial and development was suspended (Elliott, 2008). The drug did have obvious potential for abuse in sport but, to date, this hasn't materialised. There have been no adverse analytical findings for RSR13. There has been one media report of an elite Italian cyclist being in possession of RSR13 in 2001. The manufacturer, Allos Therapeutics, from Denver, Colorado, reported that sensitive and validated methods of detection exist for both human blood and urine (Paranka, 2001). Breidbach and Catlin (2001) have developed a detection method using gas chromatography and mass spectrometry.

Plasma volume expanders

Finally, plasma expanders that can be used to mask the raised Hct caused by EPO are banned as prohibited substances (S5, diuretics and other masking agents: WADA, 2010). Hydroxyethyl starch (HES, Hespan™) is a synthetic polymer derived from starch amylopectin. It has a high molecular weight and causes plasma volume expansion for 24 hours. It can be detected in plasma for 17 to 24 weeks. It has numerous side effects, including increased coagulation (American Society of Anaesthesiologists, 1999). Nevertheless, it is a drug of abuse in sport. Six top cross-country skiers from Finland were banned for using HES. In what was subsequently referred to as the 2001 Lahti doping scandal, police investigations revealed that the Finnish Ski Association had bought quantities of plasma expanders over a period of at least four years (Helsingin Sanomat, 2002). There were no adverse analytical findings in 2008 (WADA, 2008).

9.7 Actovegin

Actovegin is a deproteinized hemodialysate of calf blood and contains peptides, oligosaccharides and nucleic acid derivatives (Schaffler *et al.*, 1991). It has been the subject of clinical research since the mid-1970s. Actovegin has been shown to improve glucose tolerance in diabetics but not in patients with normal carbohydrate metabolism (Heidrich *et al.*, 1979). More specifically, Actovegin increased insulin-stimulated glucose disposal in type II diabetes (non-insulin dependent diabetes [IDDM]) (Jacob *et al.*, 1996). These authors speculated that this could have been caused by supplementation of inositol-phosphate-oligosaccharides. Actovegin improved pain-free and pain-limited walking times in patients with Fontaine stage IIb peripheral arterial occlusive disease (Streminski *et al.*, 1992). Perhaps of more immediate relevance to sport, intra-muscular injection of Actovegin reduced the time to recovery of full sports activity after acute muscle injury (Pfister and Koller, 1990). In a later placebo-controlled, double-blind study of patients with Achilles paratendinitis, Actovegin was shown to evoke a significant reduction in severe pain on full athletic activity after three weeks of treatment (Pforringer *et al.*, 1994).

It was the drug at the centre of allegations against the U.S. Postal Service cycle team. Allegedly, it was recovered from items discarded by the team during the 2000 Tour de France. Numerous national teams brought Actovegin into Australia for the 2000 Sydney Olympics. It was added to the list of banned substances by the IOC in December 2000 under the category of blood-doping agents. It was suspected of being an oxygen-carrying agent. Two months later, the IOC announced that it was unclear about the mode of action of the drug and uncertain as to whether Actovegin enhanced performance. The IOC was to await further investigations into the potential ergogenic value of Actovegin and make an announcement before the 2002 Winter Olympics in Salt Lake City. However, that did not happen and Actovegin is not currently included on the WADA prohibited list (2010). Nevertheless, the Australian Sports Anti-Doping Authority did warn athletes that intravenous injection of Actovegin is banned by WADA under prohibited methods (M2, chemical and physical manipulation) (Tsitsimpikou *et al.*, 2009).

Although the mode(s) of action of Actovegin remain unclear and any possible ergogenic value remains unproven in placebo-controlled, double-blind, cross-over trials, reports of use continue. Thus in the 2004 Summer Olympics in Athens, 22 athletes attending doping controls declared the use of haemoderivatives of which 16 reported using Actovegin. Interestingly, 59 per cent of those using Actovegin were participants in non-aerobic sports (e.g. wrestling, boxing, judo and weightlifting) (Tsitsimpikou *et al.*, 2009). Post-2004, there have been numerous media reports of the use of Actovegin in a variety of sports (e.g. Australian rugby league) and scientific papers published on the clinical use of Actovegin (e.g. in the treatment of polyneuropathy in Type 2 diabetes). Thus, it is reasonable to assume that WADA may need to revisit the status of Actovegin at some stage in the future.

9.8   Biological passports

In October 2007, the Paris Summit on Doping in Cycling was hosted by the France Minister for Health, Youth and Sport, Ms. Roselyne Bachelot-Narquin. In attendance were representatives of the UCI, the organisers of the Tour de France, representatives from WADA and pro cycling teams, race organisers and professional cyclists. At this conference, approval was granted for the introduction, in 2008, of "an innovative anti-doping project", which would become known as the biological passport (UCI, 2008) .

A biological passport is an individual, electronic record for each rider, in which the results of all doping tests are collated over a period of time (i.e. a longitudinal project or study). It contains four elements, namely:

- the results of individual urine tests
- results of individual blood tests
- a haematological profile
- a steroid profile

The collection of data began in 2008. All riders registered with a UCI pro team were tested together with all those in teams either granted wild-card entry for particular races or selected by the Steering Group of the UCI. The riders were subjected to four different categories of test:

- blood tests, of which the majority were out of competition to establish a haematological profile;
- urine tests, of which the majority were out of competition to establish a steroid profile;
- stand-alone blood tests collected in competition during specific races and not included in the haematological profile;
- additional out-of-competition tests if required, for follow-up or targeted testing.

This resulted in 8404 blood samples from 805 riders at an approximate cost of €3.887 million. The data from these tests were then analysed statistically to establish whether the profile was normal or abnormal (i.e. the values were within or without set limits or confidence intervals). Abnormal profiles were then reviewed by a panel of nine independent scientific experts. As a consequence of the 2008 programme, the UCI reported that several riders were dismissed by their teams and seven riders demonstrated abnormal profiles arising from targeted out-of-competition urine tests. The UCI also reported that the deterrent value had been very high (ANADO Blood Workshop, 2009).

In June 2009, the UCI stated that five riders had "violated the anti doping rules on the basis of information from blood profiles on their biological passports". Igor Astarloa, the 2003 World Road Race Champion, was one of those named by the UCI. "These adverse findings were a direct result of a targeted test programme conducted on Mr Di Luca using information from his biological passport's blood profile, previous test results and his race schedule," the UCI press release stated (UCI 2009).

It seems likely that detection of blood doping, in its wider definition, will be best served by a combination of deterministic and probabilistic methods as suggested by Melioli and D'Onofrio (2006).

9.9 Conclusion

This chapter has painted a rather bleak picture of the prohibited substances and methods used to enhance oxygen transport. Blood doping began almost 40 years ago and has mirrored the scientific and medical advances in the understanding and treatment of anaemia and reduced oxygen availability. However, it should be borne in mind that in 2008, the last year for which WADA data were available at the time this book was going to press, the number of adverse analytical findings (AAFs) helps to put this into perspective. In 2008, there were 5,523 AAFs of which only 106 (1.9 per cent) were for S2 (hormones and related substances). Of those 106, only 58 were for ESAs, which is just 1.05 per cent of the total number of AAFs. There were no AAFs for prohibited methods M1 (enhancement of oxygen transfer) (WADA, 2008). So although the media would suggest that abuses of EPO and blood doping are reaching epidemic proportions in endurance sports, the official data suggest that the situation might not be quite as bad as it is made out to be.

9.10 References

AFP/Expatica. (2009). Safety in question after deaths of high profile athletes. Available at http://www.expatica.com/de/news/german-news/safety-inquestion-after-deaths-of-high-profile-athletes-_49329.html (accessed 2 August 2010).

American Society of Anaesthesiologists. (1999). Blood substitutes and pharmacological alternatives. Available at http://www.asahq.org (accessed 29 March 2001).

ANADO Blood Workshop. (2009). The biological passport—The good news and bad news... Available at http://www.anado.org/documents/(Anne)%20Biological%20Passport-%20ANADO%20Blood%20work.pdf (accessed 14 September 2009).

Ashenden, M. (2004). Contemporary issues in the fight against blood doping in sport. *Haematologica* **89(8)**, 901–904.

Ashenden, M., Varlet-Marie, E., Lasne, F. and Audran, M. (2006). The effects of microdose recombinant human erythropoietin regimens in athletes. *Haematologica* **91(8)**, 1143–1144.

Austen, I. (1999). PFC. Procycling. Available at http://www.bikemagic.com/news/article/mps/uan/189 (accessed 22 August 2009).

Barrett, K.E., Barman, S.M., Boitano, S. and Brooks, H.L. (2009). *Ganong's review of medical physiology*. 23rd ed., McGraw-Hill, New York.

Baxter Pharmaceuticals. (1998). Baxter ends U.S. trauma study of Hemassist®(DCLHb). Available at http://www.baxter.com/utilities/news/releases/1998/03–31hemassist.html (accessed 29 September 2001).

Bick, R.L., Bennett, J.M., Brynes, R.K. *et al.* (1993). *Haematology: Clinical and laboratory practice*. Mosby, St Louis, Missouri.

Birkeland, K.I., Stray-Gundersen, J., Hemmersbach, P. *et al.* (2000). Effect of r-HuEPO administration on serum levels of sTfR and cycling performance. *Medicine and Science in Sports and Exercise* **32(7)**, 1238–1243.

Breidbach, A. and Catlin, D.H. (2001). RSR13, a potential athletic performance enhancement agent: detection in urine by gas chromatography/mass spectrometry. *Rapid Communications in Mass Spectrometry* **15(24)**, 2378–2382.

Cazzola, M. (2001). Erythropoietin pathophysiology, clinical uses of recombinant human erythropoietin, and medical risks of its abuse in sport. *The International Society for Laboratory Hematology (ISLH) XIVth International Symposium*, p. 21. Available at http://mmserver.cjp.com/gems/labhem/7.1.Doping.pdf (accessed 2 August 2010).

Davison, A.M. (2004). *Oxford textbook of clinical nephrology*. 2004. 3rd ed., Oxford University Press, New York.

Dine, G. (2001). Biochemical and haematological parameters in athletes. *The International Society for Laboratory Hematology (ISLH) XIVth International Symposium*, p. 24. Available at http://mmserver.cjp.com/gems/labhem/7.1.Doping.pdf (accessed 2 August 2010).

Donati, S. (2001). Curriculum vitae. Available at http://www.play-the-game.org/speeches/doping/antidoping.html (accessed 16 August 2001).

Donati, S. (2003). Sandro Donati: "Anti-doping: the fraud behind the stage". Available at http//www.ergogenics.orgdonati.htnl (accessed 8 September 2009).

Drezner, J.A, and Khan, K. (2008). Editorial: Sudden cardiac death in young athletes. *British Medical Journal* **337**, 309.

Eichner, E.R. (1987). Blood doping: Results and consequences from the laboratory and the field. *Physician and Sports Medicine* **15**, 121–129.

Eichner, E.R. (2007). Blood doping: Infusions, erythropoietin and artificial blood. *Sports Medicine* **37(4–5)**, 389–391.

Ekblom, B. (1997). Blood doping, erythropoetin and altitude. In *The clinical pharmacology of sport and exercise*, ed. T. Reilly and M. Orme, Elsevier, Amsterdam. 199–212.

Ekblom, B. and Berglund, B. (1991). Effect of erythropoietin administration on maximal aerobic power. *Scandinavian Journal of Medicine and Science in Sports* **1**, 88–93.

Elliott, S. (2008). Erythropoiesis-stimulating agents and other methods to enhance oxygen transport. *British Journal of Pharmacology* **154**, 529–541.

Fisher, J.W. (2003). Erythropoietin: Physiology and pharmacology update. *Experimental Biology and Medicine* **228**, 1–14.

Gains, P. (1998). A new threat in blood doping. *New York Times*, October 18.

Gaudard, A., Varlet-Marie, E., Bressolle, F. *et al.* (2003). Drugs for increasing oxygen transport and their potential use in doping. *Sports Medicine* **33(3)**, 187–212.

The Guardian. (2002). Italy cool about Frigo's flourish William Fotheringham. Available at http://www.guardian.co.uk/sport/2002/jul/26/tourdefrance2002.tourdefrance (accessed 20 September 2009).

The Guardian. (2009). Espanyol captain Dani Jarque dies of heart failure. Available at http://www.guardian.co.uk/football/2009/aug/09/espanyol-dani-jarque-dies) (accessed 2 August 2010).

Harrison, C. 2003. The man who knows too much. *Sports Monthly.* Available at http://www.chrisharrisonwriting.com/journalism/_3/ (accessed 18 September 2008).

Heidrich, H., Quednau, J. and Schirop, T. (1979). Reaction of blood sugar and serum insulin to intravenous long-term treatment with Actovegin. Clinical double-blind study (author's transl.). *Med Klin* **74(7)**, 242–245.

Helsingin Sonomat. (2002). Finnish skiers used plasma expanders for years prior to Lahti doping scandal. Available at http://www2.hs.fi/english/archive/news.asp?id=20020326IE14 (accessed 2 August 2010).

Hughes, G.S., Francom, S.F., Antal, E.J. *et al.* (1995). Hematologic effects of a novel hemoglobin-based oxygen carrier in normal male and female subjects. *Journal of Laboratory Clinical Medicine* **196(5)**, 444–451.

International Meeting of International Olympic Committee (IOC). (April 1990). Lausanne, Switzerland.

International Olympic Committee Medical Commission. (2000). Post-Olympic public report on doping controls at the Games of the XXVII Olympiad in Sydney (Australia). Lausanne, 14 December 2000.

International Olympic Committee Medical Commission. (2001). Prohibited classes of substances and prohibited methods. 1 September 2001.

Jacob, S., Dietze, G.J., Machicao, F. *et al.* (1996). Improvement of glucose metabolism in patients with type II diabetes after treatment with hemodialysate. *Arzneimittelforschung* **46(3)**, 269–272.

Kimmage, P. (1988). *Rough ride.* Yellow Jersey Press, London.

Lasne, F. and de Ceaurriz, J. (2000). Recombinant erythropoietin in urine. *Nature* **405**, 635.

Leigh-Smith, S. (2004). Blood boosting: A review. *British Journal of Sports Medicine* **38**, 99–101.

Leith, W. (July 1992). EPO and cycling. *Athletics*, pp. 24–26.

Lowe, K.C. (2001). Fluorinated blood substitutes and oxygen carriers. *Journal of Fluoride Chemistry* **109(1)**, 59–65.

Melioli, G. and D'Onofrio, G. (2006). Blood doping: Present procedures and detection techniques. *Expert Review of Endocrinological Metabolism* **1(6)**, 793–800.

National Health Service. (2006). Blood transfusion: Clinical standards. Available at http://www.nhshealthquality.org/nhsqis/files/bloodtrans_stnf_sep06.pdf (accessed 14 September 2009).

New Zealand Herald. (2007). Spanish footballer dies after collapse. Available at http://www.nzherald.co.nz (accessed 11 August 2009).

Pace, N. (1947). The increase in hypoxia tolerance of normal men accompanying the polycythemia induced by transfusion of erythrocytes. *American Journal of Physiology* **148**, 152–163.

Paranka, N. (2001). Haemoglobin modifiers: Is RSR 13 the next aerobic enhancer? *The International Society for Laboratory Hematology (ISLH) XIVth International Symposium*, p. 23.

Parisotto, R., Wu, M., Ashenden, M.J. *et al.* (2001). Detection of recombinant human erythropoietin abuse in athletes utilizing markers of altered erythropoiesis. *Haematologica* **86**, 128–137.

Pfister, A. and Koller, W. (1990). Treatment of fresh muscle injury. *Sportverletz Sportschaden* **4(1)**, 41–44.

Pforringer, W., Pfister, A. and Kuntz, G. (1994). The treatment of Achilles paratendinitis: Results of a double-blind, placebo-controlled study with a deproteinized hemodialysate. *Clinical Journal of Sports Medicine* **4(2)**, 92–99.

Rendell, M. (2006). *The death of Marco Pantani: A biography*. Weidenfield & Nicolson, London.

Schaffler, K., Wauschkuhn, C.H. and Hauser, B. (1991). Study to evaluate the encephalotropic potency of a hemodialysate. Controlled study using electro-retinography and visual evoked potentials under hypoxic conditions in human volunteers (preliminary communication). *Arzneimittelforschung* **41(7)**, 699–704.

Schamasch, P. (1998). EPO and PFCs: Personal view. *Olympic Review* **26(22)**, 8.

Schellekens, H. (2009). Biosimilar therapeutics—What do we need to consider? *Nephrology Dialysis Transplantation* **2 (Suppl. 1)**, i27–i36.

Schumacher, Y.O. and Ashenden, M. (2004). Doping with artificial oxygen carriers: An update. *Sports Medicine* **34(3)**, 141–150.

Streminski, J.A., de la Haye, R., Rettig, K. *et al.* (1992). Comparison of the effectiveness of physical training with parenteral drug therapy in Fontaine stage IIb peripheral arterial occlusive disease. *Vasa* **21(4)**, 392–402.

Thevis, M., Kuuranne, T. Geyer, H. *et al.* (2009). Annual banned-substance review: The prohibited list 2008—Analytical approaches in human sports drug testing. *Drug Testing and Analysis* **1**, 4–13.

Tsitsimpikou C., Tsiokanos A., Tsarouhas K. *et al.* (2009). Medication use by athletes at the Athens 2004 Summer Olympic Games. *Clinical Journal of Sports Medicine* **2009(1)**, 33–38.

UCI (2009). Press release : Commencement of first disciplinary proceedings on the basis of the biological passport http://www.uci.ch/Modules/ENews/ENewsDetails.asp?source=SiteSearch&id=NjM5OA&MenuId=MTI1ODA&CharValList=&CharTextList=&CharFromList=&CharToList=&txtSiteSearch=ASTARLOA&LangId=1 (accessed 14 September 209).

Union Cycliste Internationale (UCI). (2008). The biological passport and the UCI's anti-doping measures. Available at http://www.uci.ch/Modules/BUILTIN/getObject.asp?MenuId=MjI0NQ&ObjTypeCode=FILE&type=FILE&id=NDY4MjA&LangId=1 (accessed 14 September 2009).

Voet, W. (2001). *Breaking the chain*. Yellow Jersey Press, London.

World Anti-Doping Agency (WADA). (2008). Adverse analytical findings and atypical findings reported by accredited laboratories. Available at http://www.wada-ama.org/rtecontent/document/WADA_2008_LaboratoryStatisticsReport_Final.pdf (accessed 13 October 2009).

World Anti-Doping Agency (WADA). (2009). Technical document—TD 2009. EPO harmonization of the method for the identification of recombinant erythropoietins (i.e. epoetins) and analogues (e.g. darbepoetin and methoxypolyethylene glycol-epoetin beta) Available at http://www.wada-ama.org/rtecontent/document/TD_EPO_2009.pdf. (accessed 2 August 2010).

World Anti-Doping Agency (WADA). (2010). Prohibited list. Available at http://www.wada-ama.org (accessed 2 September 2009).

Zotter, H., Robinson, N., Zorzoli, M. *et al.* (2004). Abnormally high serum ferritin levels among professional road cyclists. *British Journal of Sports Medicine* **38**, 704–708.

Chapter 10

Prohibited methods

Chemical and physical manipulation

David R. Mottram

10.1 Current (2010) WADA regulations with respect to chemical and physical manipulation

The 2010 WADA regulations for prohibited methods involving chemical and physical manipulation state that:

1   Tampering or attempting to tamper in order to alter the integrity and validity of samples collected during doping controls is prohibited. These include but are not limited to catheterisation, urine substitution and/or alteration (e.g. proteases).
2   Intravenous infusions are prohibited except for those legitimately received in the course of hospital admissions or clinical investigations.

Clearly, there are significant legitimate circumstances where an athlete may require intravenous infusions. WADA therefore provides clarification with respect to these regulations as follows:

> Intravenous infusions are prohibited and thus require Therapeutic Use Exemption except in the management of surgical procedures, medical emergencies or clinical investigations.
>   The intent is to prohibit hemodilution, overhydration and the administration of prohibited substances by means of intravenous infusion. An intravenous infusion is defined as the delivery of fluids through a vein using a needle or similar device.

The legitimate medical uses of intravenous infusions that follow are not prohibited:

1   Emergency intervention including resuscitation;
2   Blood replacement as a consequence of blood loss;
3   Surgical procedures;
4   Administration of drugs and fluids when other routes of administration are not available (e.g. because of intractable vomiting) in accordance with good medical practice, exclusive of exercise-induced dehydration.

Injections with a simple syringe are not prohibited as a method if the injected substance is not prohibited and if the volume does not exceed 50 ml.

It is difficult to anticipate the varied and imaginative ways in which athletes may undertake chemical and physical manipulation in order to avoid detection of prohibited drug use. The next section of this chapter therefore provides illustrative case studies in which various methods have been used.

10.2   Prevalence of chemical and physical manipulation in sport

WADA statistics relating to chemical and physical manipulation

Table 10.1 shows the numbers of positive test results from WADA-accredited laboratories, relating to chemical and physical manipulation, since 2003.

It is clear that few instances have been identified. To what extent this reflects athletes' disinclination to use such techniques or an inability on behalf of the laboratories to identify such practices is difficult to establish.

Case studies of attempted chemical and physical manipulation

Katrina Krabbe, 1992

Katrina Krabbe won three gold medals at the 1990 European Athletic Championships, the last time East Germany competed in track and field athletics under its own flag. She won two gold medals for the unified German team, in the 100- and 200-metre events at the 1991 World Championships in Tokyo.

Prior to the 1992 Olympic Games, Katrina Krabbe and her teammates Grit Breuer and Silke Moeller provided allegedly identical urine samples during a test at a training camp in South Africa. All three athletes were suspended from racing, although the suspension was lifted four months later on a technicality associated with the test.

Table 10.1 Positive test results relating to chemical and physical manipulation from WADA statistics, 2003–2008

Year	Number of positive results
2003	2
2004	–
2005	–
2006	4
2007	3
2008	–

Katrina Krabbe and Grit Breuer received subsequent suspensions, having tested positive for clenbuterol prior to the 1992 Barcelona Olympic Games.

Michelle de Bruin (née Smith), 1998

At the 1996 Atlanta Olympic Games, Michelle de Bruin, somewhat unexpectedly in the minds of many observers, won three gold medals in swimming events. Her trainer had been her husband, Eric de Bruin, a former Dutch discus thrower who had served a four-year suspension for failing a drug test for testosterone.

Following the Atlanta Games, Michelle de Bruin missed at least one out-of-competition drug test and received a warning from her governing body, FINA. In January 1998 she was asked to provide a urine sample at her home in Dublin during an unannounced out-of-competition drug test administered by FINA. The sample was analysed at the IOC-accredited laboratory in Barcelona and was found to have "unequivocal signs of adulteration" according to the laboratory report.

The report stated that the concentration of alcohol present "is in no way compatible with human consumption" and that the sample showed "a very strong whiskey odor". A second test on the urine B sample was performed in May 1998, the results being compatible with the January findings. At a hearing in July 1998, a FINA doping panel found that the sample had been manipulated in an uncertain manner by de Bruin.

Michelle de Bruin was banned from national and international competition for four years. She appealed the decision at the Court of Arbitration for Sport (CAS). The hearing revealed that traces of a metabolic pre-cursor of testosterone had been found in three samples from the swimmer during tests taken between November 1997 and March 1998. The CAS upheld the ban.

Galabin Boevski, 2003

The Bulgarian weightlifters Galabin Boevski, Zlatan Vanev and Georgi Markov were suspended from competition after it was alleged that they provided identical urine samples derived from one person when tested at the World Championships in Vancouver in 2003.

Zlatan Vanev and Georgi Markov, both World Champions, were given 18-month suspensions. Galabin Boevski, who won gold at the 2000 Olympic Games in Sydney, was given an eight-year suspension as it was his second adverse analytical finding since 1995.

Rebeca Gusmão, 2007

The Brazilian swimmer Rebeca Gusmão underwent a doping control test at the 2007 Pan American Games in Rio de Janeiro, Brazil. The WADA-accredited laboratory in Rio reported the test to be negative. However, the Games were attended by a WADA independent observer (IO) team, whose role was randomly to monitor and report on all phases of the doping control and results management processes in a neutral and unbiased fashion.

The IO team reported to the international swimming federation, FINA, that Gusmão had been tested on multiple occasions prior to and over the course of the Games and that these tests had yielded some suspicious results suggestive of possible manipulation. Upon review of the steroid profiles for the swimmer it appeared that the samples were from two different people as the endogenous steroid profile was very different.

Urine samples were re-tested to compare genotypes. It was confirmed that they belonged to different donators. Gusmão denied having tampered with the samples and, furthermore, claimed invalidity of the follow-up tests. The FINA doping panel rejected her claims and instituted a lifetime ban, Gusmão having already received a previous suspension from FINA. The case was complicated by a CAS appeal hearing in which it was decided to reject an earlier finding and the suspension was reduced to two years; suspended subject continued appeals at the time of writing.

Olga Yegorova, 2008

Olga Yegorova and seven other leading Russian track and field athletes were suspended by the IAAF after being charged with manipulating urine samples. They were accused of urine substitution when samples taken at the World Championships in Osaka did not match samples taken in out-of-competition tests in May 2007. At the time of writing, these athletes were appealing to CAS.

Olga Yegorova had previously tested positive for erythropoietin at the 2001 World Championships in Edmonton but her suspension for that offence was lifted because incomplete testing procedures had taken place.

10.3   Techniques for identifying chemical and physical manipulation

The most common method of manipulation used by athletes, as determined from WADA laboratory results, has involved sharing of urine samples between fellow athletes or from other individuals. In recent years, it has been possible to individualize urine specimens using steroid and metabolic profiling. An athlete steroid profile is made by recording ratios of various urinary steroid components repeatedly, each time the athlete is tested. The steroidal ratios recorded include testosterone/epitestosterone (T/EpiT), andresterone/etiocholanolone (A/E), 5α-androstane-3α, 17β-diol/5β-androstane-3α, 17β-diol(Adiol/Bdiol) and androstane/testosterone (A/T) (Mareck *et al.*, 2008).

The successful detection of manipulation by three weightlifters is described by Thevis *et al.* (2007) where they employed steroid profiling along with common drug testing approaches, including chromatographic and mass spectrometric assays as well as DNA typing.

Adulteration of urine samples with highly oxidative chemicals has been reported (Paul, 2004). Athletes have reportedly introduced protease granules into the urethra. When flushed out into the urine sample, protease enzymes digest urinary proteins, such as erythropoietin and insulins, without affecting other urinary parameters. Testing regimes can detect increased levels of protease enzymes in the urine and also detect the absence of proteins normally excreted in the urine, such as albumin (Thevis *et al.*, 2008).

Such strategies for combating drug misuse and sample manipulation require comprehensive out-of-competition testing and intelligent targeting of athletes.

In addition to biochemical laboratory urine testing, blood sampling and longitudinal monitoring of steroid profiles a further refinement involves performance profiling (Schumacher and Pottgiesser, 2009). Although sudden increases in performance can be induced by many factors, including improved training methods and nutrition regimes, performance profiling can identify suspicious athletes.

10.4   References

Mareck, U., Geyer, H., Opfermann, G. *et al.* (2008). Factors influencing the steroid profile in doping control analysis. *Journal of Mass Spectrometry* **43**, 877–891.

Paul, B.D. (2004). Six spectroscopic methods for detection of oxidants in urine: Implication in differentiation of normal and adulterated urine. *Journal of Analytical Toxicology* **28**, 599–608.

Schumacher, Y.O. and Pottgiesser, T. (2009). Performance profiling: A role for sport science in the fight against doping? *International Journal of Sports Physiology and Performance* **4**, 129–133.

Thevis, M., Geyer, H. and Mareck, U. (2007). Detection of manipulation in doping control urine sample collection: A multidisciplinary approach to determine identical urine samples. *Anal Bioanalytical Chemistry* **388**, 1539–1543.

Thevis, M., Kohler, M. and Schänzer, W. (2008). New drugs and methods of doping and manipulation. *Drug Discovery Today* **13(1/2)**, 59–66.

Chapter 11

Gene doping

Dominic J. Wells

11.1   Introduction

Genetic manipulation as a form of performance enhancement is, at the time of writing this, still a theoretical rather than a proven issue. The possibility of advances in genetic technology being applied in sports has been recognized by the World Anti-Doping Agency (WADA) since 2001. The current 2010 regulations define gene doping as follows:

> The following, with the potential to enhance athletic performance, are prohibited:
>
> 1   the transfer of cells or genetic elements (e.g. DNA, RNA);
> 2   the use of pharmacological or biological agents that alter gene expression.
>
> Peroxisome Proliferator Activated Receptor delta (PPARδ) agonists (e.g. GW 1516) and PPARδ-AMP-activated protein kinase (AMPK) axis agonists (e.g. AICAR) are prohibited.
>   (WADA, the 2010 prohibited list, international standard)

Why is gene doping seen as such a problem for WADA? Conventional drug and protein treatments are given on an intermittent basis via oral or intravenous dosing. It is necessary to give large doses to maintain effective levels in target tissue(s) until the time of the next dose. This peak-and-trough pharmacodynamics means that there is a greater chance of detection of high levels of the prohibited drug. In contrast, gene transfer means that continuous steady-state expression is possible and so the peak level may only be close to the minimum therapeutic level, making detection harder. Secondly, as the protein is made within the body of the treated individual it is more likely to be indistinguishable from the normal endogenous protein. Finally, in many cases the gene and its product may remain within the treated tissue, for example skeletal muscle, and so is less likely to be detected by assays using urine or blood. Consequently, gene doping may be harder to detect than conventional drug doping and so may be more likely to be adopted by athletes who are seeking to gain an unfair competitive advantage.

11.2 Methods of genetic modification

There is concern that methods developed for genetic approaches to human disease (gene therapy) may be used for athletic enhancement. Although there have been 1537 human gene therapy trials approved in the past 20 years (http://www. wiley.co.uk/genmed/clinical/), very few have shown clear efficacy and no therapeutic products have been registered for human use apart from two viral products for the treatment of cancer that are licensed in China (Kim et al., 2008).

Genetic manipulation of the early embryo can be used to produce transgenic animals in which additional genes are added or where specific genes are inactivated in all cells of the body or in all cells of a specific cell type (for example, skeletal muscle cells). The technology for this early manipulation is relatively inefficient and is thus not suitable for use in humans even if such modifications were ever considered ethically acceptable. However, in animals, particularly the mouse, the effects of such manipulations can be used to understand gene function and the potential consequences of genetic manipulation at the whole body level. This technology can be used to look at the ability of different forms of a therapeutic protein to prevent disease in a mouse model of human disease, for example testing different forms of dystrophin in the *mdx* mouse model of the lethal muscle-wasting disease, Duchenne muscular dystrophy (Wells et al., 1995; Phelps et al., 1995).

Genetic material can be delivered to cells both *in vitro* (cell culture) and *in vivo* (whole animal) using transfer systems called vectors. Modified viruses are the most common form of vectors because during evolution viruses have developed highly efficient systems for introducing their genomes into cells in order to complete their life cycle and generate more viruses. By deleting part or all of the viral genes from the modified viruses they can be rendered replication-deficient and so the introduction of genetic material into the cell is not followed by the cell damage associated with viral replication. Not only does this help to prevent cell damage but it also ensures that the spread of such modified viruses is limited. The production of replication-deficient viral vectors is accomplished in specific cell lines where the genes for viral replication are introduced in a form that allows viral replication but does not allow these genes to be packaged into the viruses that are produced by the cells. The removal of viral genes from the virus also provides space for introduction of the gene(s) of choice together with the regulatory elements controlling expression. The latter can be used to ensure that the genes are only expressed in the correct tissue.

A large number of viruses have been developed as viral vectors, like adenoviruses, adeno-associated viruses (AAV), herpesviruses and retroviruses including lentiviruses and alphaviruses, such as Semliki forest virus. The retroviruses have the particular property of inserting their genomes into the host genome and this leads to a permanent modification of the host cell. In contrast most of the other viruses exist as non-integrated episomes within the nucleus and can be lost with successive rounds of cell division. All viruses have viral proteins on their surfaces and these determine the cell types that the viruses are able to enter.

This tropism can be modified by altering the viral proteins either by selecting different serotypes or by pseudotyping with proteins from other viruses. Recent advances in understanding AAV serotypes have identified minor changes in capsid protein sequences that dramatically alter the tissue targeting of the specific serotypes and these can be used to increase the efficiency and specificity of tissue targeting (Gao et al., 2002; Vandenberghe et al., 2009). Preclinical studies have shown that AAV is the viral vector of choice, particularly for targeting skeletal muscle. In rodents a number of studies have shown that it is possible to achieve body-wide genetic modification of skeletal muscle in rodents and larger species using AAV vectors of several different serotypes (e.g. Gregorevic et al., 2004; Zhu et al., 2005; Denti et al., 2006; Yue et al., 2008; Vitiello et al., 2009). However, a significant drawback with the use of viral vectors is that the presence of viral proteins on the surface leads to an interaction with the acquired immune system that can neutralize and thus block any effects of repeated administration. In the case of people exposed to the wild-type virus this can effectively block the initial administration. While it appears possible to use immunosuppression to modify the interaction with the immune system, this increases the risks associated with gene transfer.

An alternative to using viral vectors is to use plasmid DNA grown in bacteria. Plasmids are circular forms of DNA that replicate in bacteria separately from the bacterial genome. These can be isolated and highly purified so that the product is plasmid DNA without any protein contamination. When administered to animals the plasmid does not provoke an acquired immune response nor does it generate an auto-immune response. It does, however, activate the innate immune response, which produces an inflammatory reaction to DNA of bacterial origin. This inflammatory response can cause local swelling and transient non-specific flu-like symptoms but these do not prevent repeated administration of plasmid. Thus it is possible to top up the effects of previous treatments. The biggest problem with this approach is that the efficiency of cell entry is very poor. This can be improved by two methods. The first is to condense the plasmid that protects the DNA from degradation and enhances uptake by the cell. Specific ligands can be added to enhance cell uptake via receptor-mediated pathways. This approach can work very efficiently in cell culture and moderately efficiently for some tissues in vivo (e.g. Midoux et al., 2008). The alternative method of enhanced delivery is to use a physical force to drive the plasmid across the cell membrane and into the cell, mostly through transient micropores. This can be achieved by using high-volume/high-pressure force (hydrodynamic, reviewed by Herweijer and Wolff, 2007), by using a set of electrical pulses (electroporation, reviewed by Trollet et al., 2008), by firing the DNA into the cell/tissue (ballistic, reviewed by Wells, 2004) or by using ultrasound, commonly in conjunction with contrast microbubbles (reviewed by Newman and Bettinger, 2007). It is therefore not feasible to consider efficient whole body treatment with non-viral vectors and these systems are better suited to local or regional (for example, limb) treatment.

An alternative to the use of viral or non-viral vectors *in vivo* is to use cells modified *in vitro*. For example, genetically modified cells can be used to aid the repair of damaged muscle or may be used as a platform for secreting proteins. In the latter case it is possible to encapsulate the cells in an inert capsule that can prevent the immune rejection of the cells. This has the advantage that such implants can be readily removed if they fail to express the protein of interest at appropriate levels and the coating means that the cells do not need to be those of the recipient (Ponce *et al.*, 2006).

With all of the above techniques it is important to consider the regulation of gene expression. Where cells have been modified *ex vivo* they can be assessed for the level of expression of the transferred gene prior to implantation. However for *in vivo* gene transfer the efficiency of gene transfer and hence the level of expression will be variable. In some cases excess expression carries significant health risks and may decrease performance. There is a range of drug-inducible systems that would allow athletes to regulate the amount of gene expression. These include tetracycline-, rapamycin- and tamoxifen-regulated systems (e.g. Nordstrom, 2003; Rivera *et al.*, 2005; Stieger *et al.*, 2009). These not only allow control over any harm associated with excessive levels of expression but may also provide a method for avoiding doping detection in the case of systemically secreted proteins.

Temporary genetic modification can also be performed with the use of anti-sense sequences, either to reduce expression of a specific gene, most commonly using small interfering RNAs or by steric block oligonucleotides to inhibit translation, or to modify splicing of the primary transcript. The latter method has been extensively studied in the context of restoring the open reading frame in DMD and is in clinical trial at present. By preventing an exon from being spliced into the mature mRNA the reading frame can also be disrupted and this approach could conceivably be used to eliminate the open reading frame and thus prevent gene expression. A number of chemical modifications are available for oligonucleotide chemistry and such molecules can be highly gene specific and may be difficult to identify unless the testing authorities suspect they are being used.

Finally there are a number of small molecule drugs that are more or less gene specific and can be used to increase gene expression, for example by stabilising the mRNA or to allow the ribosomal apparatus to read through premature stop mutations, e.g. PTC 124 (Welch *et al.*, 2007). This list can be expanded to include agonists or antagonists that act on the expression and function of specific genes, for example GW 1516, an agonist of PPARδ, and AICAR, an agonist of AMPK (Narkar *et al.*, 2008).

11.3 Genes that might enhance athletic performance

A wide variety of different genes appear to contribute to athletic performance and fitness and studies of these genes up to and including 2007 have been recently reviewed by Bray and colleagues (2009). Although the associations have no doubt been further refined in recent studies, the authors noted 214 autosomal genes and trait loci, seven X chromosome genes and 18 mitochondrial genes. Thus there is a wide range of potential targets for genetic manipulation and this is likely to increase in the coming years. Well-known examples of genetic mutations conferring increased strength or endurance are the marked muscle hypertrophy reported in a myostatin null infant (Schuelke *et al.*, 2004) and the Finnish cross-country skier Eero Mantyranta, whose natural mutation in his erythropoietin (Epo) receptor gene led to high haemoglobin levels and, therefore, high endurance (de la Chapelle *et al.*, 1993).

A number of genetic manipulations conferring an increased athletic performance have been tested only in laboratory animals and yet the results of these studies have concerned regulatory authorities. The first of these was published in 1995 when Coleman and colleagues showed that expression of insulin-like growth factor 1 (IGF-1) in the skeletal muscle of transgenic mice led to a large increase in muscle fibre size (muscle hypertrophy). Concern was increased when Barton-Davis and colleagues (1998) showed that AAV-mediated delivery of IGF-1 to the skeletal muscles of mice increased muscle mass and strength in both young and old mice. This was a significant finding as it showed that it was possible to genetically enhance muscle in an adult animal and thus by extrapolation this could potentially be done in humans. The same group has gone on to demonstrate that gene transfer of IGF-1 can act synergistically with training to enhance muscle strength in rats (Lee *et al.*, 2004) and others have noted that IGF-1 can improve the rate of muscle repair (Schertzer and Lynch, 2006), which further adds to the allure of this method for performance enhancement.

Since the demonstration of the effects of IGF-1 over-expression, a number of other genetic manipulations have been shown to enhance muscle strength and/or endurance. These include experiments in which the myostatin gene was removed or blocked. Myostatin is a negative regulator of muscle growth, acting to reduce muscle mass when the physical demand on the muscle is reduced. Mice lacking the myostatin gene (knockout) have muscles with both a greater number of muscle fibres (hyperplasia) and larger fibres (hypertrophy) than normal mice (McPherron *et al.*, 1997). A number of natural myostatin mutants have been identified in dogs, cattle and sheep (Grobet *et al.*, 1997; Mosher *et al.*, 2007; Boman *et al.*, 2009) and in the human example quoted previously (Schuelke *et al.*, 2004). Although the complete knockout of myostatin in mice has been linked to a decrease in specific force (Amthor *et al.*, 2007), partial knockdown of myostatin due to a heterozygous genetic mutation has been clearly linked to improved muscle performance in the whippet (Mosher *et al.*, 2007). A number of studies have shown that a partial knockdown of myostatin can be performed in normal animals using a variety of approaches, including antibody blockade (Whittemore *et al.*, 2003), blockade by use of a mutant propeptide (Qiao *et al.*, 2008) and antagonism using follistatin or molecules derived from follistatin (Iezzi *et al.*, 2004; Nakatani *et al.*, 2008).

Our increasing understanding of the regulation of energy balance and fibre type determination in skeletal muscle has opened up a number of additional targets. Transgenic mice expressing peroxisome-proliferator-activated receptor-gamma (PPARδ) have been shown to have double the running endurance compared to wild-type mice (Wang et al., 2004). Gene transfer of PPARδ into rat muscle by plasmid electroporation increased IIa and decreased IIb fibres following acute gene transfer (Lunde et al., 2007). Transgenic mice expressing the PPARγ co-activator alpha (PGC-1α) develop muscles composed mostly of type I and demonstrate a high fatigue resistance (Lin et al., 2002) and improved aerobic performance (Calvo et al., 2008). Similar mice expressing PGC-1β develop muscles with a high proportion of type IIX fibres and have increased endurance at high workloads (Arany et al., 2007). Finally, transgenic mice expressing phosphoenolpyruvate carboxykinase (PEPCK) show a substantially enhanced aerobic capacity (Hakimi et al., 2007). These findings correlate with observations in elite human athletes, for example, mRNA expression of PPARα, PPARδ, PPARγ, PGC-1α and PGC-1β is naturally increased in elite human cyclists, with an increased proportion of type I slow twitch, oxidative fibres, when compared with normally active subjects (Krämer et al., 2006).

It should be noted that, apart from the study by Lunde and colleagues (2007), all the other experimental animal studies were performed in transgenic mice and therefore it is not certain that the same responses will follow gene transfer in the adult. In addition there are studies that show conflicting results. Although two reports showed improved performance in PGC-1α transgenic mice, Miura and coworkers (2006) found that over-expression of PGC-1α led to muscle atrophy and Choi and colleagues (2008) reported PGC-1α transgenics showed fat-induced insulin resistance in muscle similar to that of type 2 diabetics. In contrast, the PPARδ agonist GW 1516 raised endurance levels by 75 per cent in normal exercising mice and the PPARδ-AMP-activated protein kinase (AMPK) agonist AICAR improved exercise performance by 44 per cent following four weeks of treatment without any training (Narkar et al., 2008), which demonstrates that these pathways can be effectively manipulated.

A significant limitation to endurance in high-performance athletes is the rate of delivery of oxygen to the muscle and this can be improved by increasing the proportion of red blood cells (haematocrit), and hence the oxygen-carrying haemoglobin. Red blood cell production is governed by a hormone called erythropoietin (often shortened to EPO), which is produced in the kidneys. Recombinant EPO has a long history of abuse in endurance events, such as cross-country skiing and cycling. A number of studies in animals have demonstrated the potential of gene transfer to boost circulating levels of EPO. For example, electroporation of plasmid encoding EPO into mouse and non-human primate muscle resulted in a raised haematocrit (Fattori et al., 2005) and drug-regulated expression of EPO has been demonstrated following intramuscular delivery of AAV-encoding EPO into muscles of non-human primates (Rivera et al., 2005). In the latter study the haematocrit could be controlled by the administration of rapamycin, thus avoiding the dangers associated with an excessively high haematocrit.

11.4   Methods of detection

Doping controls were originally developed to detect approved drugs and known methods of performance enhancement such as blood doping. However there is increasing evidence of the use of non-clinically approved or designer drugs, such as the anabolic steroid tetrahydrogestrinone (THG). Emerging drugs under development that could be used for doping have recently been reviewed by Thevis and coworkers (2009). The problems posed by designer drugs are more difficult and screening for a type of action rather than for the specific drug may become an important part of the methodology, for example, screening for androgenic activity in a mammalian cell bio-assay (Houtman et al., 2009). The diagnostic challenge posed by gene therapy may be even greater. Doping detection relies on urine and blood samples and it is not currently possible to take solid tissues, which are most likely to give clear evidence of genetic manipulation. Products of gene doping that are secreted following gene transfer into ectopic sites show different patterns of post-translational modification, for example, EPO secreted from muscle is demonstrably different from the endogenous EPO secreted from the kidneys (Lasne et al., 2004).

It may also be possible to detect minute traces of gene transfer vectors using highly sensitive polymerase chain reaction–based techniques such as the recently described single-copy primer-internal intron-spanning PCR (spiPCR) procedure (Beiter et al., 2008). However, the evidence to date (reviewed by Baoutina et al., 2008) shows that the window for detection of vectors after administration is relatively small, particularly for non-viral vectors. Where regulated promoters are used, it may be possible to detect the activating molecule, such as tetracycline, rapamycin or tamoxifen, but each of these has another non-doping therapeutic action. Finally, it may be possible to detect evidence of prior administration of viral vectors by looking for evidence of an antibody response to the virus but this could be explained by inadvertent exposure to the natural infectious virus.

An alternative approach is to use indirect techniques to detect gene doping by looking for the consequence of the genetic manipulation, such as changes in patterns of target gene expression (transcriptomics), proteins (proteomics) or their metabolites (metabalomics). The transcriptomic approach has been recently reviewed (Rupert, 2009) and the use of the proteomics approach for detecting androgenic steroid abuse in racehorses is another example (Barton et al., 2009). However, these methods require the establishment of normal standards and some individuals are likely to fall outside of a normal range as a consequence of natural genetic variation. Indeed, the problem of ethnic and individual variation has been highlighted with assessment of the metabolism of testosterone (Strahm et al., 2009). A solution to this problem would be the use of an athlete's endocrinological passport based on the results of repeated tests over time (Sottas et al.,

2008) as has been done for "blood passports" for the detection of blood doping (Robinson *et al.*, 2007). This would provide testers with a lifelong "biological fingerprint" of competitors to use when comparing drug-test samples.

11.5   The practicalities and risks of gene doping

Many of the impressive studies showing increased athletic performance in experimental animals were performed with transgenic mice in which genetic modification is made to the very early embryo. This is highly unlikely to be undertaken in humans due to the low efficiency of the procedures, let alone the major ethical concerns that such manipulations raise. Relatively few of the genes in question have been modified by somatic gene transfer in adult animals and most examples have been in laboratory rodents. In these models, a single intramuscular injection is often sufficient to modify most, if not all, of one muscle. However, in larger animals the diffusion of gene transfer vectors from the site of treatment is very limited (O'Hara *et al.*, 2001) and thus multiple intramuscular injections would be needed to modify human muscle. Systemic administration of AAV vectors have been effective in treating all muscles in mice but such high efficiencies have not been noted with studies in larger animals such as dogs except after neonatal administration (Yue *et al.*, 2008), although regional perfusion in a limb temporarily isolated from the general circulation by a tourniquet has been quite successful in adult dogs (Arruda *et al.*, 2005; Qiao *et al.*, 2009). Plasmid DNA can also be delivered hydrodynamically to the temporarily isolated limb although probably with a lower gene transfer efficiency than AAV (Hagstrom *et al.*, 2004).

Intramuscular injection of either AAV or plasmid delivered by electroporation would probably be sufficient to boost the circulating EPO levels and would be quite practical using current technology. More risky but essentially feasible would be the perfusion of a limb with AAV or plasmid. Although it would not be possible to target all of the muscle fibres in a limb, transfer of genes whose products work in an autocrine or paracrine fashion, such as IGF-1, might be sufficient to marginally improve performance. The production of plasmid DNA free of major contaminants, although not at a clinical grade acceptable for legal use in humans, is relatively easy and would be within the capabilities of a small illegal laboratory. The production of large quantities of AAV is more difficult and currently would require specialist skills. However, as the methodologies continue to be refined it is becoming a more practical possibility for a well-equipped lab.

There are clear dangers associated with gene doping. Administration of large quantities of viral vectors or plasmids risks activating the innate immune system and in one trial in 1999 using an adenoviral vector this led to disseminated intravascular coagulation, organ failure and death (Raper *et al.*, 2003). Plasmid DNA can also activate the innate immune system via specific sequences that are recognised as bacterial and this can lead to inflammation and fever. However, recent developments in non-viral vector design have largely removed these sequences, which significantly reduce interaction with the innate immune system and increase longevity of expression. The use of integrating viral vectors has been associated with oncogenesis in recent human clinical trials (Hacein-Bey-Abina *et al.*, 2008) but the vectors that are more likely to be used for gene doping, AAV and plasmid, do not integrate at a significant rate and so this oncogenesis risk is relatively small.

Over-expression of genes may have harmful consequences. Excess EPO leads to polycythaemia, an excess of red blood cells that makes the blood more viscous and thus puts a greater load on the heart. This can lead to blockage of the micro-circulation, including stroke and heart failure. In addition, the production of EPO following gene transfer has been reported as causing autoimmune anaemia in macaques (Chenuaud *et al.*, 2004; Gao *et al.*, 2004). Over-expression of PGC-1a has been linked to muscle atrophy and type II diabetes in some of the transgenic mouse studies (Miura *et al.*, 2006; Choi *et al.*, 2008). IFG-1 is a potent mitogen and has anti-apoptotic effects. Consequently, over-expression following gene transfer would imply an increased risk of oncogenesis (reviewed by Perry *et al.*, 2006).

11.6   Summary

Although gene doping appears to offer the prospect of illegal improvements in athletic performance, the current state of the technology makes its use unlikely at present. The biggest threat is posed by small molecule drugs that are specifically designed to activate specific genetic targets, either by increasing the rate of RNA transcription or translation. However, as biotechnology development continues to accelerate, it is sensible to keep monitoring the field of gene therapy carefully and to be proactive in creating methods of detection. The increasing interest in the "omics" technologies and in athletic blood passports as methods for detecting novel drugs will also pay dividends in detecting gene doping.

11.7   Acknowledgements

Work in the author's laboratory is primarily focused on the development of genetic treatments for DMD and over recent years has been sponsored by the Muscular Dystrophy Campaign, the Department of Health, the Medical Research Council, the Big Lottery fund, the Wellcome Trust, Parent Project Muscular Dystrophy and the GM Trust.

11.8   References

Amthor, H., Macharia, R., Navarrete, R. *et al.* (2007). Lack of myostatin results in excessive muscle growth but impaired force generation. *Proceedings of the National Academy of Sciences USA* **104**, 1835–1840.

Arany, Z., Lebrasseur, N., Morris, C. *et al.* (2007). The transcriptional coactivator PGC-1beta drives the formation of oxidative type IIX fibers in skeletal muscle. *Cell Metabolism* **5**, 35–46.

Arruda, V.R., Stedman, H.H., Nichols, T.C. *et al.* (2005). Regional intravascular delivery of AAV-2-F.IX to skeletal muscle achieves long-term correction of hemophilia B in a large animal model. *Blood* **105**, 3458–3464.

Barton, C., Beck, P., Kay, R. *et al.* (2009). Multiplexed LC-MS/MS analysis of horse plasma proteins to study doping in sport. *Proteomics* **9**, 3058–3065.

Barton-Davis, E.R., Shoturma, D.I., Musaro, A. *et al.* (1998). Viral mediated expression of insulin-like growth factor I blocks the aging-related loss of skeletal muscle function. *Proceedings of the National Academy of Sciences USA* **95**, 15603–15607.

Baoutina, A., Alexánder, I.E., Rasko, J.E. *et al.* (2008). Developing strategies for detection of gene doping. *Journal of Gene Medicine* **10**, 3–20.

Beiter, T., Zimmermann, M., Fragasso, A. *et al.* (2008). Establishing a novel single-copy primer-internal intron-spanning PCR (spiPCR) procedure for the direct detection of gene doping. *Exercise Immunology Review* **14**, 73–85.

Boman, I.A., Klemetsdal, G., Blichfeldt, T. *et al.* (2009). A frameshift mutation in the coding region of the myostatin gene (MSTN) affects carcass conformation and fatness in Norwegian White Sheep (Ovis aries). *Animal Genetics* **40**, 418–422.

Bray, M.S., Hagberg, J.M., Pérusse, L. *et al.* (2009). The human gene map for performance and health-related fitness phenotypes: The 2006–2007 update. *Medical Sciences in Sports and Exercise* **41**, 35–73.

Calvo, J.A., Daniels, T.G., Wang, X. *et al.* (2008). Muscle-specific expression of PPARgamma coactivator-1alpha improves exercise performance and increases peak oxygen uptake. *Journal of Applied Physiology* **104**, 1304–1312.

Chenuaud, P., Larcher, T., Rabinowitz, J.E. *et al.* (2004). Autoimmune anemia in macaques following erythropoietin gene therapy. *Blood* **103**, 3303–3304.

Choi, C.S., Befroy, D.E., Codella, R. *et al.* (2008). Paradoxical effects of increased expression of PGC-1alpha on muscle mitochondrial function and insulin-stimulated muscle glucose metabolism. *Proceedings of the National Academy of Sciences USA* **105**, 19926–19931.

Coleman, M.E., DeMayo, F., Yin, K.C. *et al.* (1995). Myogenic vector expression of insulin-like growth factor I stimulates muscle cell differentiation and myofiber hypertrophy in transgenic mice. *Journal of Biological Chemistry* **270**, 12109–12116.

de la Chapelle, A., Träskelin, A.L. and Juvonen, E. (1993). Truncated erythropoietin receptor causes dominantly inherited benign human erythrocytosis. *Proceedings of the National Academy of Sciences USA* **90**, 4495–4499.

Denti, M.A., Rosa, A., D'Antona, G. *et al.* (2006). Body-wide gene therapy of Duchenne muscular dystrophy in the *mdx* mouse model. *Proceedings of the National Academy of Sciences USA* **103**, 3758–3763.

Fattori, E., Cappelletti, M., Zampaglione, I. *et al.* (2005). Gene electro-transfer of an improved erythropoietin plasmid in mice and non-human primates. *Journal of Gene Medicine* **7**, 228–236.

Gao, G.P., Alvira, M.R., Wang, L. *et al.* (2002). Novel adeno-associated viruses from rhesus monkeys as vectors for human gene therapy. *Proceedings of the National Academy of Sciences USA* **99**, 11854–11859.

Gao, G., Lebherz, C., Weiner, D.J. *et al.* (2004). Erythropoietin gene therapy leads to autoimmune anemia in macaques. *Blood* **103**, 3300–3302.

Gregorevic, P., Blankinship, M.J., Allen, J.M. *et al.* (2004). Systemic delivery of genes to striated muscles using adeno-associated viral vectors. *Nature Medicine* **10**, 828–834.

Grobet, L., Martin, L.J., Poncelet, D. *et al.* (1997). A deletion in the bovine myostatin gene causes the double-muscled phenotype in cattle. *Nature Genetics* **17**, 71–74.

Hacein-Bey-Abina, S., Garrigue, A., Wang, G.P. *et al.* (2008). Insertional oncogenesis in 4 patients after retrovirus-mediated gene therapy of SCID-X1. *Journal of Clinical Investigation* **118**, 3132–3142.

Hagstrom, J.E., Hegge, J., Zhang, G. *et al.* (2004). A facile nonviral method for delivering genes and siRNAs to skeletal muscle of mammalian limbs. *Molecular Therapy* **10**, 386–398.

Hakimi, P., Yang, J., Casadesus, G. *et al.* (2007). Overexpression of the cytosolic form of phosphoenolpyruvate carboxykinase (GTP) in skeletal muscle repatterns energy metabolism in the mouse. *Journal of Biological Chemistry* **282**, 32844–32855.

Herweijer, H. and Wolff, J.A. (2007). Gene therapy progress and prospects: Hydrodynamic gene delivery. *Gene Therapy* **14**, 99–107.

Houtman C.J., Sterk S.S., van de Heijning M.P. *et al.* (2009). Detection of anabolic androgenic steroid abuse in doping control using mammalian reporter gene bioassays. *Analytica Chimica Acta* **637**, 247–258.

Iezzi, S., Di Padova, M., Serra, C. *et al.* (2004). Deacetylase inhibitors increase muscle cell size by promoting myoblast recruitment and fusion through induction of follistatin. *Developmental Cell* **6**, 673–684.

Kim, S., Peng, Z. and Kaneda, Y. (2008). Current status of gene therapy in Asia. *Molecular Therapy* **16**, 237–243.

Krämer, D.K., Ahlsén, M., Norrbom, J. *et al.* (2006). Human skeletal muscle fibre type variations correlate with PPAR alpha, PPAR delta and PGC-1 alpha mRNA. *Acta Physiologica (Oxford)* **188**, 207–216.

Lasne, F., Martin, L., de Ceaurriz, J. *et al.* (2004). "Genetic doping" with erythropoietin cDNA in primate muscle is detectable. *Molecular Therapy* **10**, 409–410.

Lee, S., Barton, E.R., Sweeney, H.L. *et al.* (2004). Viral expression of insulin-like growth factor-I enhances muscle hypertrophy in resistance-trained rats. *Journal of Applied Physiology* **96**, 1097–1104.

Lin, J., Wu, H., Tarr, P.T. *et al.* (2002). Transcriptional co-activator PGC-1 alpha drives the formation of slow-twitch muscle fibres. *Nature* **418**, 797–801.

Lunde, I.G., Ekmark, M., Rana, Z.A. *et al.* (2007). PPAR δ expression is influenced by muscle activity and induces slow muscle properties in adult rat muscles after somatic gene transfer. *Journal of Physiology* **582**, 1277–1287.

McPherron, A.C., Lawler, A.M. and Lee, S.J. (1997). Regulation of skeletal muscle mass in mice by a new TGF-beta superfamily member. *Nature* **387**, 83–90.

Midoux, P., Breuzard, G., Gomez, J.P. *et al.* (2008). Polymer-based gene delivery: A current review on the uptake and intracellular trafficking of polyplexes. *Current Gene Therapy* **8**, 335–352.

Miura, S., Tomitsuka, E., Kamei, Y. *et al.* (2006). Overexpression of peroxisome proliferator-activated receptor gamma co-activator-1alpha leads to muscle atrophy with depletion of ATP. *American Journal of Pathology* **169**, 1129–1139.

Mosher, D.S., Quignon, P., Bustamante, C.D. *et al.* (2007). A mutation in the myostatin gene increases muscle mass and enhances racing performance in heterozygote dogs. *PLoS Genetics* **3**, e79.

Nakatani, M., Takehara, Y., Sugino, H. *et al.* (2008). Transgenic expression of a myostatin inhibitor derived from follistatin increases skeletal muscle mass and ameliorates dystrophic pathology in *mdx* mice. *FASEB Journal* **22**, 477–487.

Narkar, V.A., Downes, M., Yu, R.T. *et al.* (2008). AMPK and PPARdelta agonists are exercise mimetics. *Cell* **134**, 405–415.

Newman, C.M. and Bettinger, T. (2007). Gene therapy progress and prospects: Ultrasound for gene transfer. *Gene Therapy* **14**, 465–475.

Nordstrom, J.L. (2003). The antiprogestin-dependent GeneSwitch system for regulated gene therapy. *Steroids* **68**, 1085–1094.

O'Hara, A.J., Howell, J.M., Taplin, R.H. *et al.* (2001). The spread of transgene expression at the site of gene construct injection. *Muscle Nerve* **24**, 488–495.

Perry, J.K., Emerald, B.S., Mertani, H.C. *et al.* (2006). The oncogenic potential of growth hormone. *Growth Hormone and IGF Research* **16**, 277–289.

Phelps, S.F., Hauser, M.A., Cole, N.M. *et al.* (1995). Expression of full-length and truncated dystrophin mini-genes in transgenic *mdx* mice. *Human Molecular Genetics* **4**, 1251–1258.

Ponce, S., Orive, G., Hernández, R.M. *et al.* (2006). *In vivo* evaluation of EPO-secreting cells immobilized in different alginate-PLL microcapsules. *Journal of Control Release* **116**, 28–34.

Qiao, C., Li, J., Jiang, J. *et al.* (2008). Myostatin propeptide gene delivery by adeno-associated virus serotype 8 vectors enhances muscle growth and ameliorates dystrophic phenotypes in *mdx* mice. *Human Gene Therapy* **19**, 241–254.

Qiao, C., Li, J., Zheng, H. *et al.* (2009). Hydrodynamic limb vein injection of AAV8 canine myostatin propeptide gene in normal dogs enhances muscle growth. *Human Gene Therapy* **20**, 1–10.

Raper, S.E., Chirmule, N., Lee, F.S. *et al.* (2003). Fatal systemic inflammatory response syndrome in a ornithine transcarbamylase deficient patient following adenoviral gene transfer. *Molecular Genetics and Metabolism* **80**, 148–158.

Rivera, V.M., Gao, G.P., Grant, R.L. *et al.* (2005). Long-term pharmacologically regulated expression of erythropoietin in primates following AAV-mediated gene transfer. *Blood* **105**, 1424–1430.

Robinson, N., Sottas, P.E., Mangin, P. *et al.* (2007). Bayesian detection of abnormal hematological values to introduce a no-start rule for heterogeneous populations of athletes. *Haematologica* **92**, 1143–1144.

Rupert, J.L. (2009). Transcriptional profiling: A potential anti-doping strategy. *Scandinavian Journal of Medicine and Science in Sports* **19**, 753–763.

Schertzer, J.D. and Lynch, G.S. (2006). Comparative evaluation of IGF-I gene transfer and IGF-I protein administration for enhancing skeletal muscle regeneration after injury. *Gene Therapy* **13**, 1657–1664.

Schuelke, M., Wagner, K.R., Stolz, L.E. *et al.* (2004). Myostatin mutation associated with gross muscle hypertrophy in a child. *New England Journal of Medicine* **350**, 2682–2688.

Sottas, P.E., Saudan, C., Schweizer, C. *et al.* (2008). From population- to subject-based limits of T/E ratio to detect testosterone abuse in elite sports. *Forensic Science International* **174**, 166–172.

Stieger, K., Belbellaa, B., Le Guiner, C. *et al.* (2009). *In vivo* gene regulation using tetracycline-regulatable systems. *Advanced Drug Delivery Review* **61**, 527–541.

Strahm, E., Sottas, P.E., Schweizer, C. *et al.* (2009). Steroid profiles of professional soccer players: An international comparative study. *British Journal of Sports Medicine* **43**, 1041–1044.

Thevis, M., Thomas, A., Kohler, M. *et al.* (2009). Emerging drugs: Mechanism of action, mass spectrometry and doping control analysis. *Journal of Mass Spectrometry* **44**, 442–460.

Trollet, C., Scherman, D. and Bigey, P. (2008). Delivery of DNA into muscle for treating systemic diseases: Advantages and challenges. *Methods in Molecular Biology* **423**, 199–214.

Vandenberghe, L.H., Wilson, J.M. and Gao, G. (2009). Tailoring the AAV vector capsid for gene therapy. *Gene Therapy* **16**, 311–319.

Vitiello, C., Faraso, S., Sorrentino, N.C. *et al.* (2009). Disease rescue and increased lifespan in a model of cardiomyopathy and muscular dystrophy by combined AAV treatments. *PLoS One* **4**, e5051.

Wang, Y.X., Zhang, C.L., Yu, R.T. *et al.* (2004). Regulation of muscle fiber type and running endurance by PPARdelta. *PLoS Biology* **2**, e294.

Welch, E.M., Barton, E.R., Zhuo, J. *et al.* (2007). PTC124 targets genetic disorders caused by nonsense mutations. *Nature* **447**, 87–91.

Wells, D.J., Wells, K.E., Asante, E.A. *et al.* (1995). Expression of human full-length and minidystrophin in transgenic *mdx* mice: Implications for gene therapy of Duchenne muscular dystrophy. *Human Molecular Genetics* **4**, 1245–1250.

Wells, D.J. (2004). Gene therapy progress and prospects: Electroporation and other physical methods. *Gene Therapy* **11**, 1363–1369.

Whittemore, L.A., Song, K., Li, X. *et al.* (2003). Inhibition of myostatin in adult mice increases skeletal muscle mass and strength. *Biochemical and Biophysical Research Communications* **300**, 965–971.

Yue, Y., Ghosh, A., Long, C. *et al.* (2008). A single intravenous injection of adeno-associated virus serotype-9 leads to whole body skeletal muscle transduction in dogs. *Molecular Therapy* **16**, 1944–1952.

Zhu, T., Zhou, L., Mori, S. *et al.* (2005). Sustained whole-body functional rescue in congestive heart failure and muscular dystrophy hamsters by systemic gene transfer. *Circulation* **112**, 2650–2659.

Chapter 12

Stimulants

David R. Mottram

12.1 History of stimulant use in sport

Stimulants have a long history of use as potential performance-enhancing agents in sport. The potent, but non-selective and highly toxic stimulant strychnine was used as long ago as the end of the nineteenth century. Amphetamines, first developed in the nineteen twenties, have been a favourite of athletes in many sporting disciplines. It is not surprising that stimulants, along with narcotic analgesics, were the first classes of drugs to be included on an IOC list of prohibited substances in 1967. At that time, stimulants were divided into three classes: sympathomimetic amines, psychomotor stimulants and central nervous system (CNS) stimulants. In 1988, the IOC grouped all these classes of drugs under the heading of stimulants.

It can be seen from the prevalence statistics presented in Chapter 25 that the number of adverse findings for stimulants have been second only to anabolic agents. To what extent stimulants have been used in an attempt to enhance performance or simply as "recreational" drugs is impossible to ascertain.

There have been a number of landmark cases relating to the use of stimulants by athletes.

Case studies related to stimulants

Tommy Simpson

One of the most frequently cited cases is that of Tommy Simpson, the British cyclist who died of heat-stroke and cardiac arrest whilst climbing the infamous Mont Ventoux during stage 13 of the 1967 Tour de France. Simpson was trying to make up time lost in earlier stages, resulting from the fact that he had been suffering from a stomach bug. The postmortem found that Simpson had taken amphetamines and alcohol. The effect of these drugs was compounded by the fact that the temperatures on the mountain were extremely high on that day, the upper slopes of the mountain offered no shade from the sun and, in those days, the Tour organisers limited the fluid intake of riders during each stage, the effects of dehydration being poorly understood at that time.

Kelli White

Kelli White tested positive for modafinil at the World Athletics Championships in 2003. She claimed that her physician was prescribing modafinil for narcolepsy. Arising from the 2003 BALCO investigation, the U.S. Anti-Doping Agency also found evidence for the use of tetrahydrogestrinone (THG) and erythropoietin (EPO). Kelli White was banned for two years and stripped of her medals. The athlete had also claimed that modafinil was not on the prohibited list. However, although not included under the list of examples of stimulants, modafinil was banned as it had the pharmacological properties of a stimulant.

One group of stimulants that has consistently caused problems for athletes has been the drugs that are available over-the-counter (OTC), without a prescription. Athletes have therefore been able to purchase OTC medicines that have contained stimulants on the prohibited list. Despite the fact that the IOC used cut-off levels for these drugs, below which the athlete would not be sanctioned, it has been shown that these cut-off levels were unrealistic (Chester *et al.*, 2003). This has led to a number of high-profile cases involving elite athletes.

Andreea Raducan

At the 2000 Sydney Olympic Games, the gymnast Andreea Raducan tested positive for the drug pseudoephedrine, which was present in an OTC cough and cold product that the gymnast had taken. Despite the fact that she had taken the drug on advice from her team doctor, strict liability rules prevailed and she was stripped of her gold medal. The Romanian physician was also sanctioned, being expelled from the Games and barred from Olympic Games for four years (Hilderbrand *et al.*, 2003).

Alain Baxter

Alain Baxter won a bronze medal in the Men's Slalom Skiing event at the Winter Olympic Games in Salt Lake City in February 2002. He then tested positive for methamphetamine and was stripped of his bronze medal. Baxter had used an American product (Vicks Vapour Inhaler) as a nasal decongestant to treat a cold. This product contains levmetamfetamine, the levo isomer of methamphetamine, a relatively inactive isomer compared with the dextro form. Baxter claimed that he was unaware that the product contained a banned substance because the medicine looked the same as a similar product that Baxter had used in the UK, which did not contain levmatamfetamine. The International Ski Federation (ISF) accepted that Baxter had taken the drug inadvertently but imposed a ban of three months from all competitions. This ban was lifted by the Court of Arbitration in Sport. However, although the IOC's Court of Arbitration accepted that Baxter "did not intend to obtain a competitive advantage", it refused to overturn the medal disqualification.

These, and other similar cases, led WADA, in 2004, to remove most of the OTC stimulants from the prohibited list. These drugs have been placed on amonitoring list and their use by athletes is being recorded by WADA's accredited laboratories. It appears that athletes still do not fully understand the status and function of these OTC medicines and many consider that they should be returned to the prohibited list (Mottram *et al.*, 2008).

Martina Hingis

The A and B urine samples taken from Martina Hingis at the 2007 Wimbledon Tennis Championships both showed a positive result for cocaine. She was banned from competition for two years but announced her retirement from tennis in November 2007. Hingis claimed that she had never used cocaine and independently submitted a hair sample for testing that was negative for drugs. Furthermore she argued that the urine samples must have been handled improperly but stated that she did not wish to contest the finding or the two-year ban.

Richard Gasquet

On March 28, 2009, the French tennis player Richard Gasquet submitted a urine sample at a tournament in Florida. Both the A and B samples tested positive for cocaine. Gasquet was charged with a doping offence and banned from competition. An independent anti-doping tribunal appointed by the International Tennis Federation (ITF) held a hearing on June 29 and 30, 2009, at which Gasquet claimed his positive result was caused by cocaine entering his body when he kissed a girl who had been using cocaine at a night club. The tribunal stated that since the amount of cocaine found in Gasquet's system was "about the size of a grain of salt", he was cleared to return to competition. On August 6, 2009, the ITF announced that it was appealing to the Court of Arbitration for Sport against the tribunal's decision. At the time of writing this book, the case was still ongoing.

12.2   Types of stimulants and their modes of action

As indicated above, stimulants were classed by the IOC as sympathomimetic amines, psychomotor stimulants and central nervous system (CNS) stimulants. This classification distinguished the stimulants on the basis of their mode of action.

Figure 12.1 shows the inter-relationship between the various nervous systems of the body. Overall control of body function lies within the central nervous system (CNS). The CNS receives information about the body's environment, such as sight, sound, touch and taste, through sensory nerves. The CNS then relays information through either the motor nervous system to the skeletal muscles or through the autonomic nervous system (ANS) to control the parts of the

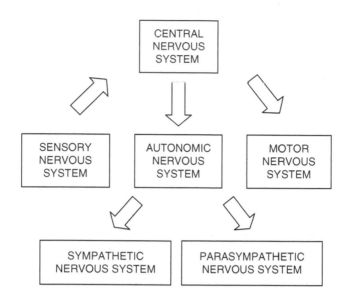

Figure 12.1 The inter-relationship between the various nervous systems of the body.

body that are not under conscious control, such as the heart, blood vessels, respiratory tract, gastrointestinal tract and various glands. The ANS is divided into the parasympathetic nervous system (PNS), which controls function under times of rest, and the sympathetic nervous system (SNS) which controls function under times of stress. The latter is augmented by the hormone adrenaline (epinephrine) under extreme stress conditions.

There are numerous neurotransmitters within the CNS and ANS. The principal neurotransmitters, through which drugs classed as stimulants on the WADA list exert their effects, are adrenaline, noradrenaline, dopamine and to a lesser extent 5-hydroxytryptamine. The effects produced are due to increasing the levels of these neurotransmitters at their site of action, either centrally or peripherally. This is achieved, variously, by increasing the release, preventing the re-uptake, reducing the metabolism or mimicking the effects of these neurotransmitters (Jones, 2008).

Sympathomimetic amines mimic or potentiate the effects of the sympathetic nervous system, which is responsible for preparing the body for stress situations, the most extreme of which is referred to as the "flight or fight" reaction. The principal neurotransmitter for the sympathetic nervous system is noradrenaline (norepinephrine), and sympathomimetics, such as ephedrine, pseudoephedrine and phenylephrine, increase the release of noradrenaline or act on the same receptors as the noadrenaline to potentiate its effect.

CNS stimulants have relatively little effect on mental function but increase the activity of the respiratory and vasomotor centres of the CNS or increase reflex excitability. There are few CNS stimulants that are used in sport. Strychnine remains on the prohibited list, having been used for more than 100 years.

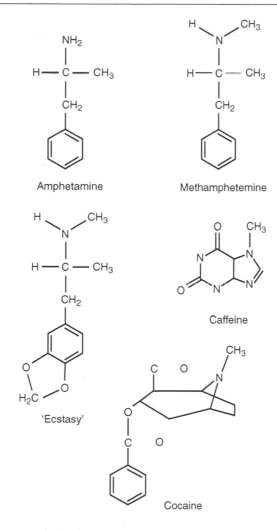

Figure 12.2 Some central stimulants.

Psychomotor stimulants have a number of effects related to mental function and behaviour. They can induce excitement and euphoria, increase motor activity or reduce fatigue. Psychomotor stimulants include amphetamine and other drugs related to amphetamine, cocaine and methylxanthines, such as caffeine (see Figure 12.2).

Amphetamines and cocaine affect a number of neurotransmitters, collectively known as catecholamines that are on the WADA prohibited list. Methylxanthines are not on the 2010 prohibited list, caffeine having been removed from the list in 2004. The effects of caffeine are discussed in Chapter 20.

Some of the drugs listed as stimulants have actions on both the central and sympathetic nervous systems. WADA provides a comprehensive list of drugs as examples of stimulants. The pharmacology of these drugs is complex. A good review of their pharmacology can be found in Docherty (2008).

Ephedrine, methylephedrine and cathine

These three drugs were retained on the WADA prohibited list when most OTC sympathomimetics, such as pseudoephedrine, phenylephrine and phenylpropanolamine were removed in 2004 and placed on a monitoring list. Their principal mode of action is as sympathomimetics, although they do exhibit some central stimulant properties.

This group of drugs is structurally related to amphetamine. They exert their effect indirectly on neurones of the sympathetic and central nervous systems, by displacing noradrenaline and possibly other monoamine transmitters from neuronal storage sites. They also exert direct effects on adrenergic α and β receptors and are weak inhibitors of monoamine uptake. They are resistant to breakdown by the enzyme monoamine oxidase, which metabolises adrenaline and noradrenaline.

Ephedrine occurs naturally in the plant genus Ephedra and has been a component of ancient Chinese medicine for many centuries. This, and other herbal sources of stimulants, has been reviewed by Bucci (2000). Ephedrine is reported to be five times less potent than amphetamine. The CNS effects of ephedrine are much less than those of amphetamine. For example, a 75 mg/70 kg body weight dose of ephedrine is required before it will cross the blood-brain barrier. This may explain why ephedrine produces less depletion of brain monoamines than amphetamine (Wadler and Hainline, 1989). The effects of ephedrines are produced within 40 minutes after administration and can last up to three hours.

Adverse effects of ephedrines are, most commonly, tachycardia, hypertension, headache and dizziness. These drugs may cause anorexia, insomnia, irritability and nervousness at low to medium doses, whereas high doses are associated with mania and a psychosis similar to that occasionally seen with amphetamines.

Cathine is derived from the plant Khat, which contains a number of active constituents, the most potent of which is cathinone, which has amphetamine-like actions (Kalix, 1992). Cathinone is not specifically mentioned as an example of a stimulant on the WADA prohibited list but would constitute an adverse finding under the rider "other substances with a similar structure or similar biological effect(s)".

Amphetamines

Several structurally related drugs are known as amphetamines and include dextroamphetamine, methamphetamine, phenmetrazine and methylphenidate. Other examples of amphetamines are listed under stimulants in the WADA prohibited list. In this chapter the word *amphetamine* will refer to dextroamphetamine, the structure of which is shown in Figure 12.2 Amphetamine is a phenyl isopropylamine and was first synthesized in 1920. It was originally prescribed for the treatment of nasal congestion. In 1935, amphetamine was used to treat the neurological condition narcolepsy, and its use in the treatment of depression, anxiety and hyperactivity in children followed from this. Amphetamine was used widely during the Second World War to reduce fatigue and increase alertness. The rapid development of tolerance to amphetamine and the occurrence of dependence have led to the drug being withdrawn from clinical use.

The mode of action of amphetamine

There are four mechanisms by which amphetamine may produce its effects. These are (1) release of neurotransmitters—dopamine (DA) noradrenaline or 5HT—from their respective nerve terminals; (2) inhibition of monoamine oxidase activity; (3) inhibition of neurotransmitter re-uptake; and (4) direct action on neurotransmitter receptors. Of these four possibilities, neurotransmitter release appears to be the most important (Brookes, 1985).

Amphetamine stimulates DA release by reversing the neuronal membrane uptake transporter (Seiden et al., 1993). It also inhibits the activity of the enzyme monoamine oxidase (Seiden et al., 1993). It seems that several major behavioural changes induced by amphetamine are most closely mimicked by stimulation of central noradrenaline-releasing neurones. Thus, the amphetamine-induced loco-motor activity and self-stimulation seen in animals and the increased alertness and elevation of mood produced in humans are closely related to increases in noradrenergic activity. Amphetamine is a potent anorectic and elevates plasma-free fatty acid levels. Body temperature is also elevated. The cardiovascular, gastrointestinal and respiratory effects of amphetamine are sympathomimetic in nature.

Pharmocokinetics

Amphetamines are readily absorbed, mainly from the small intestine, and the peak plasma concentration occurs one to two hours following administration. Absorption is usually complete within four hours and is accelerated by food intake.

The metabolism of amphetamines has been difficult to investigate because of the wide variation between species in the metabolic effects of amphetamines. The principal amphetamine metabolites are p-hydroxyephedrine and p-hydroxyamphetamine. Both these metabolites have similar pharmacological effects to the parent amphetamine. Amphetamine is lost from the blood by renal filtration.

The effect of amphetamines on human mood and performance

The desire to enhance mood or performance or both is usually the main reason for taking amphetamines. In their comprehensive review, Weiss and Laties

(1962) agreed that amphetamine does produce an enhanced performance in many tasks and does not simply normalize fatigue responses. They examined various tasks such as (a) work output by subjects on a bicycle ergometer, (b) performance on arduous military exercises, and (c) performance during flying or driving missions. Apparent improvements in athletic performance as well as a reduction in reaction time and increased co-ordination and steadiness are produced by amphetamines in events as diverse as shot put, swimming and running. Intellectual performance does not seem to be improved by amphetamines, unless the performance has been degraded by boredom and fatigue (Brookes, 1985). In the short term, amphetamine increases the speed of learning of new tasks. The effects of amphetamine on judgement are uncertain and several conflicting studies have been published (Brookes, 1985). There is general agreement that amphetamines cause a mild distortion of time perception, which may lead to misjudgement in planning manoeuvres or in manipulations such as driving a car. Active avoidance learning is facilitated by amphetamine. Although there is considerable inter-individual variation in the effects of amphetamine on mood, the general effects are of positive mood enhancement. These positive effects include an increase in physical energy, mental aptitude, talkativeness, restlessness, vigour, excitement and good humour. Subjects taking amphetamine also report that they feel confident, efficient and ambitious and that their food intake is reduced because they are less hungry. Many athletes report that they feel most aggressive when taking amphetamines and are unlikely to report or complain of injuries (Laties and Weiss, 1981).

Adverse effects of amphetamines

Some negative effects of amphetamine include anxiety, indifference, slowness in reasoning, irresponsible behaviour, irritability and restlessness, dry mouth, tremors, insomnia and, following withdrawal, depression. These effects of amphetamine on mood are dose-dependent and are thought to be produced by the stimulation of dopamine and adrenergic receptors.

Tolerance develops rapidly to many of the effects of amphetamines. Tolerance is said to be present when, over a period of time, increasing doses of a drug are required to maintain the same response. There is much evidence to show that amphetamines induce drug dependence and the amphetamine-dependent person may become psychotic, aggressive and anti-social. Withdrawal of amphetamines is associated with mental and physical depression. Tolerance to the positive effects of methamphetamine does occur over time at least in new abusers while the severity of the negative effects increases overtime (Comer *et al.*, 2001). Methamphetamine is a powerful, positive reinforcing agent in humans as well as animals (Hart *et al.*, 2001).

Other major side effects of amphetamine administration (excluding those following withdrawal) include confusion, delirium, sweating, palpitations, dilation of the pupils and rapid breathing, hypertension, tachycardia, tremors, muscle and joint pain. Though amphetamines may initially stimulate libido, chronic amphetamine use often leads to a reduced sex drive. Chronic amphetamine administration is also associated with myocardial pathology and with growth retardation in adolescents. Usually the personality changes induced by chronic low doses of amphetamine are gradually reversed after the drug is stopped. However, high chronic doses may lead to a variety of persistent personality changes. Possibly the most serious of the severe personality disorders induced by amphetamine is the so-called amphetamine psychosis described by Connell in 1958. The frightening array of psychiatric symptoms he described in patients presenting with amphetamine psychosis include many commonly found in para-noid-type schizophrenics. An important distinction between amphetamine psychosis and schizophrenia is that amphetamine induces a preponderance of symptoms of paranoia and of visual hallucinations.

Cocaine

Cocaine first became available commercially in the 1880s. Sigmund Freud took the drug to try and cure his own bouts of depression and suggested it as a "cure all" for others. The drug fell out of medical use by the 1920s, only to reappear in the 1960s as a major drug of abuse.

Pharmacology

Cocaine affects the brain in a complex way. The most obvious initial effects are a decrease in fatigue, an increase in motor activity and an increase in talkative-ness, coupled with a general feeling of euphoria and well-being. These mood changes soon subside and are replaced by dysphoria (mood lowering).

The mechanism by which cocaine produces these effects is not known fully. Animal studies show that cocaine is a powerful "reinforcer" and rewarding agent. It stimulates elements of the brain's pleasure and reward "centres", which are distributed throughout the limbic system of the brain and include the dopamine-rich mesocortical and mesolimbic systems. The evidence for the action of cocaine on these systems has been reviewed by Fibiger et al. (1992). Further evidence for the involvement of cocaine with dopamine-releasing neurones comes from stud-ies at the molecular level reviewed by Kuhar (1992). He has shown that cocaine inhibits the re-uptake of dopamine (DA) into the nerve terminals of dopamine-releasing neurones, and it has a similar though less potent effect on noradrenaline uptake in noradenergic neurones (Zhu et al., 2000). This initially leads to a poten-tiation of the action of DA at post-synaptic receptor sites. This acute effect of cocaine on the dopamine transporter has been demonstrated by many investiga-tions (Chen and Reith, 2000), but it is also exhibited by other drugs, such as methylphenidate, which do not have the same addictive potential as cocaine (Volkow et al., 1999). In chronic cocaine abusers, in vivo scanning of behaviour-ally important areas of the cerebral cortex has shown a significant reduction in dopamine D_2 receptors associated with decreased dopamine metabolism. There are also significant decreases in dopamine release in such abusers and these inter-related actions may be part of a mechanism leading to reduced activities of cerebral "reward circuits" in cocaine abuse and subsequent addiction (Volkow *et al.*, 1999). However, though dopamine receptor antagonists appear to antagonise all the actions of cocaine in rats, in humans they appear to inhibit cocaine craving but not the euphoria (Kuhar, 1992). Some investigators have linked the dysphoria and craving following a cocaine dose with an increase in post-synaptic receptor numbers (Wadler and Hainline, 1989), though this is contradicted by the studies of Volkow's group (1999).

Pharmacokinetics

Cocaine may be administered by injection, orally, intranasally or by inhalation. Oral administration produces peak effects at variable times with behavioural changes lasting up to one hour. The most popular route is via nasal "snorting", which produces peak effects from 5 to 15 mins and lasts for an hour. Inhalation of "free-base" cocaine produces peak effects in less than one minute but also has a short-lived physiological effect measured in minutes. The route of cocaine administration influences the time course and onset of other actions. Effects of the drug such as increases in heart rate and blood pressure are longer-lasting via the oral compared to the intravenous (IV) route (Smith *et al.*, 2001). Inhalation of cocaine results in the most intense cravings compared to other routes of administration (Wadler and Hainline, 1989). The frequency of cocaine administration also influences the density of brain opioid and dopamine receptors (Unterwald *et al.*, 2001). Cocaine is mainly metabolised, by plasma and liver cholinesterases, to benzoylecgonine and ecgonine methyl ester, which are excreted in the urine.

Adverse effects

Cocaine is highly addictive (more so than amphetamine) and the abuser may experience acute psychotic symptoms and undertake irrational actions in addition to the well-known adverse effects of euphoria. Chronic symptoms include a paranoid psychosis similar to that induced by amphetamine, coupled with spells of delirium and confusion. Other CNS side effects include epileptogenesis (stimulation of epileptic seizures). This adverse effect is particularly dangerous because animal studies have revealed that the epileptogenic effect increases with frequency of cocaine abuse, a process known as reverse tolerance (Smith and Perry, 1992), which is important when the powerful reinforcing properties of the drug are considered. The epileptogenic effect can be produced even by repeated small doses of the drug (Wadler and Hainline, 1989), which may be more toxic than the same total dose given less frequently (Unterwald *et al.*, 2001).

Cocaine abuse is strongly associated with cerebrovascular accidents arising either from the rupture or spasm of cerebral blood vessels. Some of these incidents may be due to pre-existing vascular pathologies but there are several cases where no predisposing cause has been found during the autopsy (Wadler and Hainline, 1989). Cocaine is also responsible for a number of cardiovascular side effects; those relating directly to exercise are discussed later. A review of the literature relating to cocaine-induced coronary disease by Benzaquen *et al.* (2001) reveals that a number of factors may influence the development of cardiovascular pathology in cocaine abusers. Original ideas that suggested a simple mismatch between myocardial oxygen supply and demand caused by cocaine-induced vasoconstriction and the resulting increased myocardial workload are too simplistic. Benzaquen *et al.* have argued that there is a more complex interaction between three key factors: coronary vasoconstriction, intra-coronary thrombosis and accelerated athero-sclerosisi may be involved, as all three can be induced by cocaine abuse. Smith and Perry (1992) have suggested that the increase in cardiovascular and cerebrovascular side effects seen in recent years is due to the rise in abuse of "crack" cocaine, which is rapidly absorbed and produces a concentrated effect on cerebral arterioles.

12.3   Stimulants and sport

Ephedrine and other sympathomimetics in sport

Ephedrine and other sympathomimetics have been promoted for weight loss as well as for enhancement of athletic performance. The first comprehensive study of the possible ergogenic effects of these drugs was carried out by Sidney and Lefcoe (1977). They examined the effect of 25 mg of ephedrine versus placebo in a double-blind crossover study using three separate athletic trials during a three-week period. In this comprehensive experiment 10 variables were measured, including strength, endurance, reaction time, anaerobic capacity and speed of recovery from effort. The results showed that though exercise heart rate and resting pulse pressure increased and post-exercise recovery rate slowed, none of the physical performance measures improved. It was also interesting that no subjective improvements in performance were noted. Bell *et al.* in Canada (2001) measured the effects of 120 mg of ephedrine on power output (electrically braked ergometer) and oxygen debt and VO_{2max} in 16 healthy volunteers. They found that, compared to placebo, ephedrine significantly increased power output during the first 10 seconds of cycle exercise but had no effect after that time. Ephedrine also had no effect on O_2 deficit or accumulated VO_2. Ephedrine treatment has been associated with increased plasma glucose levels both before and after exercise and increased plasma lactate and noradrenaline levels after exercise.

In 2003, Jacobs *et al.* carried out a control trial of ephedrine (0.8 mg/kg) alone or in combination with caffeine compared with placebo. They investigated the effects on males undertaking a weight-training circuit. The authors concluded that acute ingestion of ephedrine or ephedrine plus caffeine increased muscular endurance during the first set of resistance-training exercises. However, they concluded that the performance enhancement was attributed primarily to the effects of ephedrine, with no additive effect from the caffeine.

With respect to weight loss and enhanced performance due to ephedrine, Shekelle *et al.* (2003) undertook a meta-analysis of several trials. They showed that ephedrine can promote modest weight loss in the short term (approximately 0.9 kg/month more than placebo), for up to six months, but that the differences in the parameters used to measure performance within the various trials meant that conclusive evidence for performance enhancement could not be achieved.

Adverse effects of sympathomimetics in athletes

The adverse effects observed in athletes are similar to those seen in the general population. Recent investigations into potential side effects of ephedrine in athletes have centred on the cardiovascular system. In the study by Jacobs *et al.* (2003), systolic blood pressure was increased significantly in subjects given ephedrine. The meta-analysis of Shekelle *et al.* (2003) showed that ephedrine was associated with a two- to threefold increase in adverse effects, such as enhanced autonomic effects, including heart palpitations, and an increased risk of psychiatric and upper gastrointestinal symptoms. Haller and Benowitz (2000) have reported even more serious side effects—such as seizures, stroke and even death—from the use of ephedrine within dietary supplements.

Amphetamines in sport

Many of the studies on the effects of amphetamine on athletic performance have been carried out on cyclists. One reason for this is that there are numerous examples of fatalities arising from the use of amphetamines by cyclists, notably the incidence of death from heat-stroke. Wyndham *et al.* (1971) carried out a wide-ranging placebo-controlled biochemical and physiological investigation on two champion cyclists who exercised on a bicycle ergometer. There was no difference between amphetamine and placebo in terms of submaximal or maximal oxygen uptake, heart rate or minute ventilation. However, there were significant increases in blood lactate levels. The authors concluded that amphetamines have no effect on the ability to do aerobic work but they insignificantly increased the cyclists' ability to tolerate higher levels of anaerobic metabolism. The dangers inherent in these results are that an athlete taking amphetamine might be better able to ignore the usual internal signals of over-exertion and heat stress, which may therefore explain the incidence of heat-stroke and cardiac problems in cyclists who take amphetamines during long-distance cycling events.

Several reviewers, including Conlee (1991), have remarked on the considerable inconsistency of amphetamine effects in humans, particularly with regard to ergogenicity. A poorly explored feature of amphetamine action is its effect on fatigue. Most studies have concentrated on the central aspects of fatigue while neglecting peripheral contributions. The few studies of amphetamine effects on muscle glycogen stores before and during exercise have been contradictory (Conlee, 1991).

Because there is no significant improvement in performance associated with amphetamine use, why does it continue to be taken? The answer could be an effect on mental attitude in terms of improved mood, greater confidence and optimism and increased alertness. Amphetamines could be abused for different reasons by different athletes. Thus, baseball and football players may use them to increase alertness and concentration, whereas runners or swimmers use them to increase energy and endurance (Smith and Perry, 1992).

Several studies indicate that the effect of amphetamine on the psychological state of athletes might be self-induced and occurs as a result of the athlete expecting to perform better and be more alert. A review of the confounding influences in psychostimulant results has been presented by Clarkson and Thompson (1997). They quoted two studies carried out in the 1940s in which all the subjects on active drug (amphetamine) perceived that they had done more work on a cycle ergometer than was actually measured. In their review they also question the validity of some of the earlier experiments in terms of clinical methodological vigour (blindness), statistical inference and control.

Another feature of most studies is the failure to control for trained or untrained subjects. This is very important if we are considering that amphetamine may have an effect on motivation, as trained athletes often exhibit higher motivational levels than the untrained and the untrained therefore may not exercise fully to exhaustion (Clarkson and Thompson, 1997).

In a review of CNS stimulants, Avois *et al.* (2009) concluded that amphetamines may (1) improve reaction time when fatigued; (2) increase muscular endurance and strength; (3) increase acceleration; (4) raise lactic acid levels during maximal exercise; (5) increase aerobic endurance capacity and (6) stimulate metabolism by inducing a loss of body fat.

Adverse side effects of amphetamines in athletes

Some important side effects of amphetamine have only been revealed in individuals undertaking extremely arduous training or sporting schedules. One of the most widely publicised side effects of amphetamine, from which a number of fatalities have occurred, is heat-stroke. This has been most prominent in cyclists owing to the intensity of their exercise, the endurance required and the high ambient temperatures at which the exercise often occurs. Amphetamines cause a redistribution of blood flow away from the skin, thus limiting the cooling of the blood. As a result, two cyclists (Knud Jensen and Tommy Simpson) who had both been taking amphetamine died of heat-stroke and cardiac arrest, respectively, during gruelling road races. Jensen's death occurred in the intense summer heat of Rome, while Simpson succumbed while climbing the infamous Mont Ventoux during the 1967 Tour de France.

The side effects of amphetamine on behaviour are also important in sport. There were several accounts quoted by Golding (1981) in which the euphoric effects of amphetamines rendered the takers unaware of the errors and misjudgements they were making on the field of play.

The prescription and administration of amphetamines are strictly controlled by law in most developed countries. They produce powerful stimulating effects such as euphoria, excitation and increased aggression and alertness. These effects are achieved at the expense of judgement and self-criticism. Amphetamine administration may be followed by severe bouts of depression and dependence. Increases in athletic performance induced by amphetamine are very small and several studies have failed to show that amphetamine produces any physical advantage. Some evidence suggests that amphetamine may increase confidence before and during an event, and laboratory studies have shown that it may also reduce fatigue in isometric muscle construction. The induction of dependence and the increased susceptibility to heat-stroke and cardiac abnormalities seem to suggest that amphetamine taking is of little value as a performance-enhancing drug in the long term.

Effects of cocaine in athletes and on exercise

Cocaine was used by native South Americans for centuries to increase efficiency, vigour and physical endurance. In 1930, Theil and Essing reported that 0.1 g of cocaine administered to subjects before exercising on a cycle ergometer improved work efficiency, as determined by VO_2 measurements per unit work, and that exercise could be maintained for longer. The results were attributed to reduced CNS perception of fatigue. A second study using the same cocaine dose revealed no increase in work efficiency but a more rapid increase in recovery after exercise (Conlee, 1991). In his review of pre-1983 studies of the effects of cocaine on exercise, Conlee (1991) concluded that they were all contradictory and were usually poorly controlled and not well carried out. Many of the studies reviewed since 1983 have been in animals because of ethical considerations and these have involved rats trained to run on treadmills connected to ergometers.

Early studies demonstrated that cocaine had no beneficial effect on running times within a dose range of 0.1–20.0 mg/kg bodyweight, and at doses above 12.5 mg/kg the cocaine actually reduced running time. At all doses used, cocaine significantly increases glycogen degradation while increasing plasma lactate concentration without producing consistent changes in plasma catecholamine levels. In 1991 Conlee and colleagues demonstrated that, in rats exercising voluntarily, cocaine increases glycogen metabolism and enhances exercise-induced sympathetic responses. Conlee suggested three possible mechanisms to explain cocaine's action which could operate in parallel: (1) cocaine releases catecholamines that increase glycogenolysis and lactate production leading to early fatigue, (2) cocaine may induce skeletal muscle vasoconstriction, reducing oxygen delivery, oxidative metabolism, strength and reaction time, and thereby stimulate glycogen breakdown; and (3) cocaine may have a direct effect on muscle glycogen breakdown. Indirect evidence originally suggested that mechanism 2 is less likely because cocaine-induced reduction of myocardial bloodflow is not associated with increased myocardial glycogen breakdown. In 1994, Braiden *et al.* demonstrated a threefold increase in muscle lactate accumulation in the white vastus muscle of rats under cocaine-fueled exercise conditions.

A study of the effect of the coca leaf has been described by Spielvogel *et al.* (1996). In this experiment metabolic and hormonal changes in habitual coca chewers were compared to non-coca chewers during incremental exercise to exhaustion. The coca leaf ingestion was controlled at 12 g and this produced a mean cocaine blood concentration of 72 ng/ml. At rest, both habitual and naïve coca chewers had similar noradrenaline and adrenaline plasma levels but habitual chewers had higher free fatty acid levels. During sustained exercise, oxygen uptake and work efficiency were similar in both groups while during incremental exercise habitual chewers demonstrated lower arterial oxygen saturation, which was not due to reduced ventilatory response. Free fatty acid (FFA) levels were increased during incremental exercise in the coca chewers. This interesting study remains inconclusive as the possible "benefits" of raised FFA levels could not be determined. There were no simultaneous measurements of changes in carbohydrate metabolism or endurance. Therefore, it is unclear whether a carbohydrate-sparing "mechanism" was activated by coca chewing and because catecholamine (i.e. noradrenaline and adrenaline) plasma levels remained unaltered, the mechanism for the elevation of plasma free fatty acid was unknown. A similar increase in FFA concentration following coca chewing has been described by Favier *et al.* (1996) although they observed increased adrenaline and FFA levels during exercise, coupled with lower blood glucose concentrations. Their conclusion was that this might be evidence that cocaine might prolong work and postpone fatigue by increasing fat mobilisation and sparing glycogen utilisation, but it did not increase time to exhaustion. Clarkson and Thompson (1997) questioned the validity of experiments using coca leaves rather than pure cocaine even where the plasma cocaine concentration has been subsequently determined. The pharmacokinetics of cocaine may be altered by ingesting it via this route and also the coca leaf may contain other naturally occurring ingredients that might (a) influence cocaine metabolism and disposition; (b) affect cocaine action at receptors or transporters; or (c) have metabolic effects of their own. Habitual and naïve cocaine/coca users may exhibit different responses and experiments in rats seem to support this (Conlee *et al.*, 2000).

The effect of cocaine on catecholamine secretion could be the basis of the ergolytic effect of cocaine on exercise. Cocaine effects may not be caused by a vascular action of noradrenaline because blockade of α_1-receptors does not block the action of cocaine on glycogenolysis or lactic acid production (Conlee *et al.*, 2000). As it is quite likely that athletes abusing cocaine will be chronic abusers, a comparison was made between cocaine responses in naïve and chronic cocaine-administered rats. It was found that responses to cocaine in terms of noradrenaline and adrenaline release were greater in rats that had previously received cocaine on a regular basis (Kelly *et al.*, 1995).

It may be that cocaine's positive ergogenic effect is manifested only in activities of short duration that require a burst of high-intensity energy output or in activities associated with the drug's central stimulatory effect rather than its action on peripheral metabolism. It has been suggested that it is precisely for these central heightened arousal and increased alertness effects, achieved principally at "low" doses, that cocaine is abused in sport (Wadler and Hainline, 1989).

Adverse effects of cocaine in athletes

There have been reports of athletes combining cocaine abuse with other drugs such as alcohol and anabolic steroids. According to Welder and Melchert (1993), heavy alcohol consumption combined with cocaine abuse enhances cocaine's cardiotoxicity, possibly by the production of a unique metabolite "cocaethylene". The existence and structure of cocaethylene, as the ethyl esters of the cocaine metabolite benzoylecgonine, has been established by Farre *et al.* (1993), and its actions in animals and man have been reviewed and investigated by McCance-Katz *et al.* (1998). They have detailed the following facts: that cocaine and alcohol taken together have additive deleterious effects, that simultaneous consumption of alcohol and cocaine leads to the formation of cocaethylene, and that though cocaethylene is less potent than cocaine, it is eliminated more slowly and could thus accumulate during or following an alcohol/cocaine binge. Further dangers arise from the possibility that the increased sense of well-being produced by the cocaine/alcohol mixture would lead to further abuse leading to increased toxicity from the drugs plus the toxicity of cocaethylene. Is this relevant to sport? Most certainly it is. This may well have been the ultimate cause of death of the Canadian ice-hockey player John Kordic, who abused cocaine, alcohol and anabolic steroids. His downfall has been chronicled in detail by Scher (1992) and his games included frequent fights with opponents, teammates and officials.

12.4   Stimulants and the WADA prohibited list

Stimulants have the potential for performance enhancement during competition. They are therefore classed, by WADA, under "substances and methods prohibited in competition". Out-of-competition testing for stimulants is not considered necessary, thereby saving resources.

In 2009, WADA categorised stimulants as "specified" or "non-specified". The move was made to align the 2009 prohibited list with the more flexible sanctions set forth in the revised World Anti-Doping Code of 2009 (WADA, 2009). The objective of this flexibility was to allow enhanced sanctions for deliberate doping offenders and reduced sanctions for inadvertent cheaters or for athletes who can unequivocally establish that the substance involved was not intended to enhance performance.

"Specified" stimulants were identified taking into account:

- their potential to enhance performance in sport
- their risk to health
- their general use in medicinal products
- their legitimate market availability
- their illicit use
- their legal/controlled status in various countries
- their history and potential of abuse in sport
- their potential of addiction
- the likelihood of approval for therapeutic use
- their pharmacology
- the likelihood of a non-doping explanation.

In its 2009 prohibited list WADA gave 26 examples of specified stimulants, many of which could be obtained by athletes over-the-counter. These include ephedrine, methylephedrine, cathine, and levmetamphetamine (the drug taken inadvertently by the skier Alain Baxter, as described in the case studies earlier in this chapter). Other OTC stimulants, such as pseudoephedrine and phenylephrine, which were removed from the WADA prohibited list in 2004, are described in more detail in Chapter 21.

In 2010, WADA decided to return pseudoephedrine to the prohibited list as a result of evidence from their monitoring programme of a sustained increase in use at high concentrations and because of scientific evidence of its performance-enhancing effects at certain doses.

With respect to ephedrine, methylephedrine and cathine, WADA have introduced urinary cut-off levels. Therefore, cathine is prohibited when its concentration in urine is greater than 5 µg/ml. For ephedrine and methylephedrine, the cut-off level is 10 µg/ml. A previous study (Chester et al., 2003) has, however, questioned the levels at which such cut-offs are set. This evidence was taken into consideration when WADA re-introduced pseudoephedrine to the prohibited list in 2010 when they increased the urinary threshold to 150 µg/ml from the 25 µg/ml threshold in operation prior to 2004.

The list of non-specified stimulants includes cocaine. Athletes need to therefore avoid the possibility of passive inhalation of cocaine when in the presence of other people smoking highly volatile "crack" cocaine, although Yonamine et al. (2004) have reviewed the literature on this issue and concluded that only individuals exposed to cocaine smoke under "extremely harsh conditions" would eliminate cocaine metabolites in the urine.

Statistics on the prevalence of the use of stimulants in sport can be found in Chapter 25.

12.5   References

Avois, L., Robinson, N., Saudan, C. *et al.* (2009). Central nervous system stimulants and sport practice. *British Journal of Sports Medicine* **40(Suppl 1)**, i16–i20.

Bell, D.G., Jacobs, I. and Ellerington, K. (2001). Effect of caffeine and ephedrine ingestion on anaerobic exercise performance. *Medicine and Science in Sports Exercise* **33**, 1399–1403.

Benzaquen, B.S., Cohen, V. and Eisenberg M.J. (2001). Effects of cocaine on the coronary arteries. *American Heart Journal* **142**, 402–410.

Braiden, R.W., Fellingham, G.W. and Conlee, R.K. (1994). Effects of cocaine on glycogen metabolism and endurance during high intensity exercise. *Medicine and Science in Sports Exercise* **26**, 695–700.

Brookes, L.G. (1985). Central nervous system stimulants. In *Psychopharmacology: Recent advances and future prospects*, ed. S.D. Iverson, Oxford University Press, Oxford. 264–277.

Bucci, L.R. (2000). Selected herbals and human performance. *American Journal of Clinical Nutrition* **72**, 624S–636S.

Chen, N. and Reith, M.E.A. (2000). Structure and function of the dopamine transporter. *European Journal of Pharmacology* **405**, 329–339.

Chester, N., Mottram, D.R., Reilly, T. *et al.* (2003). Elimination of ephedrines in urine following multiple dosing: The consequences for athletes, in relation to doping control. *British Journal of Clinical Pharmacology* **57(1)**: 62–67.

Clarkson, P.M., and Thompson, H.S. (1997). Drugs and sport - research findings and limitations. *Sports Medicine* **24**, 366–384.

Comer, S.D., Hart, C.L., Ward, A.S., *et al.* (2001). Effects of repeated oral methamphetamine administration in humans. *Psychopharmacology* **155**, 397–401.

Conlee, R.K. (1991). Amphetamine, caffeine and cocaine. In Perspectives in Exercise Science and Sports Medicine 4. Ed: Lamb, D.R. Williams, M.H. New York, Brown and Benchmark pp.285–328.

Conlee, R.K., Han, D.H., Kelly, K.P. *et al.* (1991). Effects of cocaine on plasma catecholamine and muscle glycogen concentrations during exercise in the rat. *Journal of Applied Physiology* **70**, 1323–1327.

Conlee, R.K., Kelly, K.P., Ojuka, E.O. *et al.* (2000). Cocaine and exercise: alpha-1 receptor blockade does not alter muscle glycogenolysis or blood lactacidosis. *Journal of Applied Physiology* **88**, 77–81.

Connell, P.H. (1958). *Amphetamine psychosis*. London, Chapman and Hall.

Docherty, J.R. (2008). Pharmacology of stimulants prohibited by the World Anti-Doping Agency (WADA). *British Journal of Pharmacology* **154**, 606–622.

Farre, M., De La Tour, R., Llorente, M. *et al.* (1993). Alcohol and cocaine interactions in humans. *Journal of Pharmacology and Experimental Therapeutics* **266**, 1364–1373.

Favier, R. Caceres, E. and Koubi, H. (1996). Effects of coca chewing on metabolic and hormonal changes during prolonged submaximal exercise. *Journal of Applied Physiology* **80**, 650–655.

Fibiger, H.C., Phillips, A.G. and Brown, E.E. (1992). The neurobiology of cocaine-induced reinforcement. In *Cocaine: scientific and social dimensions*, ed. G.E.W. Wolstenholme, Ciba Foundation Symposium 166, John Wiley, Chichester. 96–124.

Golding, L.A. (1981). Drugs and hormones. In *Ergogenic aids and muscular performance*, ed. W.P. Morgan, Academic Press, New York. 368–397.

Haller, C.A. and Benowitz, N.L. (2000). Adverse cardiovascular and central nervous system events associated with dietary supplements containing ephedra alkaloids. *New England Journal of Medicine* **343(25)**, 1833–1838.

Hart, C.L., Ward, A.S., Harvey, M. *et al.* (2001). Methamphetamine self-administration by humans. *Psychopharmacology* **57**, 75–81.

Hilderbrand, R.L., Wanninger, R. and Bowers, L.D. (2003). An update on regulatory issues in antidoping programs in sport. *Current Sports Medicine Reports* **2**, 226–232.

Jacobs, I., Pasternak, H. and Bell, D.G. (2003). Effects of ephedrine, caffeine and their combination on muscular endurance. *Medicine and Science in Sports and Exercise* **35(6)**, 987–994.

Jones, G. (2008). Caffeine and other sympathomimetic stimulants: Modes of action and effects on sports performance. *Drugs and Ergogenic Aids to Improve Sport Performance* **44**, 109–123.

Kalix, P. (1992). Cathinone, a natural amphetamine. *Pharmacologicol Toxicology* **70**, 77–86.

Kelly, K.P., Han, D.H., Fellingham, G.W. *et al.* (1995). Cocaine and exercise: Physiological responses of cocaine-conditioned rats. *Medicine Science in Sports Exercise* **27**, 65–72.

Kuhar, M.J. (1992). Molecular pharmacology of cocaine: A dopamine hypothesis and its implications. *Cocaine: scientific and social dimensions*, ed. G.E.W. Wolstenholme, Ciba Foundation Symposium 166, John Wiley, Chichester. 81–95.

Laties, V.G. and Weiss, B. (1981). The amphetamine margin in sports. *Federation Proceedings* **40**, 2689–2692.

McCance-Katz, E.F., Kosten, T.R. and Jatlow, P. (1998). Concurrent use of cocaine and alcohol is more potent and potentially more toxic than use of either alone—A multi-dose study. *Biological Psychiatry* **44**, 250–259.

Mottram, D., Chester, N., Atkinson, G. *et al.* (2008). Athletes' knowledge and views on OTC medication. *International Journal of Sports Medicine* **29**, 851–855.

Scher, J. (1992). Death of a goon. *Sports Illustrated* **76**, 112–116.

Seiden, L.S., Sabol, K.E. and Ricaurte, G.A. (1993). Amphetamine: Effects on catecholamine systems and behaviour. *Annual Review of Pharmacology and Toxicology* **32**, 639–677.

Shekelle, P.G., Hardy, M.L., Morton, S.C. *et al.* (2003). Efficacy and safety of ephedra and ephedrine for weight loss and athletic performance. A meta analysis. *Journal of the American Medical Association* **289(12)**, 1537–1545.

Sidney, K.H. and Lefcoe, W.M. (1977). The effects of ephedrine on the physiological and psychological responses to submaximal and maximal exercises in man. *Medicine and Science in Sports* **9**, 95–99.

Smith, B.J., Jones, H.E., and Griffiths, R.R. (2001). Physiological, subjective and reinforcing effects of oral and intravenous cocaine in humans. *Psychopharmacology* **156**, 435–444.

Smith, D.A. and Perry, P.J. (1992). The efficacy of ergogenic agents in athletic competition. Part II: Other performance-enhancing agents. *Annals of Pharmacotherapy* **26**, 653–659.

Spielvogel, H., Caceres, E., Karbritt, B. *et al.* (1996). Effects of coca chewing on metabolic and hormonal changes during graded incremental exercise to maximum. *Journal of Applied Physiology* **80**, 643–649.

Theil, D. and Essing, B. (1930). Cocaine und muskelarbeit I. Der einfluss auf leistung und gastoffwechsel. *Arbeitsphysiologie* **3**, 287–297.

Unterwald, E.M., Kreek, M.J. and Cuntapay, M. (2001). The frequency of cocaine administration impacts cocaine-induced receptor alteration. *Brain Research* **900**, 103–109.

Volkow, N.D., Fowler, J.S. and Wang, G.J. (1999). Imaging studies on the role of dopamine in cocaine reinforcement and addiction in humans. *Journal of Psychopharmacology* **13**, 337–343.

Wadler, G.A. and Hainline, B. (1989). *Drugs and the athlete*. F.A. Davies, Philadelphia.

Weiss, B. and Laties, V.G. (1962). Enhancement of human performance by caffeine and the amphetamines. *Pharmacological Reviews* **14**, 1–36.

Welder, A.A. and Melchert, R.B. (1993). Cardiotoxic effects of cocaine and anabolic-androgenic steroids in the athlete. *Journal of Pharmacology and Toxicological Methodology* **29**, 61–68.

World Anti-Doping Agency (WADA). (2009). World Anti-Doping Code 2009. Available at http://www.wada-ama.org (accessed March 2009).

Wyndham, G.H., Rogers, G.G., Benade, A.J.S. *et al.* (1971). Physiological effects of the amphetamines during exercise. *South African Medical Journal* **45**, 247–252.

Yonamine, M., Garcia, P.R. and de Moraes Moreau, R.L. (2004). Non-intentional doping in sports. *Sports Medicine* **34(1)**, 697–704.

Zhu, M.Y., Shamburger, S., Li, J. *et al.* (2000). Regulation of human dopamine transporter by cocaine and amphetamine. *Journal of Pharmacology and Experimental Therapeutics* **295**, 951–959.

Chapter 13

Narcotic analgesic drugs

Peter N. Elliott

13.1 Introduction

The administration of many drugs to sportsmen and sportswomen is banned as there is the potential for achieving enhanced levels of performance, which is widely considered to be cheating. With some drugs, the potential to induce unnecessary harm to the user is also an issue. The use of some drugs without prescription is also illegal in many countries. Many drugs are effectively banned from use by participants of competitive sports. The list of banned substances includes narcotic analgesic drugs.

As described in Chapter 22, inflammation is a key response to sports injuries. Obviously one of the key components of inflammation is pain. Pain is an important, protective cue to the individual that all is not well. It is a stimulus that promotes rest, an important adjunct to recovery. It is also associated with a learning process that encourages the individual to avoid a repetition of the incident. Pain is unpleasant and, at a moderate to severe level, frequently requires alleviation.

Because the pain associated with a sports injury will inevitably be associated with a traumatic inflammatory reaction there is a strong case for using anti-inflammatory drugs to reduce the overall scale of the body's reaction to trauma as well as reduce the level of pain. In some circumstances, however, the level of pain associated with a serious injury will require the use of more powerful analgesic drugs such as the narcotic analgesic drugs (possibly in association with non-steroidal anti-inflammatory drugs [NSAIDs]). Narcotic analgesic drugs such as morphine, codeine and dihydrocodeine are very effective drugs that can alleviate pain more profoundly than NSAIDs (or paracetamol). The mechanism of action for narcotic analgesics is fundamentally different from that of the aspirin-like drugs. Where NSAIDs reduce pain, at least in part by a peripheral mechanism involving a reduction in inflammation with a consequent lowering of pain, the narcotic analgesics seem to affect the brain's appreciation of pain.

Morphine is the most common analgesic component of the opium poppy. Its potency can be significantly enhanced by acetylation to diamorphine (heroin), which has the convenience of greater solubility. Codeine (3-methylmorphine) has only one-fifth the potency of morphine but is more reliably absorbed from the gastrointestinal system. Dihydrocodeine is similar in potency to codeine when given orally, though it is about twice as potent when injected.

Given that one of the barriers to extreme performance is pain, there has been much speculation over many years as to whether powerful analgesic drugs could raise levels of performance. There is no convincing evidence that narcotics can provide such an enhancement, but they are nevertheless banned substances in competition. They are, however, generally permissible outside of competition periods.

13.2   Pain and nociception

Pain and nociception are not one and the same thing. Nociception is the appreciation of something untoward affecting the body. We are generally acutely aware that we have suffered an injury and often have an intuitive knowledge of its severity. Pain is a much more subjective phenomenon and the scale of pain depends on many factors apart from the severity of an injury. Pain is subjective and is notoriously difficult to measure. It is undoubtedly affected by mood and is likely to be affected by a knowledge of the implications of the source of the pain. Undiagnosed chest pain in an average man in his fifties is likely to cause more distress than it would if he knew for certain that it was due to reflux oesophagitis ("heart burn"). The undiagnosed condition may seem more painful because the subject thinks he may be suffering a heart attack.

As a student, I observed experiments designed to measure the effectiveness of narcotics. The model involved measuring the narcotic-induced increase in duration of tolerance in mice placed on a mildly hot surface. For an inexperienced technician, defining the point of reaction is quite difficult. In an attempt to overcome this uncertainty, the technician raised the hot-plate about 30 cm above the bench in the hope that the end point could be unequivocally recorded as the time at which the mouse made a conscious decision to jump down from the hot-plate. It was hoped that narcotics would increase the endurance of the mouse. In reality the exact opposite happened! Treated mice jumped off, immediately after they were placed on the hot-plate. The apparent reason for this was that the narcotic rendered the mice unconcerned about jumping from height. An obvious and important additional conclusion is that the narcotic did not inhibit the ability of the mice to sense the mildly unpleasant heat sensation. The moral of this tale is, perhaps, that narcotics do indeed affect perception in complex ways.

As this unusual experiment suggests, morphine-like drugs are not just analgesics. It is clear from a variety of sources that they exhibit multiple activities including respiratory depression, emesis and smooth muscle relaxation. In addition they have profound effects on perception. It can be argued that their analgesic effect has more to do with a change in concern about pain than with a "physical" reduction of pain. Euphoria is a common experience, too. Whilst attitude is a very difficult human trait to measure, the highest competitive performances require a single-mindedness that is almost certain to be a casualty of narcotic usage.

13.3   Mechanism of action of narcotic analgesics

Turning to the mechanisms by which these drugs induce analgesia we see that their impact is on both nociception and the appreciation of pain. In the 1970s, it was discovered (Kosterlitz and Hughes, 1977; and Simantov and Snyder, 1976, independently) that the body produces neuropeptides called endorphins, which stimulate neural receptors, resulting in a reduction of nociception and inducing a sense of well-being. Narcotic analgesics stimulate the same receptors and induce similar or more profound levels of analgesia and euphoria.

Pain sensation is transmitted by several distinct types of nerves. C fibres are not myelinated and transmit nerve impulses relatively slowly. Nerves in this category provide information on a wide range of sensations including burning, itching, and cramping. A fibres, which are myelinated, give the sensation of acute, localised pain in response to mechanical trauma. The sensory nerves pass from their point of origin in the tissues to the dorsal horn of the spinal column where they terminate and interact with the dorsal horn neuron. From there, nerve impulses pass up the spinal canal to the thalamus of the brain from whence the information is relayed to the cortex of the brain. There are a number of neural pathways that can moderate the sensation of pain. These include, most notably, nerve impulses descending from the thalamus to inhibit the activity of the dorsal horn neuron.

Narcotic analgesics relieve most types of pain, including that associated with traumatic injuries. Their analgesic effect is achieved by a variety of concomitant activities. They inhibit the generation of nerve impulses in the peripheral pain fibres, inhibit transmission of impulses in the dorsal horn neuron and stimulate the descending inhibitory pathway (which also suppresses the activity of the dorsal horn neuron).

13.4   Side effects of narcotic analgesics

Narcotic analgesics are powerful drugs that produce a significant number of side effects. These range from troublesome constipation to respiratory depression. However, narcotics have achieved notoriety due to their propensity towards tolerance and psychic and physical dependence, when used regularly. Tolerance is the need for an increased dose of the drug to produce the same pharmacological effect. Psychic dependence is characterised by the continued desire or craving for a substance. Physical dependence is observed when a substance is no longer administered and physical withdrawal symptoms are experienced.

13.5   The use of narcotic analgesics in sport

Indirect enhancement of performance

Whilst it is now generally accepted that narcotic analgesics are unlikely to enhance performance in a competition, there is some evidence that they may serve to enhance preparation.

Cycling

Cycling has been the subject of several narcotic abuse cases in recent years. To be successful in long-distance cycling races, a cyclist must be able to overcome pain barriers. A mixture of drugs including a narcotic analgesic, such as heroin, and stimulants, such as amphetamines and cocaine, was nicknamed the Belgian Mix or "pot Belge". Its use has certainly not been limited to cyclists in Belgium but it is this country that may well have been its original source. Cycling is a very popular sport in that country and even amateurs can gain significant financial reward from success in sponsored, unregulated races at local levels.

In the 1998 Tour de France, a French team was suspended when its physio-therapist, Willy Voet, was found to have a large number of drugs, including narcotics, in his possession. The Belgian cyclist Christophe Brandt tested positive for methadone in the 2004 Tour de France. Methadone is a drug that shares many of the properties of morphine. It is used as a heroin substitute for heroin addicts in some countries.

Perhaps the most significant case involving the use of narcotics in cycling was the infamous "Cahors Affair". Emanating from 2004, its associated trial opened in 2005 and culminated in 2006 with 23 convictions relating to the illicit use of performance-enhancing drugs, including "pot Belge". Some of the convictions included custodial sentences. Those testifying and those mentioned in testimonies read like a who's who of European cycling. The former French professional cyclist Laurent Roux intimated that some teams spent more on "doctors" than on riders.

Cycling, particularly road-racing, has been in a sad state of affairs. The impact of the cases described here and others (not all including narcotics) has been enor-mous. The sport has been shaken to the core. The triumph of the Team GB cyclists in the 2008 Beijing Olympics has at last done something to restore the sport's image.

Long-distance running

Other endurance events have also been tarnished by narcotic usage. The Ethiopian runner Ambesse Tolossa, who had already experienced success in marathon events, won the December 2007 Honolulu marathon. He was subsequently dis-qualified because of a positive test for morphine and his prize money of $40,000 was withheld. Despite Tolossa's insistence that he had no idea how the drug came to be in his body, he also received a two-year ban because of the strict liability policy associated with Olympic events. The race was awarded instead to second-placed Jimmy Muindi, his sixth win of the Honolulu Marathon.

As a measure of the seriousness with which governing bodies are now taking illegal drug abuse, even when dealing with drugs not generally considered as performance enhancing, one only has to consider the case of the British runner Kate Reed. Kate, who was part of the 2008 Beijing Olympics team, had suffered an injury to her leg, and had apparently joked with teammates about taking morphine for the pain. Shortly afterwards, her room was searched for drugs by British Olympic Association officials. Luckily, none were found and she duly passed a doping test.

Runner's high

It has been suggested that strenuous activity can lead to the production of endorphins in the brain. This is most evident at the threshold of endurance. Endorphins may help the athlete to persevere beyond the point where pain is otherwise unbearable. This may correspond with the exhaustion of muscle stores of glycogen and a build-up of lactate. This concept is not universally approved.

Equestrian sport

The abuse of narcotics is not restricted to humans. In 2002, twenty British-owned or -trained racehorses tested positive for morphine. The most celebrated horse involved in this scandal was Be My Royal, winner of the 2002 Hennessy Cognac Gold Cup at Newbury. Despite appeals by the trainer, Willie Mullins, the horse was disqualified from the race. It was claimed that the horse was fed with contaminated feed.

World Anti-Doping Agency statistics

The World Anti-Doping Agency published data that show that the presence of narcotics in analysed samples remains at a consistently low level. In 2005, 2006, 2007 and 2008, there were 17, 16, 21 and 28 cases of narcotic detection in samples, respectively. This represents an incidence of 0.4 per cent of all drugs detected in samples tested.

Therapeutic Use Exemption

There has been a significant increase in the number of Therapeutic Use Exemption (TUE) applications for single-dose use of narcotics. This is only possible when the drug is prohibited in competition but not in training. In the UK, a TUE is only required by UK Sport if the athlete will be in competition within seven days of the administration of the narcotic. Detailed background information, including medical records, is required. These applications are considered by an independent panel of three medical experts.

13.6   References

Kosterlitz, H.W. and Hughes, J. (1977). Peptides with morphine-like action in the brain. *British Journal of Psychiatry* **130**, 298–304.

Simantov, R. and Snyder, S.H. (1976). Morphine-like peptides in mammalian brain: Isolation, structure elucidation, and interactions with the opiate receptor. *Proceedings of the National Academy of Sciences USA* **73(7)**, 2515–2519.

World Anti-Doping Agency (WADA). (2005, 2006 and 2007). Adverse analytical findings. Laboratory statistics. Available at http://www.wada-ama.org/en/dynamic. ch2?pageCategory.id=335 (accessed July 2009).

Chapter 14

Cannabinoids

David R. Mottram

14.1 What are cannabinoids?

The source of cannabinoids

Cannabinoids are defined, chemically, as aryl-substituted meroterpenes. They are derived principally from the plant *Cannabis sativa*. This plant contains approximately more than 400 chemical constituents. Of these constituents, more than 60 are chemically classed as cannabinoids. The most potent of these cannabinoids that produces psychoactive effects is Δ^9-tetrahydrocannabinol (Δ^9-THC). Other plant cannabinoids include cannabinol and cannabidiol, which, along with other cannabinoids, produce complex pharmacological actions and interactions when herbal cannabis is smoked (Ashton, 2001).

The Δ^9-THC content varies to a great extent depending on the source of the plant and how the drug is taken (Ashton, 2001). New varieties of cannabis plant have been bred in recent years, leading to more potent products than those that were available in the 1960s and 1970s (Ashton, 1999).

The cannabis plant, when used for recreational purposes, is processed in various ways in order to derive the effects of the active constituents. The two most common are cannabis resin (hashish) and marijuana, which is normally associated with the dried and ground leaves, flower and other parts of the plant prepared for smoking (Campos *et al.*, 2003). When inhaled, in addition to the cannabinoids, the smoke from cannabis contains many of the constituents of tobacco smoke (Ashton, 1999).

Tetrahydrocannabinol-like derivatives, such as dronabinol and nabilone, have been synthesised and are prescribed in some countries to treat weight loss and nausea and vomiting associated with cancer therapy (Campos *et al.*, 2003).

Mode of action of cannabinoids

Specific receptors for cannabinoids have been identified in humans. These are termed CB_1 receptors and they are located in the plasma membrane of nerve endings in the brain. Stimulation of these receptors inhibits transmitter release, particularly acetylcholine within the hippocampus, the area of the brain responsible for learning and memory, and noradrenaline in the cerebral cortex and cerebellum, responsible for alertness and motor coordination (Pertwee, 1997). They are amongst the most numerous receptors in the brain. A second type of receptor, termed CB_2, is mainly found peripherally, associated with the immune system.

The discovery of cannabinoid receptors led to a search for endogenous mediators, of which a number have been identified. The two well-established endocannabinoids are anandamide and 2-arachidonoyl glycerol (Porter and Felder, 2001). Anandamide has a high affinity for CB_1 receptors and has most of the actions of Δ^9-THC (Ashton, 2001).

When cannabis is smoked, the effects of cannabinoids are perceived within minutes. Oral cannabis results in the absorption of around 25–30 per cent of the amount of cannabinoids obtained by smoking and the onset of effects is between 30 minutes to 2 hours, although the duration of action may be more prolonged by the oral route (Maykut, 1985). Following absorption, cannabinoids are rapidly and widely distributed throughout the body. They tend to accumulate in fatty tissue from where they are slowly released over extended periods of time. Complete elimination from the body may take as long as 30 days (Huestis *et al.*, 1995), which may have consequences with respect to dope testing. Another reason for the extended period of elimination is that the metabolites are only partially excreted in the urine (approximately 25 per cent) whereas most (65 per cent) is excreted into the gastrointestinal tract from where they are re-absorbed into the body, a process that continues over a considerable period of time (Ashton, 2001).

Effects and side effects of cannabinoids

It is difficult to distinguish between the effects and side effects of cannabinoids as the desired effect in one individual under one set of circumstances may be perceived as an undesired effect by another person under different conditions.

Cannabinoids produce both physical and psychological effects, the extent of which will vary depending on patterns of use. Therefore, isolated or infrequent use can lead to mild intoxication, drowsiness and sedation, slower reaction times and memory deficiency. Regular consumption can lead to social detachment and psychological dependence (Saugy *et al.*, 2006).

Cannabinoids affect almost any system in the body and combine many of the properties of alcohol, tranquillizers, opiates and hallucinogens. They are therefore anxiolytic, sedative, analgesic and psychedelic in their action (Ashton, 2001).

The main central effects of cannabinoids are impairment of short-term memory, learning tasks and motor coordination, along with catalepsy, hypothermia, analgesia, an increase in appetite and an anti-emetic action. The main peripheral effects are tachycardia, bronchodilation, vasodilation and a reduction of intra-ocular pressure (Rang *et al.*, 2007). Users of cannabis develop a mild form of tolerance and dependence to the drug.

The incidence of serious, acute toxic side effects due to cannabinoids is low and no deaths directly attributable to acute cannabis use have been reported (Ashton, 1999). However, Ashton (1999, 2001) has found a number of significant adverse effects of cannabinoids on the cardiovascular and respiratory systems as well as on the central nervous system.

Cannabis use in society

There is no doubt that cannabis use in society as a whole has increased in recent years, with figures up to 16 per cent being quoted for use by young adults in Europe and the USA (Saugy et al., 2006). Even higher figures of prevalence have been reported in a review by Ashton (2001). It is not, therefore, surprising that a similar trend has happened in sport (Mottram, 1999). Cannabinoids are now the third most frequently recorded class of substances on WADA's prohibited list, according to the annual statistics from WADA-accredited laboratories.

14.2 History of cannabis in sport

Addition to the prohibited list

The International Olympic Committee (IOC) first included cannabis on its list of prohibited substances in 1989, under the heading "classes of prohibited substances in certain circumstances". Unfortunately, at that time, not all international sports federations (ISFs) included cannabis on their respective prohibited lists. This led to confusion within the minds of athletes, as exemplified in the case studies below. A study in 1999 by Venema et al. illustrated the inconsistency that persisted for many years in the attitude of ISFs with respect to whether they considered cannabis to be performance enhancing or not. This inconsistent attitude undermined athletes' belief in a fair judgement of "positive" cannabis cases.

WADA removed the doubt, in 2004, by placing cannabinoids on their prohibited list for all athletes in all sports, within competition. Whether that decision was rational remains open to debate.

Case studies relating to cannabinoids

Ross Ribagliati, 1998

Ross Ribagliati, a Canadian snowboarder, won the inaugural men's giant slalom event at the 1998 Winter Olympic Games in Nagano. Immediately after the event, he tested positive for cannabinoids and was stripped of his gold medal. He claimed that he had not taken marijuana himself but that he was a victim of passive smoking. Regardless of the veracity of this claim, he had his medal re-instated three days later. Although the IOC had marijuana on its prohibited list, Ribagliati's governing body, the International Ski Federation, did not prohibit the use of the drug at that time. This landmark case further highlighted the inconsistency in the application of rules between sporting organisations at the time.

Tomas Enge, 2002

In August 2002, Tomas Enge, a Czech motor racing driver, tested positive for cannabinoids after a Formula 3000 race in Hungary. He was conditionally suspended from racing for 12 months by his governing body, the International Automobile Federation (Campos *et al.*, 2003).

Michael Phelps

A photograph of Michael Phelps, the holder of 14 Olympic gold medals, smoking marijuana at a party in South Carolina was published by a British newspaper in January 2009. Although this incident was not the result of a dope-test violation, USA Swimming decided to suspend Michael Phelps from competition for three months.

14.3   Cannabinoids in sport

The use of cannabinoids within sport

There are no studies relating to the use of cannabinoids in elite athletes. The few studies that have been undertaken have been with student athletes.

A study by Lorente *et al.* (2005), involving French university sports students, suggested that around 12 per cent of students had used cannabis in an attempt to enhance "performance". The authors noted that using cannabis to improve performance in a recreational manner can lead to its use in an attempt to refine sporting performance. These authors also showed that cannabis use to enhance sport performance was positively related to the level of competition and to particular sports such as "sliding sports" (skiing, snowboarding, surfing, windsurfing and sailing).

Another study on college student athletes revealed that 28.4 per cent of US National Collegiate Athletic Association students used marijuana (Green *et al.*, 2001).

Are cannabinoids performance enhancing?

The balance of evidence suggests that cannabinoids, in most sports, are ergolytic rather than ergogenic (Eichner, 1993). Recreationally, cannabis use produces a feeling of euphoria and reduces anxiety. These properties may be beneficial in alleviating the stress induced through competition, either pre- or post-event. However, cannabis smoking impairs cognition and psychomotor and exercise performance (Saugy *et al.*, 2006). When compared with control subjects, marijuana was shown to reduce maximal exercise performance (Renaud and Cornier, 1986).

Adverse effects of cannabinoids in sport

The adverse effects of cannabinoids on physical and psychological function means that cannabis consumption can be dangerous in sports that rely on clear thinking, quick reactions and split-second timing (Campos *et al.*, 2003). Particular adverse effects include somnolence, dizziness, and feelings of paranoia. Anxiety and tachycardia may also occur. All these effects are incompatible with most athletic endeavours (Campos *et al.*, 2003).

The consequences of cannabinoid use for other competitors

If cannabinoids do not confer significant performance enhancement for the majority of users, does their use pose a threat to fellow competitors? This probably depends on the sport. Menetrey *et al.* (2005) assessed driving capability under the influence of cannabinoids and concluded that they have a negative effect, which would impair alertness and reflexes in motor sports, leading to danger for both the user and their fellow competitors.

14.4   Cannabinoids and the WADA prohibited list

WADA regulations with respect to cannabinoids

The 2009 WADA prohibited list states that cannabinoids are prohibited in all sports but that an adverse analytical finding is only reported if a positive urine sample is detected in competition. Furthermore, cannabinoids are classed as "specified substances", which allows for more flexible sanctions to be applied in the case of an adverse finding. WADA laboratories undertake urine analysis, using gas chromatography/mass spectrometry, of 11-nor-delta 9-tetrahydrocannabinol-9-carboxylic acid (carboxy-THC), the principal metabolite of Δ^9-THC, in either its free or conjugated form. If the sum of the concentration of free and conjugated carboxy-THC is greater than 15 ng/ml, an adverse analytical finding is reported by the laboratory (WADA, 2009).

Prevalence of adverse findings for cannabinoids

Statistics from WADA-accredited laboratories showed a significant rise in the annual number of adverse findings for cannabinoids in the period from 1993 to 2004, rising from 48 to 518 (Mottram, 2005). Since then, the annual figure has remained at more than 500 per year, making cannabinoids the third most frequently cited class of substances and methods on the WADA prohibited list, behind anabolic agents and stimulants (see Chapter 25). It is worth noting that cannabinoids are only tested in competition; therefore, any positive results found in urine samples taken out of competition are not reported by laboratories. The extent of cannabis use by athletes could therefore be significantly higher than that indicated by the WADA statistics.

Further analysis of WADA statistics from 2004 to 2008 shows that adverse analytical findings for cannabinoids have varied from laboratory to laboratory. The mean number of findings from Ghent in Belgium, Paris in France and Los Angeles in the USA have consistently, in each year, been greater than the mean results for all countries.

Passive ingestion of cannabinoids

The WADA Anti-Doping Code states that urinary levels of carboxy-THC must exceed a threshold of 15 ng/ml in order to trigger an adverse analytical finding. This has been established in part to distinguish between active consumers of cannabinoids and those athletes who may have been exposed, passively, to cannabis smoke (Campos et al., 2003).

Several studies have been conducted to determine the likelihood of passive inhalation of cannabinoids sufficient to trigger an adverse analytical finding (Yonamine et al., 2004). The extent of passive inhalation depends on factors such as the size of the room and the effectiveness of the room's ventilation as well as the number of marijuana cigarettes being smoked and the concentration of Δ^9-THC within the cigarettes. The conclusion reached was that an individual could produce urinary levels of carboxy-THC sufficient to exceed the 15 ng/ml threshold only after "extremely severe" conditions of passive exposure to marijuana smoke (Yonamine et al., 2004).

The threshold limit also reduces the chance of an adverse test result after the consumption of food products that may contain traces of cannabinoids (Saugy et al., 2006). In this context, there has been an increase in the sale of hemp-containing products, such as cakes, cookies and brownies or of hemp-seed oil products (Yonamine et al., 2004). However, research into the chances of exceeding urinary threshold levels when consuming such products reveals very variable and inconsistent results (Cone et al., 1988; Bosy and Cole, 2000; Leson et al., 2000).

Should cannabinoids be on the WADA prohibited list?

There are arguments for and against removing cannabinoids from the WADA prohibited list. The principal argument for retaining the substances relates to the fact that cannabinoids produce a wide range of psychological and physical effects within the body that, far from being performance enhancing in most cases, intoxicate the consumer. This may have significant consequences for fellow competitors.

Arguments for removing cannabinoids from the list include the fact that, in most countries, possession and consumption of cannabis products is illegal. Is it therefore appropriate for WADA to impose a further level of legislation? Of course, this argument is flawed because the laws relating to cannabis use are not universally in place or rigorously applied.

Other arguments for removing cannabinoids relate to the possibility of passive consumption, although this is countered by the presence of a threshold level for carboxy-THC and the classification of cannabinoids as specified substances, which allows athletes to prove that they had not intended to use cannabinoids for performance-enhancing purposes. It should be noted, however, that the elimination of carboxy-THC from the body is a slow and individually variable process, making it difficult to prove intent or otherwise (Saugy et al., 2006).

14.5   References

Ashton, C.H. (1999). Adverse effects of cannabis and cannabinoids. *British Journal of Anaesthesia* **83(4)**, 637–649.

Ashton, C.H. (2001). Pharmacology and effects of cannabis: A brief review. *British Journal of Psychiatry* **178**, 101–106.

Bosy, T.Z. and Cole, K.A. (2000). Consumption and quantitation of Δ^9-tetrahydrocannabinol in commercially available hemp seed oil products. *Journal of Analytical Toxicology* **24**, 562–566.

Campos, D.R., Yonamine, M. and de Moraes Moreau, R.L. (2003). Marijuana as doping in sports. *Sports Medicine* **33(6)**, 395–399.

Cone, E.J., Johnson, R.E., Paul, B.D. *et al.* (1988). Marijuana-laced brownies: Behavioural effects, physiologic effects and urinalysis in humans following ingestion. *Journal of Analytical Toxicology* **12**, 169–175.

Eichner, E.R. (1993). Ergolytic drugs in medicine and sport. *American Journal of Medicine* **94(2)**, 205–211.

Green, G.A., Uryasz. F.D., Petr, T.A. *et al.* (2001). NCAA study of substance use and abuse habits of college student-athletes. *Clinical Journal of Sports Medicine* **11(1)**, 51–56.

Huestis, M.A., Mitchell, J.M. and Cone, E.J. (1995). Detection times of marijuana metabolites in urine by immunoassay and GC-MS. *Journal of Analytical Toxicology* **19(6)**, 443–449.

Leson, G., Pless, P., Grotenhermen, F. *et al.* (2000). Evaluating the impact of hemp food consumption on workplace drug tests. *Journal of Analytical Toxicology* **25**, 691–698.

Lorente, F.O., Peretti-Watel, P. and Grelot, L. (2005). Cannabis use to enhance sportive and non-sportive performances among French sport students. *Addictive Behaviours* **30**, 1382–1391.

Maykut, M.O. (1985). Health consequences of acute and chronic marijuana use. *Progress in Neuropsychopharmacology and Biological Psychiatry* **9**, 209–238.

Menetrey, A., Augsburger, M., Favrat, B. *et al.* (2005). Assessment of driving capability through the use of clinical and psychomotor tests in relation to blood cannabinoid levels following oral administration of 20mg dronabinol or of a cannabis decoction made with 20 or 60mg delta 9-THC. *Journal of Analytical Toxicology* **29**, 327–338.

Mottram, D.R. (1999). Banned drugs in sport: Does the International Olympic committee (IOC) list need updating? *Sports Medicine* **27(1)**, 1–10.

Mottram, D.R. (2005). Prevalence of drug misuse in sport. In *Drugs in sport*, 4th ed., ed. D.R. Mottram, Routledge, London. 357–380.

Pertwee, R.G. (1997). Pharmacology of cannabinoid CB1 and CB2 receptors. *Pharmacological Therapeutics* **74(2)**, 129–180.

Porter, A.C. and Felder, C.C. (2001). The endocannabinoid nervous system: Unique opportunities for therapeutic intervention. *Pharmacological Therapeutics* **90**, 45–60.

Rang, H.P., Dale, M.M., Ritter, J.M. *et al.* (2007). Cannabinoids. In *Rang and Dale's Pharmacology*, 6th ed., Churchill Livingstone, London. 248–255.

Renaud, A.M. and Cornier, Y. (1986). Acute effects of marijuana smoking on maximal exercise performance. *Medicine and Science in Sports and Exercise* **18(6)**, 685–689.

Saugy, M., Avois, L., Saudan, C. *et al.* (2006). Cannabis and sport. *British Journal of Sports Medicine* **40(Suppl 1)**, i13–i15.

Venema, H., de Boer, D., Horta, L. *et al.* (1999). Different anti-doping policies of International Sport Federations towards the ban of the use of cannabis. In *Fifth World Congress of Sports Sciences: Book of abstracts*, Sports Medicine Australia, Canberra. 218.

World Anti-Doping Agency (WADA). (2009). WADA laboratory standards. Available at www.wada-ama.org (accessed May 2009).

Yonamine, M., Garcia, P.R. and de Moraes Moreau, R.L. (2004). Non-intentional doping in sports. *Sports Medicine* **34(11)**, 697–704.

Chapter 15

Glucocorticosteroids

Peter N. Elliott

15.1 Introduction

As discussed in the chapter on non-steroidal anti-inflammatory drugs (Chapter 22), inflammation is the major response of the body to sports injuries. Moderation of the inflammatory response may be beneficial, certainly in terms of improving the comfort of the injured subject but also in accelerating the restoration of a competitor to fitness. In this chapter an alternative therapeutic approach using steroidal anti-inflammatory drugs will be considered. Whilst the use and approach to treatment of these drugs differ from the non-steroidal anti-inflammatory drugs (NSAIDs) the underlying issues are essentially the same.

15.2 The functions and side effects of glucocorticosteroids

Many of the body's natural hormones are based on the four-ring steroid structure. The precise activity of a steroid depends on which of a small number of substitutions are made to the structure (Figure 15.1).

Some steroids (oestrogens, progesterones and testosterones) have powerful effects on sex-related attributes and activities. Others, such as the glucocorticosteroids (glucocorticoids) or mineralocorticoids, influence the metabolic activities or fluid balance of the body. The activities of steroids are seldom completely specific and often overlap each other. Of interest here are some of the most powerful anti-inflammatory agents known to human kind, the glucocorticoids. These are drugs that are based on the chemical structure of the steroids produced by the cortex of the adrenal gland and are generally referred to as corticosteroids.

It is important to appreciate that glucocorticoids and anabolic steroids are both steroids and that the term steroid is ubiquitously used. However, glucocorticoids exhibit no practical anabolic activity.

These corticosteroids were first used to treat inflammatory conditions in the late 1940s (Hench *et al.*, 1949). They represented an exciting and, possibly, fundamental new approach to the treatment of inflammatory disease. Initial optimism waned rapidly, however, as it quickly became apparent that these

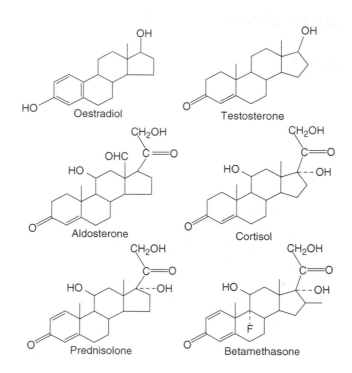

Figure 15.1 Structures of endogenous and exogenous steroids.

substances were not curative and that they were subject to considerable numbers of side effects. The anti-inflammatory activity of these steroid hormones appears to be secondary to their glucocorticoid function, as despite the severe metabolic derangement that accompanies adrenal gland insufficiency (Addison's disease) there is no general precipitation of inflammatory reactions. It would appear, therefore, that these steroids only inhibit inflammation induced by trauma or other challenge; they do not have a role to prevent inflammation being triggered without cause.

Glucocorticoids affect the way the metabolic processes provide energy for the body. In general, they promote gluconeogenesis, in particular, the conversion of certain amino acids to glucose. There has been much speculation, over many years, as to whether glucocorticoids could enhance performance by improving the availability of energy sources but no convincing evidence has emerged to support this concept. Indeed the few trials that have examined the effect of glucocorticoids on performance have failed to demonstrate any increase in performance (Soetens *et al.*, 1995, Arlettaz *et al.*, 2008).

Of course, the activation of such metabolic pathways will lead to the breakdown of functional proteins including those present in muscle. This catabolic effect of glucocorticoids on skeletal muscle may be disastrous for an athlete.

Weakness of muscles in the arms and legs can occur soon after treatment is started, even with quite modest doses of these drugs. Experiments with rats have shown that very significant reductions in muscle weight can occur within seven days (Bullock *et al.*, 1971). The most useful property that this category of drug offers the athlete is as an anti-inflammatory, which may be useful when treating an injury.

Many attempts have been made to increase the anti-inflammatory activity of these steroids. A large number of anti-inflammatory steroids are now available, many of which are an order of magnitude more potent than cortisol (the most abundant steroid secreted by the human adrenal cortex). All of these steroids have significant glucocorticoid activity. Inevitably, long-term use of these drugs will affect the general metabolic activity of the body and is likely to provoke symptoms similar to those seen when the adrenal cortex is hyperactive (Cushing's syndrome). It is, therefore, important that a distinction is made between the long-term, systemic use of anti-inflammatory steroids and their use in acute situations. Long-term use may lead to a number of side effects, such as muscle-wasting, which could be particularly unfortunate for an athlete. Osteoporosis is another frequently encountered response to corticosteroid therapy. This serious weakening of the skeletal structure affects, principally, those bones with the most trabecular structure, such as the ribs and vertebrae. Vertebral compression fractures are a frequent complication of steroid therapy. Long-term use of a drug that may cause degeneration of muscles and weaken bone structure of an individual (whose sporting activities may subject that structure to greater than normal stress) should not be contemplated lightly.

If long-term, systemic steroid treatment is initiated it must be realised that the desired anti-inflammatory effect may be achieved but the administered drug will largely take over the glucocorticoid role of the natural adrenal hormone. Due to negative feedback mechanisms operating in both the hypothalamus and the anterior pituitary, the releases of corticotrophin-releasing factor and adrenocorticotrophic hormone, respectively, are inhibited and so the adrenal cortex is not stimulated to produce its own glucocorticoids normally. Over a period of time the adrenal cortex regresses to a state such that the adrenal gland can no longer produce sufficient quantities of glucocorticoid to support the body if the drug treatment is stopped suddenly. It is important, therefore, that after long-term treatment with a steroid the drug is withdrawn gradually by progressively lowering the daily dose.

Steroids are double-edged weapons in the armoury of anti-inflammatory therapy. They are powerful, anti-inflammatory drugs but, unfortunately, they cause a great many side effects. The direct application of these drugs to an affected site such that a high concentration of the steroid is achieved locally but without the attainment of significant systemic levels offers the possibility of gaining the maximum usefulness of steroids with minimal toxicity. Direct application of steroids to the skin is not an entirely satisfactory method as, although they are generally well absorbed, large proportions of the active drug will be transported away by the blood and, therefore, accumulation in affected muscle or connective tissue is limited. Additionally topical application of steroids tends to cause thinning of the skin and delayed wound healing.

Mechanisms of action of glucocorticoids

Corticosteroids exhibit profound effects on leucocytes. Unlike other hormones and cell-signalling substances, steroids exert their effects by an intracellular mechanism, generally resulting in a modification to the nature of DNA transcription. Many leucocyte activities are depressed including, very significantly, the expression of cell adhesion molecules. This should result in a significant reduction in the recruitment of inflammatory cells, such as polymorphonuclear leucocytes, to the inflamed tissue as the binding of these cells to the endothelial cells lining the blood vessels will be inhibited.

Glucocorticoids bind to specific receptors in the cytoplasm, which then bind to glucocorticoid response elements on genes. Modification to transcription may ultimately result in an increase in the synthesis of natural anti-inflammatory proteins such as lipocortin-1 (anti-inflammatory, anti-proliferative), interleukin-10 (inhibits the activity of various pro-inflammatory cytokines) and interleukin-1 receptor antagonist (which is a natural antagonist to the activities of interleukin 1). An inhibition of the pro-inflammatory transcription factor, Nuclear Factor-κB, may also be seen. The expression of cyclo-oxygenase-2 is also inhibited by glucocorticoids.

15.3   Local steroid injections

The local injection of a corticosteroid preparation does offer considerable advantages in the treatment of an inflammatory condition restricted to a small area of the body. The achievement of therapeutic levels of the drug at the affected site may provide substantial relief without the instigation of the significant side effects associated with systemic administration. Early attempts to inject steroids locally were not particularly successful because these highly soluble drugs were rapidly removed from the site and redistributed around the body. The development of less soluble esters of hydrocortisone and prednisolone to give fairly insoluble micro crystalline preparations, which are injected as suspensions, has markedly improved the success of this particular technique. A single dose of an insoluble steroid preparation will provide relief for several days or even several weeks. If necessary these local injections can be repeated to extend the period of effectiveness. When injections of steroids are given, great care must be taken to minimise the introduction of infective agents. This is especially the case where injections have to be administered intra-articularly to improve mobility and restrict damage of an affected joint. In the case of intra-articular injection, the use of a long-acting preparation such as triamcinolone hexacetonide is indicated so that repeated injections are required less frequently.

Local injection of corticosteroids may also be valuable for the treatment of soft tissue injuries. They may be injected into the interior of a bursa (the fibrous sac, filled with synovial fluid, which may be found between muscles or between a tendon and bone and which facilitates frictionless movement between the surfaces that it separates); they may also be injected into a tendon sheath to reduce the inflammation of an affected tendon or infiltrated around the area of an inflamed ligament.

Tendinitis of the elbow (tennis elbow) is a classic example of the type of injury that responds well to local corticosteroid injection. About a fifth of all injuries to football players involve sprained ankles. Sprained ankles are a common feature of many other sports and are particularly prevalent amongst basketball players. The anterior talofibular is the most commonly affected ligament. A double lesion with the calcaneofibular ligament also being affected is common, too. Where there is no evidence of a complete tear, and early treatment is possible, the local injection of a steroid suspension can be very effective in reducing the symptoms of inflammation.

Steroids do delay the wound-healing process. Particular care should be taken when using them in situations where extensive new tissue will have to be produced (as may be the case, for example, where a collision on the sports field has resulted in an open wound). In this instance the use of steroids to reduce inflammation may not be appropriate.

Nichols (2005) reviewed 25 selected studies (involving almost a thousand subjects) on the use of corticosteroids in the treatment of athletic injuries. Complications from treatment were usually minor and typically included tendon and fascial ruptures following corticosteroid injection. More serious issues such as tibial stress fractures and multifocal osteonecrosis were reported in some subjects treated with systemic corticosteroids.

15.4   Other uses of glucocorticoids

Glucocorticoids are, as has been pointed out already, very powerful anti-inflammatory drugs. Their use in many pathological conditions is widespread. As well as their use for the treatment of musculo-skeletal disorders, these steroids are also routinely utilized for inflammation of a variety of gastrointestinal disorders (such as ulcerative colitis), a range of skin conditions (including eczema and contact dermatitis) and asthma. In diseases such as ulcerative colitis, steroids are generally used systemically, for a short period of time, to treat the more aggressive phases of the disease and to bring it into remission for treatment with other drugs. In skin conditions and asthma the steroids are generally administered in relatively small quantities to problem areas. For skin, it would be in the form of creams or ointments; for asthma, oral inhalation is used.

The use of other inhaled drugs to treat asthma is dealt with elsewhere in this book (Chapter 6). The use of a glucocorticoid inhaler requires a declaration. If it is necessary to use oral glucocorticoids to treat asthma then a Therapeutic Use

Exemption must be obtained. There have been very few studies on the effects of inhaled glucocorticosteroids on asthma in athletes, particularly in elite athletes (Carlsen *et al.*, 2008). The significant side effects of this group of drugs were highlighted by these authors, particularly side effects suffered by young sportspersons.

15.5   WADA regulations for the use of glucocorticosteroids

The World Anti-Doping Agency (WADA) 2010 prohibited list states that all glucocorticosteroids are prohibited when administered by oral, rectal, intravenous or intramuscular routes.

In accordance with the International Standard for Therapeutic Use Exemptions (TUEs), a declaration of use must be completed by the athlete for glucocorticosteroids administered by intra-articular, periarticular, peritendinous, epidural, intradermal or inhalation routes.

Topical preparations when used for auricular, buccal, dermatological (including iontophoresis/phonophoresis), gingival, nasal, ophthalmic and perianal disorders are not prohibited and require neither a TUE nor a declaration of use.

Of course, the interpretation of analysed urine samples showing the presence of glucocorticoids is complicated by this mix of regulations. A low concentration of such a steroid could be due to legitimate use of small amounts of the drug to treat asthma or eczema but could, equally, be due to the use of a larger quantity at an earlier point in time.

WADA data for 2005, 2006, 2007 and 2008 show 325, 282, 288 and 316 instances of glucocorticosteroid detection, respectively. Of all drug detection, this represents 7.6, 6.5, 5.9 and 5.7 per cent, respectively, and in the most recent (2008) data set this category of drugs was the sixth most-reported class category. However, it should be noted that these figures include samples from athletes who had been granted TUEs.

15.6   References

Arlettaz, A., Collomp, K., Portier, H. *et al.* (2008). Effects of acute prednisolone administration on exercise endurance and metabolism. *British Journal of Sports Medicine* **42**, 250–254.

Bullock, G.J., Carter, E.E., Elliott P. *et al.* (1971). Relative changes in the function of muscle ribosomes, and mitochondria during the early phase of steroid-induced catabolism. *Biochemical Journal* **127**, 881–892.

Carlsen, K.H., Anderson, S.D., Bjermer, L. *et al.* (2008). Treatment of exercise-induced asthma, respiratory and allergic disorders in sports and the relationship to doping: Part II of the report from the Joint Task Force of European Respiratory Society (ERS) and European Academy of Allergy and Clinical Immunology (EAACI) in cooperation with GA^{2}LEN. *Allergy* **63**, 492–505.

Hench, P.S., Kendall, E.C., Slocumb, C.H. *et al.* (1949). The effect of a hormone of the adrenal cortex (17-hydroxy-11-dehydrocorticosterone: compound E) and of pituitary adrenocorticotropic hormone on rheumatoid arthritis. *Proceedings of staff meetings at the Mayo Clinic* **24**, 181–197.

Nichols, A.W. (2005). Complications associated with the use of corticosteroids in the treatment of athletic injuries. *Clinical Journal of Sports Medicine* **15(5)**, 370–375.

Soetens, E., De Meirleir, K., and Hueting, J. (1995). No influence of ACTH on maximal performance. *Psychopharmacology* **118**, 260–266.

World Anti-Doping Agency (WADA). Laboratory statistics. Available at http://www.wada-ama.org/en/dynamic.ch2?pageCategory.id=335 (accessed October 2009).

Chapter 16

Alcohol

Thomas Reilly

16.1 Introduction

Throughout civilisation and up to the present day human ingenuity has found various ways of coping with the stresses of daily life. Sometime these methods include a drug-induced escape into an illusory world to eschew temporary troubles. Fermented beverages were used in ancient Egypt and in China. Alcohol can bring a transient euphoric uplift from pressing matters of the day. These strategies are perhaps truer today than they were in historic Dionysian cultures, exceptions being those countries where alcohol is taboo for religious reasons. Stress-induced illness is not just a phenomenon of contemporary urban civilization, as heavy consumption of alcohol is also found in rural communities.

Amongst athletes, participation in sports brings its own unique form of stress, not only before important contests but also due to frequent competitive events. Though a certain amount of pre-competition anxiety is inevitable, the anxiety response varies enormously between individuals, with some people coping extremely poorly. Many find their own solutions to attenuate anxiety levels, without exogenous aids. Anxiety may adversely affect performance, especially in activities highly demanding of mental concentration and steadiness of limbs. This likely impairment has prompted the use of anti-anxiety drugs, although some are not permitted in many sports.

Those individuals who can tolerate competitive stress still need to relax following competition or at times of a series of important competitions. The same applies to athletes in team sports gathered together in training camps for a sustained period. In these cases drinking alcohol is a frequent method of facilitating relaxation among athletes. The practice is sometimes condoned by the team's management as a means of "bonding" among the players. Alcohol use is more prevalent among participants in team sports than in non-participants in American school populations (Garry and Morrissey, 2000). Sports such as Rugby Union have a convention of drinking alcohol after matches between club teams. Indeed, victories are celebrated and defeats accepted by post-event drinking in many sports. Advertisements for alcohol appear at sports facilities and drinking is promoted by sponsorship of sports events by various breweries. Bar-room sports such as billiards, darts and snooker take place on licenced premises and drinking

Table 16.1 Alcohol and energy content of different beverages

I litre beer
~ 40 g alcohol
280 kcal (1172 kJ)
I litre bottle of wine
~ 120 g alcohol
840 kcal (3516 kJ)
I litre whiskey
~ 400 g alcohol
2800 kcal (11721 kJ)

alcohol is a feature of the sport for both participants and spectators. Furthermore, sports participants at all levels are social beings and drinking in social settings facilitates interactions among individuals.

Among the general population of adults aged 19–64 in the United Kingdom, the contribution of alcoholic drinks to the total energy intake amounts to 8.1 per cent for men and 6.7 per cent for women (National Diet and Nutrition Survey, 2003). The survey indicated that 38 per cent of the men and 24 per cent of the women who drank alcohol were consuming amounts greater than the maximum recommended for safe drinking by the government's Department of Health. The guidelines represent 3–4 units (a unit corresponds to 8 g ethanol; see Table 16.1 for alcoholic content of different drinks) of alcohol per day for men and 2–3 units for women; the guidelines set down by the Department of Agriculture in the USA suggest lower amounts.

The association of alcohol with cancer is apparent at lower amounts than for cardiovascular disease. The World Cancer Research Fund has concluded that drinking more than two units a day increases the risk of bowel cancer by 20 per cent and liver cancer by 18 per cent. Alcoholism can result from chronic drinking, the number of dependents on alcohol in the country being estimated to be 1 in every 13 adults (Ibrahim and Gilvarry, 2005), a prevalence that places an enormous burden on healthcare services. The progression towards dependency is outlined in Table 16.2.

In this chapter the relationship between anxiety and sport performance is first explored. The next section concentrates on alcohol, its metabolism in the body and its effect on the central nervous system. Next, the interactions between alcohol and health are considered. Its impact on physiological responses to exercise and its uses in aiming sports (such as archery, billiards, darts, pistol shooting and snooker) are then examined. Finally, the relationships between alcohol and sports accidents are addressed.

16.2 Anxiety and performance

The psychological reaction to impending sports competition is variously referred to as anxiety, arousal, stress or activation. Though these concepts are not synonymous,

Table 16.2 Warning signs for alcohol abuse and dependency

- Drinking alone or secretively
- Using alcohol deliberately and repeatedly to perform or get through difficult situations
- Discomfort at social occasions where no alcohol is available
- Escalating alcohol consumption beyond an already-established drinking pattern
- Heavy consumption in risky situations – e.g. before driving
- Getting drunk regularly or more frequently than in the past
- Drinking in the morning or at unusual times

their relationships to performance have sufficient similarities to group them together for generic purposes. Anxiety suggests worry or emotional tension, arousal denotes a continuum from sleep to high excitement, stress implies an agent that induces strain in the organism and activation refers to the metabolic state in the "flight or fight" reaction. Irrespective of which concept is adopted, the effects of the biological responses on performance are generally assumed to fit an inverted-U curve. A moderate level of anxiety about a forthcoming activity is desirable to induce the right levels of harnessed motivation for action. The simpler the task the higher is the level of anxiety that can be tolerated before performance efficiency begins to fall (Figure 16.1).

Although the inverted-U model is somewhat simplistic, it does illustrate that over-anxiety has a detrimental effect on the physical and psychomotor elements that make up sports performance. In such instances anxiety-reducing strategies will have an ergogenic effect. The athlete or mentor may have to choose between mental relaxation techniques or drugs to alleviate anxiety. Where alcohol is used to reduce stress in over-anxious individuals, the benefits must be balanced against any adverse effects on physical and neuromotor performance that might be introduced.

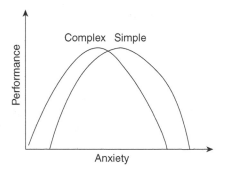

Figure 16.1 The relationship between level of anxiety and performance efficiency for simple and complex tasks.

There are various indices that the behavioural scientist employs in measuring anxiety in field conditions, such as sport, especially prior to competition. These include hand tremor, restlessness or other subjective estimates of "tension", paper and pencil tests and so on. Linked to these are physiological indices that demonstrate increased sympathetic tone. These measures include muscular tension as indicated by electromyography, tachycardia, galvanic skin response or skin conductance and elevated concentrations of stress hormones or their metabolites in blood or in urine. These variables may be important to consider if the mechanisms by which the ergogenic or adverse effects of anxiety-reducing agents operate are to be understood.

High levels of anxiety generally militate against performance and so favour attempts to reduce anxiety. Anxiety level depends very much on the nature of the sport as well as on the individual concerned. High anxiety is mostly associated with brief and high-risk activities. The highest anxiety responses before beginning an activity, as reflected in emotional tachycardia, show motor-racing, ski-jumping and downhill skiing to be at the top of the list (Reilly, 1997). Among soccer players, goalkeepers tend to be more anxious than outfield players because an error on their part is often punished by conceding a goal to the opposition. There is a habituation effect to stress in high-risk activities. Reilly et al. (1985) demonstrated a reduction in tachycardia with successive rides on an adventure park's acceleration track.

Avoiding over-anxiety may be important for game players for reasons of safety. Anxiety has been found to correlate with joint and muscle injuries in soccer; the more anxious players tend to get injured most often. This mechanism of injury proneness is probably lack of commitment or hesitancy in events such as tackling that might promote injury (Sanderson, 1981). The beneficial effects on inhibition might be countered by a more aggressive attitude in tackling. Traditionally, some soccer players used to take a nip of whisky immediately prior to going on to the pitch, the communal bottle being euphemistically referred to as "team spirit". The inhibiting effects of alcohol used to be exploited by tournament rugby players, not averse to drinking beer in between rounds of "rugby sevens" competitions, for example. Drinking the night before competing can have adverse consequences for performance due to the hangover effect the next day.

There is a thin line to tread between, on one hand, reducing anxiety to enhance well-being and mental states prior to competing and, on the other hand, impairing performance because of a disruption in motor co-ordination accompanying the treatment. The outcome depends on the concentrations of the drink, the timing of ingestion and individual susceptibility to it. Residual effects may carry over to the following day, affecting training or subsequent competitive performance. There are also possibilities of tolerance to the drug with chronic use or of drug dependence developing. These aspects are now considered in the context of alcohol in sport and exercise.

16.3   Metabolism of alcohol

The alcohols are a group of chemicals, most of which are toxic. The most common is ethanol or ethyl alcohol, which is obtained by the fermentation of sugar. It is non-toxic, except in large and chronic doses and has been enjoyed as a beverage for many centuries.

Ethyl alcohol is both a drug and a food, accounting for about 100 kcal (420 kJ) of energy per adult of the UK population each day. Its energy value per unit weight (kcal/g) is 7 compared with a value of 9 for fat but is higher than the value of 4 for both carbohydrates and protein. Wine contains about 12 per cent alcohol, and a litre bottle contains about 120 g with a calorific content of 840 kcal (3516 kJ). The value of alcohol as food is limited, because it is metabolized mainly in the liver and at a fixed rate of about 100 mg per kg body weight per hour. For a 70-kg individual this amounts to 7 g of alcohol hourly. The energy is not available to active skeletal muscle and consequently it is not possible to exercise oneself to sobriety. The diuretic effect of drinking beer makes it less than the ideal agent of rehydration after hard physical training.

Alcohol is a polar substance that is freely miscible in water. This property is due to the fact that alcohol molecules are held together by the same sort of intermolecular forces as water, namely hydrogen bonds. The alcohol molecule is also soluble in fat, is small and has a weak charge. (As the lipophilic alkyl group becomes larger and the hydrophilic group smaller, the alcohol molecules associate preferentially with other alcohol, hydrocarbon or lipid molecules rather than water.) The alcohol molecule easily penetrates biological membranes and can be absorbed unaltered from the stomach and more quickly from the small intestine. The rate of absorption is influenced by the amount of food in the stomach, whether there are gas molecules in the drink and the concentration of alcohol in the drink. Absorption is quickest if alcohol is drunk on an empty stomach, if gas molecules are present in the drink and if the alcohol content is high. Intense mental concentration, lowered body temperature and physical exercise tend to slow the rate of absorption.

From the gastrointestinal tract the alcohol is transported to the liver in the hepatic circulation. The activity of the enzyme alcohol dehydrogenase, present chiefly in the liver, governs the disappearance of alcohol from the body. In the liver, alcohol dehydrogenase converts the alcohol to acetaldehyde; it is then converted to acetic acid or acetate by aldehyde dehydrogenase. About 75 per cent of the alcohol taken up by the blood is released as acetate into the circulation. The acetate is then oxidized to carbon dioxide and water within the Krebs (or citric acid) cycle. An alternative metabolic route for acetate is its activation to acetyl co-enzyme A and further reactions to form fatty acids, ketone bodies, amino acids and steroids. Many of the effects of alcohol are related to the excess production of both NADH and acetaldehyde during these steps, acetaldehyde being thought mainly responsible for the adverse effects of alcohol.

Ethyl alcohol is distributed throughout the body by means of the circulatory system and enters all the body water pools and tissues, including within the central nervous system. Its distribution amongst the body fluids and tissues depends on several factors, such as blood flow, mass and permeability of the tissue. Organs such as the brain, lungs, liver and kidneys reach equilibrium quickly, whilst skeletal muscle with its relatively poorer blood supply attains its peak alcohol concentration more slowly. Initially, alcohol moves rapidly from blood into the tissues. When absorption is complete, arterial alcohol concentration falls and alcohol diffuses from the tissues into the capillary beds. This means that alcohol concentrations remain high in the peripheral venous blood due to the slower rates of metabolism and excretion.

The metabolism of alcohol in the liver is unaffected by its concentration in the blood. Some alcohol is eliminated in the breath, but this is usually less than 5 per cent of the total amount metabolized. This route is utilized in assessing safe levels for driving, forming the basis of the breathalyser tests. Small amounts of alcohol are excreted in urine and also in sweat if exercise is performed whilst drunk. Higher excretion rates through the lungs, urine and sweat are produced at high environmental temperatures and at high blood alcohol levels.

With a single drink the blood alcohol level usually peaks about 45 minutes after ingestion. This is the point where any influence on performance will be most evident. Effects on performance are generally greater on the ascending limb than for a corresponding value on the descending limb of the blood alcohol curve; the rate of change and the direction of change of the alcohol concentration in blood are more crucial factors than is the length of time alcohol is in the bloodstream. The peak is delayed about 15 minutes if strenuous exercise precedes ingestion due to the reduction in blood flow to the gut that accompanies exercise, the increased blood flow to skeletal muscle and the needs of the thermoregulatory system post-exercise.

Besides the exogenous ethanol in body fluids, trace amounts are synthesized endogenously. Endogenous ethanol is thought to arise both from bacterial fermentation in the gut and from the action of alcohol dehydrogenase on acetaldehyde derived from pyruvate. Blood levels of endogenous alcohol in humans are very low, ranging only up to about 7.5 mg in total.

Studies on alcohol and exercise are notoriously difficult to control, as most subjects will recognize the taste of the experimental treatment. Most experimenters use vodka in orange juice: the placebo can include enough vodka to taste but not enough to produce a measurable blood alcohol concentration. Another strategy is to put a noseclip on the subject, who is then given anaesthetic throat lozenges. Subjects vary in their responses to alcohol, as does the same subject from day to day, making inferences from laboratory studies tentative. As the effects of alcohol differ with body size, dosage is usually administered according to body weight. Effects also vary with the level of blood alcohol induced, but there is not general international agreement on acceptable maximum levels for day-to-day activities such as driving. Alcohol doses that render subjects intoxicated or drunk have little practical relevance in exercise studies and so experimental levels are usually low to moderate. Additionally, experiments that entail alcohol ingestion should be approved by the local human ethics committee, and high alcohol dosages are unlikely to gain acceptance in experimental protocols where ensuring the safety of participants until they become sober again is important.

16.4   Action of alcohol on the nervous system

The effects of ethanol administration on central nervous tissue are due to direct action rather than to acetaldehyde, its first breakdown product. Following ethanol ingestion, very little acetaldehyde crosses the blood-brain barrier, despite elevated levels in the blood. Alcohol has a general effect on neural transmission by influencing axonal membranes and slowing nerve conductance. The permeability of the axonal membrane to potassium and sodium is altered by the lowering of central calcium levels that results from ingesting alcohol (Wesnes and Warburton, 1983). Alcohol has differential effects on the central neurotransmitters, acetylcholine, serotonin, noradrenaline and dopamine.

Alcohol blocks the release of acetylcholine and disrupts its synthesis. As a result, transmission in the central cholinergic pathways will be lowered. The ascending reticular cholinergic pathway determines the level of cortical arousal and the flow of sensory information to be evaluated by the cortex. The lowering of electro-cortical arousal reduces the awareness of stressful information and the ability of the individual to attend to specific stimuli. These de-arousing changes are reflected in alterations in the electroencephalogram with moderate to large doses of alcohol. Consequences include impairments in concentration, attention, simple and complex reaction times, skilled performance and, eventually, short-term memory.

Alcohol decreases serotonin turnover in the central nervous system by inhibiting tryptophan hydroxylase, the enzyme essential for serotonin's biosynthesis. Activity in the neurones of serotonergic pathways is important for the experience of anxiety; output of corticosteroid hormones from the adrenal cortex increases the activity in these neurones. Alcohol has an opposing action and so may reduce the tension that is felt by the individual in a stressful situation.

Alcohol can increase activity in central noradrenergic pathways. This is transient and is followed, some hours later, by a decrease in activity. Catecholaminergic pathways are implicated in the control of mood states; activation of these pathways promotes happy and merry states. The fall in noradrenaline turnover as the blood alcohol concentration drops ties in with the reversal of mood that follows the initial drunken euphoric state. This is exacerbated by large doses of alcohol as these tend to give rise to depression.

The small alcohol molecules penetrating the blood-brain barrier stimulate the brain to release dopamine. Dopamine is regarded as a pleasure-related hormone and its release is triggered in the limbic system. Stimulation of sweat glands also affects the limbic system whilst cerebral cortical activity is depressed.

Pain sensors are numbed and later the cerebellum is affected, causing difficulty with balance. The reduction of pain was the reason for the classical use of alcohol as an anaesthetic in field conditions.

Alcohol also affects cerebral energy metabolism by increasing glucose utilisation in the brain. Because glucose is the main substrate furnishing energy for nerve cells, the result is that the lowered glucose level may induce mental fatigue. This will be reflected in declines in cognitive functions, mental concentration and information processing. It is unlikely that exercise, per se, will offset these effects.

The disruption of acetylcholine synthesis and release means that alcohol acts as a depressant, exerting its effect on the reticular activating system, whose activity represents the level of physiological arousal. It also has a depressant effect on the cortex. Alcohol first affects the reasoning centres in the frontal lobes and sedates inhibitory nerves; at higher levels of blood alcohol, the centres for speech, vision and motor control are affected and eventually awareness is lost. In smaller doses it inhibits cerebral control mechanisms, freeing the brain from its normal inhibition. This release of inhibition has been blamed for aggressive and violent conduct of individuals behaving out of character when under the influence of alcohol. Alcohol has been a factor in crowd violence and football hooliganism on the terraces in many countries. The association led to the banning of alcohol at football and cricket grounds in Britain in the mid-1980s. These restrictions were extended to other sporting events in the years that followed.

The deleterious effects of alcohol on the nervous system will have consequences for athletes in sports that require fast reactions, complex decision making and highly skilled performance. Alcohol also impacts hand-eye coordination; tracking tasks, such as driving; and vigilance tasks such as long-distance sailing. An effect on tracking tasks is that control movements lose their normal smoothness and precision and become more abrupt or jerky. In vigilance tasks, some studies have shown a deterioration in performance with time on task (Tong et al., 1980). At high doses of alcohol, meaningful sport becomes impractical or even dangerous. Progressive effects of alcohol at different blood alcohol concentrations are summarized in Table 16.3. An important effect of alcohol, not listed, is that it diminishes the ability to process appreciable amounts of information arriving simultaneously from two different sources.

The most frequently cited study that reported facilitatory effects of alcohol on human performance was the classical experiment of Ikai and Steinhaus (1961). They showed that in some cases moderate alcohol doses could improve isometric muscular strength. This result was similar to that obtained by cheering and loud vocal encouragement. They explained the effect on the basis of central inhibition of the impulse traffic in the nerve fibres of the skeletal muscles during maximal effort. This depression of the inhibitory effect of certain centres in the central nervous system may allow routine practices to proceed normally without any disturbing effects. This finding has not generally been replicated when other aspects of muscular performance are considered.

Table 16.3 Demonstrable effects of alcohol at different blood alcohol concentrations

Concentration level (mg/100 ml blood)	Effects
30 (0.03 per cent)	Enhanced sense of well-being; retarded simple reaction time; impaired hand-eye coordination
60 (0.06 per cent)	Mild loss of social inhibition; impaired judgement
90 (0.09 per cent)	Marked loss of social inhibition; coordination reduced; noticeably "under the influence"
120 (0.12 per cent)	Apparent clumsiness; loss of physical control; tendency towards extreme responses; definite drunkenness is noted
150 (0.15 per cent)	Erratic behaviour; slurred speech; staggering gait
180 (0.18 per cent)	Loss of control of voluntary activity; impaired vision

16.5   Alcohol and health

The effects of alcohol on health are usually viewed in terms of chronic alcoholism. Persistent drinking leads to addiction. Most physicians emphasize that alcoholism is a disease or a behavioural disorder rather than a vice, and devise therapy accordingly. The result of excessive drinking is ultimately manifested in liver disease: cirrhosis, a serious hardening and degeneration of liver tissue, is fatal for many heavy drinkers. Cancer is also more likely to develop in a cirrhotic liver. There is evidence of increased susceptibility to breast cancer in women who drink alcohol regularly (Willett et al., 1987). Cancers of the bowel, pharynx, larynx and oesophagus have also been linked to alcohol consumption. Cardiomyopathy, or damage to the heart muscle, can result from years of heavy drinking. Other pathological conditions associated with alcohol abuse include generalized skeletal myopathy and pancreatitis. Impairment of brain function also occurs, with alcoholic psychoses being a common cause of hospitalization in psychiatric wards.

Alcohol was formerly used as an anaesthetic until it was realized that it was too dangerous to supply in large quantities for that purpose. The result of applying alcohol to living cells is that the protoplasm of the cells precipitates due to dehydration. Long-term damage to tissue in the central nervous system may be an unwanted outcome of habitual heavy drinking. There are also potentially fatal consequences of "binge" drinking where excessive amounts of alcohol are drunk in one session.

Heavy drinking is not compatible with serious athletics. For the athlete, drinking is usually done only in moderation, an infrequent respite from the ascetic regimens of physical training, though the odd end-of-season binge may be customary. Nevertheless, drinking is a social convention in many sports, such as rugby, squash and water polo, where there may be peer-group pressure to drink alcohol following training or competition or at club social functions. Indeed, a few high-profile footballers in the English Premier league in the late 1990s admitted to an alcohol addiction. The sensible athlete drinks moderately and occasionally, avoiding alcohol for at least 24 hours before competing. Hangovers may persist for a day and disturb concentration in sports involving complex skills. The attitude of the retired athlete may be very different. If his or her active career is terminated abruptly and the free time that retirement releases is taken up by social drinking, the result may well be a gradual deterioration in physical condition, with body weight increasing and fitness declining. In this context, the effect of alcohol on the ex-athlete may be quite harmful.

Various institutions within sports medicine have addressed the problems of alcohol and exercise. In 1982 the American College of Sports Medicine set out a position statement on alcohol, which was unequivocally against any indulgence. It underlined the adverse effects of alcohol on health and condemned the use of alcohol by athletes. Its estimate was that there were 10 million adult problem drinkers in the United States and an additional 3.3 million in its 14- to 17-year-old age group. No evidence for any potentially beneficial aspects of alcohol was mentioned.

Alcohol use modulates the immune system and impairs host defence mechanisms. Van der Horst Graat et al. (2007) reported an association between alcohol intake and frequency of respiratory infections in apparently healthy elderly people. Alcohol taken with a meal increases post-prandial lipaemia, an effect that is the opposite of response to exercise. The suppression of fat oxidation would increase the propensity for weight gain and increased abdominal adiposity (Suter and Schutz, 2008). Alcohol may impair absorption of minerals and vitamins. Vitamin D was deficient in 90 per cent of the men and 76 per cent of the female alcoholics studied by Malik et al. (2008): the link between alcohol consumption and osteoporosis was more evident in men, because raised levels of oestradiol provided a degree of protection for women. Alcohol decreases resting levels of testosterone and cortisol; it also blunts the cortisol and growth hormone responses to submaximal exercise, factors that could impair performance. It also causes alterations in oxytoxin and prolactin among women, which parallel the feelings of drunkenness induced (Mennella and Pepino, 2006).

Despite these adverse effects, there is a belief that moderate drinking has some positive benefits for health. Small amounts increase the flow of gastric juices and thereby stimulate digestion: in large doses, alcohol irritates the stomach lining, causing gastritis and even vomiting of blood. A national survey of lifestyles in England and Wales provided support for the view that healthy people tended to drink a little. Amongst men under 60, the likelihood of high blood pressure was found to increase with the amount of alcohol consumed. For older men and for women, light drinking was associated with lower blood pressure, even when effects due to body weight were taken into account (Stepney, 1987).

It is thought also that moderate drinking provides a degree of protection against coronary heart disease. This belief may have been nurtured originally in the vineyards of France where a habitually modest consumption of wine is associated with a low incidence of heart disease. Myocardial infarction rates were found to be lower in moderate drinkers than in non-drinkers (Willett *et al.*, 1980). Goldberg *et al.* (2001) reported a 25–40 per cent reduction in risk of cardiovascular events when moderate amounts of alcohol were consumed. In a prospective cohort study over 20 years in Denmark, Pedersen *et al.* (2008) showed that engaging in physical activity was linked to a 25–30 per cent decrease in risk of death from heart disease; moderate alcohol intake was also linked to a smaller reduction, with the risk of death from heart disease reduced by 17 per cent in men and 24 per cent in women. High-density lipoprotein particles remove cholesterol from the tissues and transfer it into other particles in the blood; low-density lipoprotein, on the other hand, obtains its cholesterol from these other particles and transfers it to the tissues. A high ratio of high-density to low-density lipoprotein fractions is found in well-trained endurance athletes, a low ratio being indicative of poor cardiovascular health. The effect is apparent in autopsies of alcoholics whose blood vessels are in good condition despite pathological changes in other tissues. The mechanism by which alcohol raises the high-density lipoprotein cholesterol has not been fully explained. Other possible mechanisms are a reduction in hypertension induced by the feeling of freedom from stress. Moderate alcohol consumption may also help haemostasis by balancing the processes of coagulation and fibrinolysis. Inflammatory biomarkers may provide another mechanism. Wang *et al.* (2008) reported a positive effect of moderate alcohol consumption on high-sensitivity c-reactive protein and fibrinogen.

For a healthy athlete in a good state of training, occasional moderate drinking will have little adverse effect. It is important to emphasize that any such occasional bouts of drinking should be restrained and should follow rather than precede training sessions, whose training stimulus is likely to be lowered by the soporific influence of drinking alcohol before strenuous exercise.

16.6   Alcohol and physiological responses to exercise

Alcohol ingestion lowers muscle glycogen at rest compared with control conditions. As pre-start glycogen levels are important for sustained exercise at an intensity of about 70–80 per cent VO_{2max}, such as marathon running, taking alcohol in the 24 hours before such endurance activities is ill-advised. Effects of alcohol on the metabolic responses to submaximal exercise seem to be small. Alcohol does not impair lipolysis or free fatty acid utilization during exercise but may decrease splanchnic glucose output, decrease the potential contribution of energy from liver gluconeogenesis, cause a more pronounced decline in blood glucose levels and decrease the leg muscle uptake of glucose towards the end of a prolonged (up to three-hour) run (Juhlin-Dannfelt *et al.*, 1977). The impairment in glucose production by the liver would lead to an increased likelihood of developing hypoglycaemia during prolonged exercise.

Some studies have shown an increase in oxygen uptake (VO_2) at a fixed submaximal exercise intensity after alcohol ingestion. This may be due to a poorer co-ordination of the active muscles as the decrease in mechanical efficiency, implied by the elevation in VO_2, is not a consistent finding. Related to this is an increase in blood lactate levels with alcohol; metabolism of alcohol shunts lactate away from the gluconeogenic pathway and leads to an increase in the ratio of lactate to pyruvate. The elevated blood lactate concentrations during exercise, after taking alcohol, may reflect impairment in clearance of lactate as well as an increase in production by the exercising muscles. A failure to clear lactate would militate against performance of strenuous exercise.

Alcohol does not seem to have adverse effects on maximum oxygen consumption (VO_{2max}) or on metabolic responses to high-intensity exercise approaching VO_{2max} levels. At high doses (up to 200 mg per cent, i.e 0.20 per cent blood alcohol level) athletes may feel disinclined towards maximal efforts that elicit VO_{2max} values and a reduction in peak VE is usually observed (Blomqvist *et al.*, 1970). Similarly, they may be poorly motivated to sustain high-intensity exercise for as long as they would normally do. In middle-distance running events with an appreciable aerobic component, performance was found to be detrimentally affected in a dose-related manner, with increasing blood alcohol concentration (BAC) levels from 0.01 to 0.10 per cent (McNaughton and Preece, 1986).

Impairment in carbohydrate synthesis post-exercise would delay the restoration of muscle glycogen stores and adversely affect endurance performance. Burke *et al.* (2003) showed that alcohol delayed glycogen re-synthesis the day following strenuous exercise but not when carbohydrate intake was high. The variability in individual responses and the relatively high energy content of alcohol suggest that some athletes may not restore their liver and muscle glycogen depots as a result of consuming alcohol following competitions. Alcohol consumed post-match can account for up to 9.6 per cent of the total energy intake for the day of competition in some Premier League soccer players, with alcohol being consumed on only one other day of the week (Reilly, 1994). Maughan (1997) reported an individual value that exceeded 10 per cent of total energy intake in a Scottish Premier League player, although many of the players studied eschewed alcohol and average consumption in the first team of two clubs was 2–3 per cent of total energy intake. The pattern of drinking is broadly analogous to binge drinking displayed by young adults.

Although it has not been shown conclusively that alcohol alters VE (minute ventilation), stroke volume and muscle blood flow at submaximal exercise levels, it does decrease peripheral vascular resistance. This response is because of the vasodilatory effect of alcohol on the peripheral blood vessels, which would increase heat loss from the surface of the skin and cause a drop in body temperature. This consequence would be dangerous if alcohol is taken in conjunction with exercise in cold conditions. Sampling whisky on the ski slopes may bring an immediate feeling of warmth but its disturbance of normal thermoregulation may put the recreational skier at risk of hypothermia. Frost-bitten mountaineers especially should avoid drinking alcohol as the peripheral vasodilation it induces would cause the body temperature to fall further. In hot conditions, alcohol is also inadvisable as it acts as a diuretic and would exacerbate problems of dehydration.

Studies of maximum muscular strength, in the main, show no influence of moderate to medium doses of alcohol on maximum isometric force. Similar results apply to dynamic functions, such as peak torque measured on isokinetic dynamometers. Muscular endurance is generally assessed by requiring the subject to hold a fixed percentage of maximum for as long as possible. Here, too, the influences of moderate alcohol doses are generally found to be non-significant. This may be because the tests represent gross aspects of muscular function and, as such, are insensitive to the effects of the drug.

16.7   Alcohol in aiming sports

In aiming sports, a steady limb is needed to provide a firm platform for launching the missile at its target or to keep the weapon still. Two pistol shooters were disqualified during the 1980 Olympics due to taking alcohol in an attempt to improve their performance. There are also aiming components in sports such as fencing and modern pentathlon, especially in the rifle-shooting discipline of the latter. In some of these sports alcohol levels are now officially monitored, whilst in others, notably darts, drinking is a conventional complement of the sport itself.

The Grand National Archery Society in the UK has not banned the use of alcohol in its competitions, and so alcohol is taken in small doses in the belief that it relaxes the archer, thereby steadying the hands as well as the nerves. In order to avoid fluctuating blood alcohol concentrations, the archer, like the dart thrower, tries to keep topping up the levels to prevent reaching the descending limb of the curve.

To understand how alcohol might affect the archer, it is useful to look at the task *in toto*. The competitive player has to shoot three dozen arrows at a target placed up to 90 m away. Technological improvements in bow design have helped to produce outstanding scores, leaving the gap to perfection solely due to human factors. The modern bow has two slot-in limbs that insert into a magnesium handle section and stabilizers that help to minimize vibration and turning of the bow. Muscle strength is needed to draw the bow, whilst muscle endurance is required to hold it steady, usually for about eight seconds for each shot, while the sight is being aligned with the target. Deflection of the arrow tip by 0.02 mm at 90 m causes the arrow to miss the target, which gives some idea of the hand steadiness required. The archer, before release (or loose), pulls the arrow towards and through the clicker (a blade on the side of the bow which aids in measuring draw length). The archer reacts to the sound of the clicker hitting the side of the bow handle by releasing the string, which, in effect, shoots the arrow. Archers are coached to react to the clicker by allowing the muscles to relax; a slow reaction to the clicker is generally recognized as hesitation. This affects the smoothness of the loose and is reflected in muscle tremor, causing a "snatched loose". For these reasons, the effects of alcohol on reaction time, arm steadiness, muscle strength and endurance, and the electromyogram of one of the arm muscles were selected as appropriate parameters to study under experimental conditions (Reilly and Halliday, 1985).

Nine subjects underwent a battery of tests under four conditions: sober, placebo, 0.02 per cent blood alcohol level and 0.05 per cent blood alcohol level. The alcohol doses were administered in three equal volumes to total 500 ml over 15 minutes, 45 minutes being allowed for peak blood alcohol levels to be attained. The doses to elicit the desirable blood alcohol levels were calculated according to the formula of Hicks (1976), which was shown to be effective:

$$A = \frac{(454)(W)(R)(BAC + 0.0002)}{(0.8)(0.95)}$$

where
- A = ml 95 per cent ethanol
- W = body weight (lb)
- R = distribution coefficient of 0.765
- BAC = desired blood alcohol concentration (0.05 per cent = 0.0005)

The results for the performance measurement appear in Table 16.4 and the main observations are summarised in Table 16.5.

Alcohol had no effect on the muscular strength and muscular endurance measures; the holding time in the endurance test was about the same time as the archer normally holds the bow drawn before shooting, so that this test turned out to be reasonably realistic. Reaction time was significantly slowed by the lower

Table 16.4 Effects of alcohol treatments on four experimental tests (mean ± S.D.) (from Reilly and Halliday, 1985)

Variables	Sober	Placebo	0.02% BAC	0.05% BAC
Arm steadiness:				
Time-off-target(s)	2.64 ± 0.89	3.05 ± 0.74	3.24 ± 1.01	8.17 ± 1.49
Isometric strength(N)	546 ± 48	560 ± 37	541 ± 56	523 ± 78
Muscular endurance(s)	11.4 ± 2.1	12.0 ± 2.5	12.0 ± 2.0	10.8 ± 2.0
Reaction time (ms)	211 ± 6.5	209 ± 8.5	223 ± 9.6	226 ± 11.2

Table 16.5 The main observations on the effects of alcohol doses on tasks related to archery

1. Holding time pre-loose was extended and a clearer loose was found at the moderate BAC treatment.
2. Muscle activity was elevated post-loose at high BAC, though tremor pre-loose was reduced at both BAC values.
3. Deleterious effects of alcohol were most pronounced in arm steadiness at the higher level of BAC induced.
4. Significant slowing of RT was produced by moderate doses of alcohol.
5. Alcohol had no appreciable effect on muscle strength or muscular endurance.
6. Alcohol has differential effects on tasks related to archery, depending on the concentrations, the criteria and the subjects.

alcohol dose, a further small delay occurring at the higher blood alcohol dose. The more sensitive response of auditory reaction time to alcohol would mean, in practice, a slower reaction to the clicker and a faulty loose. Another adverse effect noted was the impairment in steadiness of the extended arm. Performance was degraded, especially at the 0.05 per cent level, and the variability in arm steadiness also increased with alcohol. This effect contradicts the conventional wisdom in archery and may have been due to the high load on the arm muscles when holding the bow drawn. It is possible that alcohol only operates to advantage in steadying the limb in contexts more competitive than laboratory experiments.

Some benefits were noted in the electromyographic profile (Figure 16.2). A clearer loose was observed at the low alcohol levels, which would be valuable in promoting a smoother release. This positive effect was supplemented by a tendency towards a reduced tremor in the muscle with both alcohol treatments. Together, these effects would indicate a greater muscle relaxation, tremor being normally associated with a snatched loose. These factors were partly offset by the longer holding time prior to loose induced by the alcohol treatments. The overall conclusion was that alcohol has differential effects on tasks related to archery, depending on the concentrations, the components of the performance analysed and individual reactivity to the drug.

The deleterious effects of alcohol on some aspects of archery would not apply to other aiming sports, such as darts and pistol shooting. In these the loading on the arm muscles is light, so a greater arm steadiness is likely to be induced by the drug. Another consideration is that the timing of the release is at the discretion of the subject and also is unaffected by a retarded reaction time. Reactions will have importance where the target is moving: it is noteworthy that the discipline of clay-pigeon shooting, for example, is not steeped in a history of alcohol use.

Bar-room sports, such as snooker, billiards and darts, have the alcohol industry as an adjunct to their matches. At the highest level of competition these sports are popular television spectacles. Although it is widely thought that the top

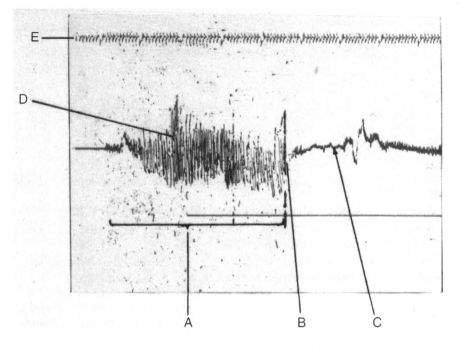

Figure 16.2 The electromyographic profile of an arm muscle whilst holding the bow down: (a) holding time; (b) the point of loose; (c) post-loose muscular activity; (d) tremor; (e) the time-scale of events marked in 100 ms.

performers swig large quantities of alcohol, this is not the case. Imbibition is regular but in small doses so that a moderate blood alcohol level is continually maintained (needless to say, at high blood alcohol levels, 0.15 per cent or more, whole-body stability and mental concentration would be degraded and any possible erogenic effect would be swamped).

A study of the effects of elevating blood alcohol levels on tasks related to dart throwing (Reilly and Scott, 1993) confirmed the finding in archery. Whilst there were negative effects from the light blood alcohol concentration (BAC 0.02 per cent) on hand-eye coordination, effects were positive for balance and dart-throwing score. A higher level of 0.05 per cent led to a fall-off in performance on all tasks. Results indicated some improvement with a light dose of alcohol for dart throwers, but performance deteriorated when BAC levels reached 0.05 per cent.

In some sports beta blockers have replaced alcohol to counter the unwanted effects of stress on performance. In a study of beta blockers in the British national pistol shooting squad, Antal and Good (1980) found significant improvement in shooting scores was restricted to the slow-fire events. The ergogenic effect of 80 mg of oxprenolol was slightly greater than for a 40-mg dose. The effect of 40 mg of oxprenolol was matched by an effect of alcohol equivalent to a half-pint

(284 ml) of beer (S'Jongers *et al.*, 1978). A substantial placebo effect applied equally to alcohol and beta blockers.

In those sports that discourage alcohol for competition, there is a disharmony in standards for what constitutes legality. (Alcohol is banned in several sports, for example, modern pentathlon [shooting events], archery and aeronautics.) The legal limit for driving differs between countries: in Norway and Greece the limit is 50 mg/100 ml, in Ireland it is twice that level. In the UK, France and Germany the safety limit is intermediate at 80 mg/100 ml. In Sweden the legal limit is 20 mg/100 ml, whilst in Turkey any measurable alcohol level is illegal. These values refer to alcohol in blood: the corresponding (to 80 mg/100 ml) levels for breath and for urine are 35 mg/100 ml and 107 mg/100 ml, respectively. The Amateur Fencing Association in Britain adopted the Norwegian value as its limit for competition and incorporated dope testing at its contests since 1984. At the request of the international governing body for fencing, alcohol tests have been carried out at the Olympic Games, although it is generally accepted that alcohol abuse is not a major problem in this sport.

Testing for alcohol is also performed on competitors in the shooting event of the modern pentathlon. Here, participants are disadvantaged by any tremor in settling down to prepare for taking their shots. Although alcohol might help competitors to relax whilst taking aim, it has little ergogenic benefit in the other disciplines of the pentathlon. For various reasons, tranquillizers and beta-blocking agents have been preferred.

16.8   Alcohol and sports accidents

It has been recommended that alcohol should be outlawed prior to aquatic activities because of the potential for catastrophic accidents in the water. Alcohol is a significant factor in spinal injuries occurring in recreational water sports. In scuba diving the potential for fatal nitrogen narcosis increases at shallower depths when alcohol is consumed. Of 752 drowning victims studied in North Carolina, 53 per cent were positive for alcohol and 38 per cent had blood alcohol values of 0.10 per cent or greater (see Reilly, 1997). In their review of alcohol-related drowning in recreational boating, Driscoll *et al.* (2004) concluded that a blood alcohol level of 0.10 g/100 ml increased the risk of fatality tenfold compared with no alcohol.

Peak effects on motor performance following administration of alcohol are typically observed 45–60 min later but impairment is evident for up to three hours after dosing (Kelly *et al.*, 1993). This could render the drinker susceptible to accidents if alcohol is imbibed after sports competitions before driving the journey home. Even at blood alcohol concentrations within the legal limit (about 0.03 per cent), accident risk is increased when driving after sleep restricted to four hours the previous night (Vakulin *et al.*, 2007) or after a prolonged period (18–21 hours) awake (Howard *et al.*, 2007).

There is evidence also of impaired exercise performance the morning after a bout of nocturnal drinking, adverse effects being observed in aerobic performance (O'Brien, 1993). This finding has implications for the behaviour of players the night before either competition or serious training. The subjective symptoms of hangover are attributed to a combination of factors that include dehydration, acid-base disturbances, disruption of cytokine and prostaglandin pathways and alterations in glucose metabolism (Maughan, 2006).

Alcohol can compound the hangover effects of some sleeping tablets and is likely to disturb complex skills more than simpler motor tasks performed on the morning of the next day (Kunsman et al., 1992). Attention and reaction time tasks were impaired by concentrations of temazepam and ethanol in combinations that alone did not cause decrements in performance. Subjects tend to be unaware of their reduced performance capabilities when taking these drugs in combination, a factor likely to increase injury risk. Of 402 victims of ski accidents, 20 per cent were positive for alcohol, 8.5 per cent had taken benzodiazepines and 2.5 per cent were positive for both drugs. Subjects positive for both drugs tended to be older than the other accident victims (Barnas et al., 1992). There is also a diurnal variation in the effects of alcohol, as drinking at lunch time has a more detrimental effect on psychomotor performance than alcohol taken in the evening (Horne and Gibbons, 1991). Consequently recreational skiers place themselves at increased risk of injury by drinking at lunch time rather than solely après ski.

16.9   Overview

Stress and anxiety are inescapable corollaries of contemporary professional activities and participation in top-level sport. Indeed, a high degree of competitiveness seems to be a prerequisite for success in both spheres, and those without the essential coping mechanism fail to climb to the top of the ladder. The relationship between sport and anxiety is paradoxical because sport, as a recreational activity, offers release from occupational cares, whilst at a highly competitive level it becomes a strong stressor. Indeed, exercise is effective therapy for highly anxious individuals, and behaviour modification strategies, either as a replacement for or complement to anti-anxiety drugs, are common in treating anxiety in competitive sports contexts. Where alcohol is used for relaxation purposes and eventually habitual use leads to addiction in active or retired athletes, the health of the individual becomes a major concern. Behaviour modification methods have a role in correcting the abuse here also and a 12-week progamme of aerobic exercise at moderate intensity has been claimed to be an important adjunct intervention for alcohol-dependent patients (Brown et al., 2009).

In recent decades, sports officials and governing bodies in sport have assumed increasing responsibility for attempts to eliminate the use of drugs for ergogenic purposes. The process of adding new pharmacological products to the list of banned substances is likely to continue despite ongoing attempts by some practitioners prepared to grasp at any means of improving their performances. The risks and benefits of anti-anxiety drugs demonstrate that regulations for their use in sport must be set down with care and circumspection. Legislation must ensure that, for the sport in question, participants especially prone to anxiety are not endangered by being deprived of their genuine prescriptions, whilst at the same time allowing fair competition to all entries. Alcohol is the most abused drug in society at large and athletes are not immune to the social conventions of using alcohol to relax and reduce stress. Alcohol is used as an ergogenic aid in a limited number of sports but its use in social contexts is pervasive. Its acute and chronic effects have implications for the health of the nation and for the health of the individuals who drink it.

16.10   References

Antal, L.C. and Good, C.S. (1980). Effects of oxprenolol on pistol shooting under stress. *The Practitioner* **224**, 755–760.

Barnas, L., Miller, G.H., Sperner, G. *et al.* (1992). The effects of alcohol and benzodiazepines on the severity of ski accidents. *Acta Psychiatry Scandinavia* **86**, 296–300.

Blomqvist, G., Saltin, B. and Mitchell, J. (1970). Acute effects of ethanol ingestion on the response to submaximal and maximal exercise in man. *Circulation* **62**, 463–470.

Brown, R.A., Abrantes, A.M., Read, J.P. *et al.* (2009). Aerobic exercise for alcohol recovery: Rationale, programme description and preliminary findings. *Behavioural Modification*, **33**, 220–249.

Burke, L.M., Collier, G.R., Broad, E.M. *et al.* (2003). Effect of alcohol intake on muscle glycogen storage after prolonged exercise. *Journal of Applied Physiology* **95**, 983–990.

Driscoll, T., Harrison, J. and Steenkamp, M. (2004). Review of the role of alcohol in drowning associated with recreational aquatic activity. *Injury Preview* **10**, 107–113.

Garry, J.P. and Morrissey, S.L. (2000). Team sports participation and risk-taking behaviours among a biracial middle school population. *Clinical Journal of Sports Medicine* **10**, 185–190.

Goldberg, I.J., Mosca, L., Piano, M.R. *et al.* (2001). AHA science advisory: Wine and your heart. *Circulation* **103**, 472–475.

Hicks, J.A. (1976). An evaluation of the effect of sign brightness and the sign reading behaviour of alcohol impaired drivers. *Human Factors* **18**, 45–52.

Horne, J.A. and Gibbons, H. (1991). Effects on vigilance performance and sleepiness of alcohol given in the early afternoon (post lunch) vs. early evening. *Ergonomics* **34**, 67–77.

Howard, M.E., Jackson, M.L., Kennedy, G.A., *et al.* (2007). The interaction effects of extended wakefulness and low-dose alcohol on simulated driving and vigilance. *Sleep* **30**, 1334–1340.

Ibrahim, F. and Gilvarry, E. (2005). Alcohol dependence and treatment strategies. *British Journal of Hospital Medicine* **66**, 462–465.

Ikai, M. and Steinhaus, A.H. (1961). Some factors modifying the expression of human strength. *Journal of Applied Physiology* **16**, 157–161.

Juhlin-Dannfelt, A., Ahlberg, G., Hagenfelt, L. *et al.* (1977). Influence of ethanol on splanchnic and skeletal muscle substrate turnover during prolonged exercise in man. *American Journal of Physiology* **233**, E195–E202.

Kelly, T.H., Fultin., R.W., Emurian, C.S. *et al.* (1993). Performance based testing for drugs of abuse: Dose and time profiles of marijuana, amphetamine, alcohol and diazepam. *Journal of Analytical Toxicology* **17**, 264–272.

Kunsman, G.W., Manno, J.B., Przekop, M.A. *et al.* (1992). The effects of temazepam and ethanol on human psychomotor performance. *European Journal of Clinical Pharmacology* **43**, 603–611.

Malik, P., Gasser, R.W., Kemmler, G. *et al.* (2008). Low bone mineral density and impaired bone metabolism in young adolescent patients without cirrhosis: A cross-sectional study. *Alcoholism: Clinical and Experimental Research* **33**, 375–381.

Maughan, R.J. (1997). Energy and macronutrient intakes of professional football (soccer) players. *British Journal of Sports Medicine*, **31**, 45–47.

Maughan, R.J. (2006). Alcohol and football. *Journal of Sports Science* **24**, 741–748.

McNaughton, L. and Preece, D. (1986). Alcohol and its effect on sprint and middle-distance running. *British Journal of Sports Medicine* **20**, 56–59.

Mennella, J.A. and Pepino, M.Y. (2006). Short-term effects of alcohol consumption on the hormonal milieu and mood states of nulliparous women. *Alcohol* **38**, 29–36.

National Diet and Nutrition Survey. (2003). Available at http://www.food.gov.uk/multimedia/pdfs/ndnsv2 (accessed 2 January 2009).

O'Brien, C. (1993). Alcohol and sport: Impact of social drinking on recreational and competitive sports performance. *Sports Medicine* **15**, 71–77.

Pedersen, J.O., Heitmann, B.L., Schnoir, P. *et al.* (2008). The combined influence of leisure-time physical activity and weekly alcohol intake on fatal ischaemic heart disease and all-cause mortality. *European Heart Journal* **29**, 204–212.

Reilly, T. (1994). Physiological aspects of football. *Biology of Sport* **11**, 3–20.

Reilly, T. (1997). Alcohol: Its influence in sport and exercise. In *The clinical pharmacology of sport and exercise*, ed. T. Reilly and M. Orme, Amsterdam, Elsevier. 281–290.

Reilly, T. and Halliday, F. (1985). Influence of alcohol ingestion on tasks related to archery. *Journal of Human Ergology* **14**, 99–104.

Reilly, T. and Scott, J. (1993). Effects of elevating blood alcohol levels on tasks related to dart throwing. *Perceptual Motor Skills* **77**, 25–26.

Reilly, T., Lees, A., MacLaren, D. *et al.* (1985). Thrill and anxiety in adventure leisure parks. In *Proceedings of the Ergonomics Society's conference*, ed. D. Oborne, Taylor and Francis, London. 210–214.

Sanderson, F.H. (1981). The psychology of the injury-prone athlete. In *Sport fitness and sports injuries*, ed. T. Reilly, Wolfe, London. 31–36.

S'Jongers, J.J., Willain, P., Sierakowski, J. *et al.* (1978). Effet d'un placebo et de faibles doses d'un bêta-inhibiteur (oxprenolol) et d'alcool éthylique, sur la précision du tir sportif au pistolet. *Bruxelles-Medical* **58**, 395–399.

Stepney, R. (1987). *Health and lifestyle: A review of a national survey*. Health Promotion Research Trust, Cambridge.

Suter, P.M. and Schutz, P. (2008). The effect of exercise, alcohol or both combined on health and physical performance. *International Journal of Obesity (London)* **32 (Suppl. 6)**, 548–552.

Tong, J.E., Henderson, P.R. and Chipperfield, G.A. (1980). Effects of ethanol and tobacco on auditory vigilance performance. *Addictive Behaviours* **5**, 153–538.

Vakulin, A., Baulk, S.D., Catcheside, P.G., *et al.* (2007). Effect of moderate sleep deprivation and low-dose alcohol on driving simulator performance and perception in young men. *Sleep* **30**, 1327–1333.

Van der Horst Graat, J.M., Terpstra, J.S., Kok, F.J. *et al.* (2007). Alcohol, smoking and physical activity related to respiratory infections in elderly people. *Journal of Nutrition Health and Aging* **11**, 80–85.

Wang, J.J., Tung, T.H., Yin, W.H. *et al.* (2008). Effects of moderate alcohol consumption on inflammatory biomarkers. *Acta Cardiology* **63 (1)**, 65–72.

Wesnes, K. and Warburton, D.M. (1983). Stress and drugs. In *Stress and fatigue in human performance*, ed. R. Hockey, John Wiley, Chichester. 203–243.

Willett, W., Hennekens, C.H., Siegel, A.J. *et al.* (1980). Alcohol consumption and high-density lipoprotein cholesterol in marathon runners. *New England Journal of Medicine* **303**, 1159–1161.

Willett, W., Starnpfer, M.J., Colditz, G.A. *et al.* (1987). Moderate alcohol consumption and the risk of breast cancer. *New England Journal of Medicine* **316**, 1174–1179.

Chapter 17

Beta blockers

David R. Mottram

17.1   What are beta blockers?

Beta blockers were first synthesised by the pharmaceutical industry in 1958. They have become one of the most frequently prescribed classes of drugs providing therapeutic support for a wide range of clinical conditions, principally associated with the cardiovascular system.

Mode of action of beta blockers

Beta blockers antagonise beta receptors, one of the subclasses of receptors that nordadrenaline (norepinephrine) and adrenaline (epinephrine) act upon.

Noradrenaline and adrenaline are found in both the central nervous system (CNS), where they act as neurotransmitters, and in the periphery, where noradrenaline is a neurotransmitter in the sympathetic nervous system and adrenaline is a hormone, released from the adrenal medulla during conditions of stress.

Both noradrenaline and adrenaline act through receptor sites known as adrenoceptors. These are subclassified into two major classes: alpha (α) and beta (β). The β-adrenoceptors are further subclassified into at least three types of receptor: β_1, β_2, and β_3. These receptors are found in a variety of tissues and organs in the body; the main ones are shown in Table 17.1, which also shows the principal effects that occur when beta blockers affect these receptors. It can be seen, therefore, that the effects of beta blockers are wide ranging.

Over the years, the pharmaceutical industry has developed beta blockers that act selectively on particular subclasses of β-adrenoceptors, in an attempt to target their therapeutic action more precisely and to reduce unwanted side effects. Table 17.2 lists some of the more common beta blockers, indicating their respective selectivity for beta receptor subclasses.

In addition to receptor selectivity, there are a number of other characteristics that distinguish one beta blocker from another. Some beta blockers, such as oxprenolol, pindolol, acebutolol and celiprolol possess intrinsic sympathomimetic activity (ISA), or partial agonist activity, which represents the capacity of these beta blockers to stimulate as well as block adrenergic receptors. They tend

Table 17.1 The main tissues and organs of the body (other than the brain) that contain β-adrenoceptors and the pharmacological effects of beta blockers

Organ	Receptor type	Principal effects of beta blockers
Heart	β_1	Decrease rate and force of beating
Blood vessels		
Arteries	β_2	Constriction
Veins	β_2	Constriction
Respiratory tract	β_2	Bronchoconstriction
Gastrointestinal tract	β_2	Increase motility
Bladder	β_2	Contraction of the bladder wall
Kidneys	β_1	Inhibition of rennin secretion
Skeletal muscle	β_2	Reduction in tremor
		Reduction of glycogenolysis
Liver	β_2	Reduction of glycogenolysis
Fat tissue	β_3	Reduction of lipolysis

Table 17.2 Some of the more common beta blockers and their receptor specificity

Non-selective beta blockers
Alprenolol
Carteolol
Levobunolol
Metipranolol
Nadolol
Oxprenolol
Pindolol
Propranolol
Sotalol
Timolol

Selective beta blockers (cardioselective for β_1-adrenoceptors)
Acebutolol
Atenolol
Betaxolol
Bisoprolol
Celiprolol
Esmolol
Metoprolol
Nevibolol

Combined beta blocker and alpha blocker
Carvedilol
Labetalol

to produce less bradycardia than other beta blockers and may also reduce coldness of extremities, a common side effect of beta blockers (Head, 1999).

Beta blockers have variable degrees of solubility between lipid and water phases. Atenolol, celiprolol, nadolol and sotalol are the most water soluble. They are less likely to enter the brain, across the blood-brain barrier, and are therefore less likely to cause centrally mediated side effects (Turner, 1983).

Effects of beta blockers

The main clinical uses for beta blockers are shown in Table 17.3.

Many of these uses relate to the effects of beta blockers on the cardiovascular system. Blocking the β_1-adrenoceptors in the heart reduces cardiac rate and force of beating. It was this pharmacological effect that prompted the search for effective drugs to treat patients with angina pectoris. This condition is characterised by severe chest pain due to insufficient oxygen reaching cardiac muscle, during exertion, in patients with compromised cardiac arteries. Beta blockers do not treat the symptoms of angina but, by reducing heart rate, they act prophylactically to prevent the onset of an anginal attack by improving exercise tolerance.

Blockade of β_1-adrenoceptors in the heart is important in the management of some types of cardiac dysrhythmias, particularly supraventricular tachycardias, and heart failure. Bisoprolol and carvedilol are particularly useful in stable heart failure.

Blockade of β_1-adrenoceptors in the heart is also used to therapeutic advantage by reducing blood pressure in hypertensive patients. Other pharmacological actions of beta blockers that contribute to their antihypertensive action include alteration of baroreceptor reflex sensitivity, depression of rennin secretion and possibly central effects, particularly with those beta blockers with lipid solubility that can easily cross the blood-brain barrier.

Beta blockers have been effective in preventing secondary heart attacks in patients who have experienced a myocardial infarction, although for some

Table 17.3 The main clinical conditions for which beta blockers are used

Cardiovascular
  Hypertension
  Angina pectoris
  Cardiac dysrhythmias
  Heart failure
  Prevention of secondary myocardial infarction
Other uses
  Phaeochromocytoma (benign cancer of the adrenal medulla)
  Migraine
  Glaucoma
  Anxiety
  Essential tremor

patients with co-morbidities such as uncontrolled heart failure, bradyarrhythmias or obstructive airways disease, beta blockers are contraindicated.

Phaeochromocytoma is a benign cancer of the adrenal medulla, leading to increased release of the hormone adrenaline. Beta blockers as well as alpha blockers are used to block the systemic effects of over-production of adrenaline.

Migraine is a condition that is treated by beta blockers through their effects on blood vessels. Not all migraine sufferers respond to beta blockers and more effective treatment regimes are available.

Glaucoma, a condition characterised by increased intra-ocular pressure in the eye, is treated by beta blockers. Although their mode of action is not fully understood, beta blockers are one of the first-line classes of drugs for this condition.

A more unusual clinical use for beta blockers is in the management of anxiety. The most widely used class of drugs to treat anxiety, the benzodiazepines, treat the psychological symptoms of anxiety, such as worry, tension and fear, mediated through the CNS. Beta blockers, on the other hand, treat the symptoms of anxiety mediated through the peripheral autonomic nervous system. They decrease heart rate by blocking β_1-adrenoceptors, thereby reducing palpitations, and reduce hand tremor mediated through β_2-adrenoceptors in skeletal muscle (Bowman and Anden, 1981).

The sympathetic nervous system, operating through β-adrenoceptors, produces metabolic effects, including the breakdown of glycogen (glycogenolysis) in the liver and in skeletal muscle and lipolysis in fat tissue. These effects produce increased glucose levels that are required when sympathetic stimulation is increased during conditions of stress. Beta blockers decrease the rate of glycogenolysis and lipolysis. There are no major clinical conditions where beta blockers are used therapeutically to inhibit these metabolic effects.

Essential tremor is a condition characterised by an involuntary rhythmic shaking of a part of the body, most commonly the arms, hands and head. Beta blockers, by blocking the β_2-adrenoceptors in skeletal muscle, can reduce the severity of tremor, particularly in the hands.

Side effects of beta blockers

Common side effects associated with beta blockers are fatigue, due to reduced cardiac output and reduced muscle perfusion in exercise, and coldness in the extremities (hands and feet), due to peripheral vasoconstriction and sleep disturbances (Cruickshank, 1981). Those beta blockers with associated ISA are less likely to produce cold extremities whilst those that are water-soluble are less likely to produce sleep disturbances such as nightmares, insomnia and occasionally depression.

Beta blockers are contraindicated in certain patients because of their wide range of pharmacological effects. In asthmatic patients beta blockers are especially contraindicated because they block the β_2-adrenoceptors in the respiratory tract, leading to bronchoconstriction with associated airways resistance. This effect is less pronounced in those beta blockers that have selectivity for β_1-adrenoceptors (see Table 17.2) but it should be noted that at higher doses these beta blockers lose their cardioselectivity.

Hypoglycaemia is associated with beta blocker use. Glucose release in response to adrenaline is important to diabetic patients and to other patients prone to hypoglycaemic attacks. Hypoglycaemia triggers symptoms to warn patients of the urgent need for carbohydrates. Beta blockers reduce these symptoms, therefore beta blockers are contraindicated in patients with poorly controlled diabetes.

17.2   History of beta blockers in sport

Beta blockers were, for many years, first-line drugs for the treatment of a number of cardiovascular diseases such as angina and hypertension. Under this pretext, a number of high-ranking professional snooker players tested positive for beta blockers at the 1987 World Professional Snooker Championships, as had occurred a few years earlier by competitors in shooting events in the 1984 Olympic Games (Reilly, 2005). The argument that beta blockers were indispensable drugs for these conditions was, however, unsustainable as other, equally effective first-line drugs were available to treat the cardiovascular conditions in question.

Beta blockers were added to the IOC prohibited list in 1985, as one of the major classes of prohibited substances. It was clear that the pharmacological effects of beta blockers would have a deleterious, rather than enhancing, effect on performance in most sports. This led the IOC Medical Commission to test for beta blockers only in high-risk sports where beta blockers may be used for their anti-anxiety effect or in sports where hand steadiness was important. This policy was adopted at the Summer and Winter Olympic Games from 1988 to 1993 (Reilly, 2005). Thereafter the IOC re-classified beta blockers from section I, doping classes, to section II, class of drugs subject to certain restrictions, where they were only prohibited in specified sports. This policy continued when WADA took over responsibility for the prohibited list and beta blockers were classed as classes of prohibited substances in certain sports.

17.3   Beta blockers and the WADA prohibited list

WADA regulations with respect to beta blockers

The 2010 WADA prohibited list classes beta blockers under "substances prohibited in particular sports". The list of sports in which beta blockers were banned in 2010 is shown in Table 17.4.

For most of these sports, beta blockers are prohibited in competition only. However, in archery and shooting, beta blockers are also prohibited out of competition.

Table 17.4 List of sports in which beta blockers are prohibited according to the 2010 WADA prohibited list

Aeronautics	Motorcycling
Archery	Modern pentathlon (for disciplines involving shooting)
Automobile	Ninepin and tenpin bowling
Billiards and snooker	Powerboating
Bobsleigh	Sailing (for match helms only)
Boules	Shooting
Bridge	Skiing/snowboarding (in ski jumping, freestyle aerials/halfpipe
Curling	and snowboard halfpipe/big air)
Golf	Wrestling
Gymnastics	

Prevalence of adverse findings for beta blockers

Annual statistics from WADA-accredited laboratories show that there are few adverse analytical findings for beta blockers. Table 17.5 shows the annual occurrence for individual drugs within the class, and the annual statistics ranged from 25 to 42 over the period from 2003 to 2008.

Results are unremarkable and probably reflect the international prescribing patterns of the respective drugs. It is interesting to note that cardioselective and non-cardioselective beta blockers are used equally.

Table 17.5 WADA statistics for the number of positive results for substances classed as beta blockers (2003–2008)

	2003	2004	2005	2006	2007	2008
Beta blockers						
Atenolol	9	8	6	9	3	6
Bisoprolol	7	5	10	2	6	5
Metoprolol	5	5	5	6	6	4
Acebutolol	4	–	1	–	–	2
Propranolol	4	6	16	6	8	9
Carteolol	1	–	–	–	1	–
Sotalol	–	1	–	–	–	–
Carvedilol	–	–	4	3	2	1
Timolol	–	–	–	2	1	–
Betaxolol	–	–	–	–	–	3
Labetalol	–	–	–	–	–	1
Total	30	25	42	28	27	31

17.4   The use of beta blockers in sport

Adverse effects of beta blockers in sport

Beta blockers produce metabolic effects including a decrease in the rate of glycogenolysis in skeletal muscle. This may have implications for performance at submaximal levels. Similarly, in sustained exercise, the inhibition of glycogenolysis in the liver will affect performance by reducing blood glucose levels (Reilly, 2005). These effects on glycogenolysis are mediated through blockade of β_2-adrenoceptors and are more evident with non-selective beta blockers such as propranolol, although the cardioselective beta blocker atenolol produced adverse effects at higher doses, when selectivity is reduced (Kaiser, 1982). Prolonged exercise may be adversely affected by the inhibition of lipolysis that is produced by beta blockers. The availability of free fatty acids is reduced, thereby causing an earlier onset of fatigue. Opie (1986) suggested that impairment of metabolic responses to exercise and effects on peripheral circulation were responsible for the reduction in physiological adaptation to exercise training, induced by propranolol. A thorough description of the metabolic effects of beta blockers in exercise can be found in a review paper by Head (1999).

A study by Rusko et al. (1980) examined the effect of beta blockers on short-term, high-intensity exercise. In order to compare the beta blocker oxprenolol with placebo control, a series of anaerobic tasks was performed by subjects. Oxprenolol reduced power output on a cycle ergometer with a concomitant reduction in heart rate and peak blood lactate. The drug had no effect on isometric strength of leg extension, stair running or vertical jumping. In a study on alpine skiers, it was reported that short-term maximal muscle power, recorded during a 30-second submaximal cycling test, was reduced by beta blockers (Karlsson et al., 1983). Beta blockers have been shown to reduce maximal oxygen uptake (VO_{2max}) (Head, 1999). It would be expected that cardioselective beta blockers would have less of an adverse effect as they have a reduced effect on β_2-adrenoceptors. This supposition was confirmed by Gordon et al. (1987), although little or no difference has been observed by other investigators (Tesch and Kaiser, 1983). Reduction in VO_{2max} due to beta blockers is more likely to occur in highly trained endurance athletes than in untrained individuals (Wilmore, 1988).

Potential benefit of beta blockers in sport

Stress and anxiety are common responses to competitive sport. Therapeutically, benzodiazepines are widely used as tranquillizers and anti-anxiety drugs. They exert their effect in the CNS through inhibition of the release of a number of neurotransmitters, most notably serotonin (Reilly, 2005). However, beta blockers are usually preferred as anti-anxiety agents in sport as they exert their effects peripherally rather than centrally and do not possess the addictive properties of benzodiazepines. Because beta blockers can reduce tremor in the extremities, a study on the effect of oxprenolol on pistol shooting found a significant improvement in shooting scores but only in slow-firing events (Antal and Good, 1980).

In 1986, Kruse *et al.* showed that there was a clear improvement in the shooting performance of pistol shooters with metoprolol compared with placebo control. The most skilled marksmen showed the greatest improvement. No correlation was found between shooting improvement and cardiovascular variables, such as heart rate and blood pressure, leading the authors to conclude that the improvement was caused by an effect of metoprolol on hand tremor.

Golf has been associated with high levels of anxiety and a specific term now describes a phenomenon experienced by golfers: the "yips" (Smith *et al.*, 2003). This has been defined as a motor phenomenon of involuntary movements associated with high stress levels and performance anxiety. The physical symptoms of the yips are tremor, jerks or freezing of the hands and forearms, particularly associated with putting strokes. For this reason, some golfers have used alcohol and/or beta blockers to alleviate the symptoms. It is only recently, in 2009, that WADA added golf to the list of sports in which beta blockers are prohibited within competition, at the request of the International Golf Federation.

17.5   References

Antal, L.C. and Good, C.S. (1980). Effects of oxprenolol on pistol shooting under stress. *Practitioner* **224**, 755–760.

Bowman, W. and Anden, N. (1981). Effects of adrenergic activators and inhibitors on the skeletal muscles. In *Adrenergic activators and inhibitors*, ed. L. Szekeres, Springer-Verlag, Berlin. 47–128.

Cruickshank, J.M. (1981). β-blockers, bradycardia and adverse effects. *Acta Therapeutica* **7**, 309–321.

Gordon, N.E., Van Rensburg, J.P., Van Den Heever, D.P. *et al.* (1987). Effect of dual beta blockade and calcium antagonism on endurance performance. *Medicine and Science in Sport and Exercise* **19**, 1–6.

Head, A. (1999). Exercise metabolism and β-blocker therapy. *Sports Medicine* **27(2)**, 81–96.

Kaiser, P. (1982). Running performance as a function of the dose-response relationship to beta-adrenoceptor blockade. *International Journal of Sports Medicine* **3**, 29–32.

Karlsson, J., Kjessel, T. and Kaiser, P. (1983). Alpine skiing and acute beta-blockade. *International Journal of Sports Medicine* **4(3)**, 190–193.

Kruse, P., Ladefoged, J., Nielsen, U. *et al.* (1986). Beta-blockade used in precision sports: Effect on pistol shooting performance. *Journal of Applied Physiology* **61(2)**, 417–420.

Opie, L.H. (1986). Biochemical and metabolic responses to beta-adrenergic blockade at rest and during exercise. In *Biochemical aspects of physical exercise*, ed. G. Benzi, L. Packer and N. Siliprandi, Elsevier, Amsterdam. 423–433.

Reilly, T.R. (2005). Alcohol, anti-anxiety drugs and sport. In *Drugs in sport*, 4th ed., Ed. D.R.Mottram, Routledge, London. 258–287.

Rusko, H., Kantola, H., Luhtanen, R. *et al.* (1980). Effect of beta-blockade on performances requiring force, velocity, coordination and/or anaerobic metabolism. *Journal of Sports Medicine and Physical Fitness* **20**, 139–144.

Smith, A.M., Adler, C.H. Crews, D. *et al.* (2003). The "yips" in golf. A continuum between a focal dystonia and choking. *Sports Medicine* **33(1)**, 13–31.

Tesch, P.A. and Kaiser, P. (1983). Effects of beta-adrenergic blockade on O_2 uptake during submaximal and maximal exercise. *Journal of Applied Physiology* **54**, 901–905.

Turner, P. (1983). β-blockade and the human central nervous system. *Drugs* **25(Suppl. 2)**, 262–273.

Wilmore, J.H. (1988). Exercise testing, training and beta-adrenergic blockade. *Physician and Sports Medicine* **16**, 45–51.

Substances and methods permitted in sport

Chapter 18

Supplements for high intensity exercise

Creatine and other ergogenic aids

Don MacLaren

18.1 Introduction

The focus of this chapter is to explore the potential for ergogenic aids to improve high intensity exercise performance, and with this in mind it is necessary to understand the likely fatigue factors impacting on such performance. This chapter examines the role of creatine, alkalinisers, and beta-alanine as potentially useful supplements because the abundance of evidence portrays them as such. In spite of the more recent wealth of information pointing to the efficacy of caffeine for such activities, this is covered in another chapter.

18.2 Energy metabolism and fatigue

Energy is supplied by adenosine triphosphate (ATP) during any form of biological work. The hydrolysis of ATP to produce energy for muscle contraction is catalysed by the enzyme myosin ATPase, and the reaction is represented as follows:

$$ATP + H_2O \rightarrow ADP + P_i + Energy$$
$$\uparrow$$
myosin ATPase

However, the stores of ATP in muscle are small and need continuous replenishment if activity is to continue beyond a few seconds. Consequently, ATP is resynthesised by at least three energy systems:

1   PCr/Cr – ADP + PCr $\rightarrow$ ATP + Cr;
2   Glycolysis – ADP + Glycogen $\rightarrow$ ATP + Lactic acid;
3   Aerobic ADP + Glucose/Glycogen/Fatty Acids $\rightarrow$ ATP + CO_2 + H_2O.

The first two energy systems occur in the cytosol rather than in the mitochondria, do not require the use of oxygen, and so are deemed anaerobic. Furthermore, these sources of energy are rapidly generated and are the major sources of

ATP restoration during exercise of maximal intensity. Indeed the use of phosphorylated creatine (PCr) is maximal in the first second of high intensity exercise and thereafter decreases over 30 seconds as first glycolysis and then aerobic sources predominate. It has been demonstrated that during a six-second sprint on a cycle ergometer, PCr contributed approximately 50 per cent of the total ATP production (Boobis, 1987). Furthermore, the increase in the concentration of muscle lactic acid after 6 s or 30 s of intense activity is around 250 per cent to nearly 1000 per cent respectively from resting values. The aerobic energy system, although relatively important during or following intense exercise, will not be explored in this chapter.

Fatigue as a consequence of high intensity exercise is a complex phenomenon. In essence, fatigue is based on the inability to sustain the necessary power output, which means a reduction in ATP cycling caused by some factors. These include the likelihood of depletion of PCr stores in type IIx (fast twitch) fibres, increases in P_i, and/or increases in H^+ concentration in the muscle causing acidosis. The increase in H^+ is a subject of debate as to whether it arises mainly from dissociation of lactic acid or other acid sources. The net result is that any ergogenic aid likely to have an impact on muscle fatigue during intense exercise should focus on elevating PCr, and/or reducing muscle H^+, and/or enhancing muscle buffer capacity to cope with the reduction in pH. On the basis of these likely fatigue factors, three supplements—creatine, sodium bicarbonate (or any alkalinising agent), and beta-alanine—appear to fit the bill.

18.3   Creatine

Creatine (Cr) has been known as a constituent of food for more than 150 years. However, it was not until the early 1990s that significant research examined the effects of creatine supplementation on sports performance. Creatine, or methyl guanidine-acetic acid, is a naturally occurring nitrogenous molecule (Figure 18.1) found mainly in the skeletal muscles of vertebrates. It is also found in smaller amounts in the liver, kidneys, and brain. Although found mainly in skeletal muscle, Cr is metabolised in the liver and then transported to muscle. This is due to the fact that most tissues lack several of the enzymes involved in creatine synthesis.

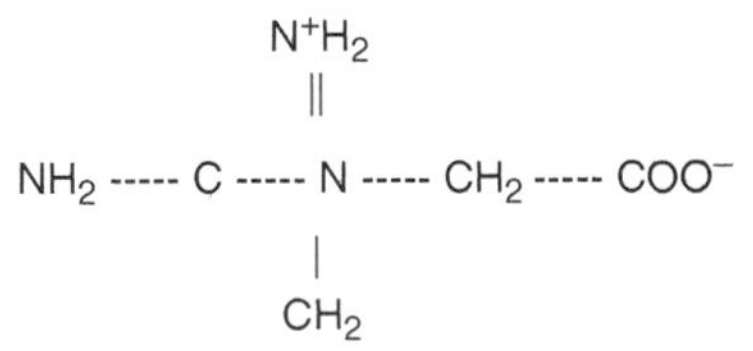

$$N^+H_2$$
$$\|$$
$$NH_2 \text{-----} C \text{-----} N \text{-----} CH_2 \text{-----} COO^-$$
$$|$$
$$CH_2$$

Figure 18.1 Structure of creatine.

Three amino acids are involved in the synthesis of creatine; they are arginine, glycine, and methionine. De novo synthesised Cr is transported from the liver to skeletal muscle where it is taken up by active transport using a Na^+-dependent transporter. Once inside the muscle cell, the Cr is "trapped" by being converted to PCr, which is unable to pass through the membrane. It is also possible that Cr is bound to an intracellular component and/or that restrictive cellular membranes exist to stop efflux of Cr from muscle to blood. Approximately 70 per cent of the creatine in muscle is in the phosphorylated form (PCr), the other 30 per cent being free Cr.

Creatine is constantly degraded to creatinine, which is its sole end product, via a non-enzymatic irreversible reaction. The creatinine diffuses through the muscle membrane and is taken to the kidneys where it is excreted in a passive process before being voided in urine. The daily urine creatinine excretion is relatively constant, although it varies between individuals due to differences in muscle mass. For a more detailed examination of creatine and creatinine metabolism, the reader should consult Wyss and Kaddurah-Daouk (2000). The daily turnover of Cr to creatinine in humans is about 2 g/day for a 70 kg person and is replaced by endogenous synthesis and exogenous sources in the diet. Synthesis is regulated by the exogenous intake through a feedback mechanism.

About 95 per cent of the Cr pool can be found in skeletal muscle, although significant amounts can also be found in the heart, spermatozoa, brain, seminal vesicles, macrophages, and photoreceptor cells of the retina. Low levels are present in the kidneys, liver, spleen, and lungs. The stores of Cr exist in both the free (Crf) and phosphorylated (PCr) forms. Total muscle Cr concentration is approximately 120 mM/kg dm in muscle. Note that total Cr concentration includes the phosphorylated form.

Factors such as age, sex, and diet influence muscle Cr concentration. Resting PCr levels have been shown to be lower in older (60-year-old) compared with younger (30-year-old) subjects (Smith et al., 1998), although there is no significant difference in the total Cr concentration. In this instance it is possible that the degree of inactivity in the older subjects may have led to the attenuated PCr levels. Females have been reported to have an elevated Cr concentration compared with males (Forsberg et al., 1991). Diet can significantly influence muscle Cr concentration. However, it should be noted that since the exogenous source of Cr is via consuming foods containing meat and fish, vegetarians may have lower concentrations because their only source is de novo synthesis. Studies have shown that vegetarians have marginally lower muscle Cr concentrations than those who eat meat and fish (Delanghe et al., 1989; Harris et al., 1992).

Another influence on muscle Cr is that of training. The results from training studies have been equivocal, although Bernus et al. (1993) established that sprint-trained athletes had elevated levels of PCr when compared with endurance athletes. In this instance the differences could be due to the muscle fibre composition of the athletes, although the effect of training cannot be overlooked. Results from longitudinal training studies that have employed sprinting or resistance modes have failed to show elevated levels of PCr or Cr (Nevill *et al.*, 1989; Sharp *et al.*, 1986).

Muscle creatine loading

Muscle Cr is restored at a rate of approximately 2 g/day by a combination of dietary Cr ingestion from sources such as meat and fish, and from endogenous synthesis. Muscle creatine content has been found to increase significantly following creatine ingestion (Harris *et al.*, 1992). In this study, ingestion of 5 g of Cr four to six times a day for two days resulted in an increase in total Cr from 127 to 149 mmol/kg. These increases were individual responses, in which some subjects increased significantly and others less so. The terms "responders" and "non-responders" apply in this instance, and a relationship between the initial resting level and the level of increase was established. Two vegetarians in the study possessed the lowest initial resting levels and responded with significant increases. Furthermore, Harris *et al.* (1992) were also able to demonstrate that whereas on the first two days the Cr storage was approximately 30 per cent of that ingested, the amount stored in the following two days was diminished to around 15 per cent of the Cr ingested.

Studies have shown that muscle Cr concentrations can be significantly enhanced using lower daily doses for a prolonged time period. Hultman *et al.* (1996) reported that Cr ingestion of 3 g/day over a four-week period produced muscle Cr concentrations similar to those found when 20 g/day were ingested over a five-day period. Most recent studies have employed a regimen in which 5 g of Cr are administered in a warm solution during four equally spaced time intervals through a day.

There is considerable variation between subjects to the extent muscle Cr concentrations are elevated following supplementation, although it appears that there is an upper limit of 160 mmol/kg dry muscle. In order to achieve this level, creatine should be ingested in combination with at least 370 g of simple carbohydrates in a day (Green *et al.*, 1996). This regimen promotes Cr stores to around 160 mmol/kg, even in the non-responders. Interestingly, the data from these studies showed that whereas previously there was an inverse relationship between initial muscle Cr and the level of loading when Cr alone was ingested, no such relationship existed when Cr was combined with carbohydrates.

It seems likely that the increase in muscle Cr stores when taken with carbohydrates results from insulin action. Hyperinsulinaemia results in enhanced muscle Cr storage, probably by stimulating the Na^+-dependent muscle Cr transporter activity. A specific, saturable, Na^+-dependent transporter responsible for Cr uptake across the plasma membrane has been described for skeletal muscle, heart, brain, kidneys, intestine, and red blood cells, but not for liver.

Following the Cr-loading phase of 20 g/day for five days, recommended maintenance doses are considerably lower. Most studies have used doses ranging from

2 to 5 g/day during the maintenance phase. Hultman *et al.* (1996) recommend a maintenance dose of 0.03 g/kg body mass per day, which for a 70-kg person amounts to approximately 2 g/day. When an athlete stops ingesting creatine, the muscle Cr levels diminish to normal levels after four weeks (Greenhaff, 1997; Hultman *et al.*, 1996).

Creatine and performance

The theoretical benefits of creatine supplementation are related to the role of Cr and PCr in the energetics of muscle contraction, and also to the potential for buffering increases in [H^+] as a consequence of raised intramuscular lactic acid concentrations. Specifically, mechanisms purported to provide an ergogenic effect of creatine include the fact that supplementation results in elevated PCr levels in muscle and hence a greater immediate source of generation of ATP, that increased levels of Cr would facilitate an enhanced rate of PCr resynthesis in recovery bouts, and that there is enhanced buffering of H^+.

Intramuscular stores of ATP and PCr are limited, and it has been estimated that these phosphagen stores could supply sufficient energy for high intensity exercise for not more than 10 seconds (Balsom *et al.*, 1994). Furthermore, Sahlin (1998) has suggested that the maximum rate of PCr hydrolysis decreases as PCr content of muscle decreases, and complete depletion is not necessary to cause a reduction in power production. In fact, a number of researchers have concluded that PCr availability is a limiting factor during high intensity exercise (Greenhaff, 1997; Balsom *et al.*, 1995).

Creatine supplementation, by increasing both Cr and PCr, particularly in the FG fibres, should prolong either single bouts of high intensity exercise and in particular repeated bouts of high intensity exercise. Probably the first two studies that reported on Cr supplementation and intense exercise were those of Greenhaff *et al.* (1993) and Balsom *et al.* (1993). Greenhaff and colleagues (1993) employed five bouts of 30 maximal isokinetic knee extensions with 1 minute of recovery between the bouts. When subjects were loaded with 20 g/day of Cr for five days, peak muscle torque was significantly enhanced in the final 10 contractions during the first bout, and during the whole of the next four bouts. The authors concluded that Cr supplementation accelerated PCr resynthesis and that the increased availability of PCr was responsible for the higher peak torque production.

Balsom *et al.* (1993) used ten six-second bouts of high intensity cycling with 30 seconds of recovery between the tests. Subjects were expected to maintain a pedal rate of 140 rpm with a resistance set so that they could complete six seconds. The test was undertaken by a placebo group and a creatine group in a random, double-blind design. Creatine loading entailed six days of 20 g/day of Cr. The creatine-loaded group were able to maintain 140 rpm in the last two seconds of each of the bouts, whereas those on placebo failed to do so after the fourth bout of cycling. Indeed, at the ninth and tenth bouts, the placebo group was averaging 125 rpm as opposed to 138 rpm for the creatine-loaded group.

Since these early reports, in excess of 300 studies have been published in peer-reviewed articles. The majority of these studies highlight the effectiveness of Cr supplementation for enhancing sports performance (Bemben and Lamont, 2005) and for being of potential use for aging athletes, too (Tarnopolsky, 2008). These studies have examined the effects on high intensity exercise (both single bouts and repeated bouts), strength and power, field-based activities and endurance (Deldicque and Francaux, 2008). Other studies have purely examined the effects of supplementation on lean body mass and body composition, although many of the other studies have also reported data on body mass changes. Recent reviews on creatine and performance (Bemben and Lamont, 2005; Hespel and Derave, 2007; Deldicque and Francaux, 2008) provide a broader exploration of studies.

Creatine and single bouts of high intensity exercise

In spite of the fact that Cr supplementation leads to increases in muscle Cr and PCr, it would be expected that single bouts of high intensity exercise produce enhanced performance. In general, this is not the case. Some studies have shown significant improvements in sprint running (Goldberg and Bechtel, 1997; Kendall et al., 2009; Law et al., 2009; Noonan et al., 1998) and vertical jump performance (Stout et al., 1999), whereas the majority of studies using single bouts of running, cycling, swimming, and jumping have failed to show significant improvements. It appears that the possibility of elevated Cr stores in muscle being available to maintain a short, sharp burst of activity when not fatigued does not happen. Interestingly a study in which a single bout of 10 seconds of sprint cycling was assessed following five bouts of 6 s sprinting with a 30 s recovery between bouts, an increase in power was observed (Balsom et al., 1995). So when there is an element of fatigue due to previous activity, creatine may help to improve single bouts of intense exercise.

Creatine and repeated bouts of high intensity exercise

Since enhanced stores of Cr and PCr result from creatine loading, there is the possibility that during recovery phases of repeated bouts of exercise the elevated Cr will be more rapidly phosphorylated. Enhanced performance may then result in subsequent bouts of exercise. Positive ergogenic effects of Cr loading have been exhibited for repeated bouts of high intensity cycling (Balsom et al., 1993; Earnest et al., 1995), running (Aaserud et al., 1998), swimming (Peyrebrune et al., 1998) and vertical jumping (Bosco et al., 1997). In most cases, the significant effects are noted in the later bouts of exercise and not usually in the first bout. Furthermore, the effects are normally associated with mean power or total work done rather than peak power values. All in all, these findings support the notion of greater rephosphorylation in the recovery period when Cr stores have been enhanced.

It should be noted, however, that not all studies have reported significant effects. Some studies on repeated sprint cycling have shown no significant effect of Cr ingestion (Barnett *et al.*, 1996; Cooke *et al.*, 1995). Similar non-responses were obtained for investigations using repeated running (Smart *et al.*, 1998), and swimming (Leenders *et al.*, 1999).

It is difficult to fathom the reasons why the majority of studies highlight positive ergogenic effects whereas a significant, though smaller, number find no such differences. Examination of the dose of Cr ingested and whether carbohydrates were ingested in addition, together with the types of subjects used (i.e. level of training), the sex of the subjects, the dietary habits of the subjects, the number of subjects employed, and variations in the mode of testing are all possible confounding variables. On balance, Cr supplementation results in an approximate 4–10 per cent improvement in repeated high intensity activities. Even some of the studies that reported no significant findings have reported 2–4 per cent improvements in performance, but they produced non-significant results due to the low power of the experimental design.

Creatine and strength

Phosphocreatine and ATP are likely to be the major energy sources during strength-based activities that are isometric, isotonic, or isokinetic. In the cases of isotonic or isokinetic exercise, the activity is repeated in either fast or slow modes, whereas isometric activity involves either an all-out fast action or a hold of the tension for a period of time. The majority of studies in which some form of strength has been assessed have shown positive ergogenic effects. Such studies include the use of isometric (Maganaris and Maughan, 1998), isotonic (Earnest *et al.*, 1995; Noonan *et al.*, 1998) or isokinetic (Greenhaff *et al.*, 1993; Vandenberghe *et al.*, 1996) modes of testing. Improvements of between 6 and 28 per cent in strength were reported in the above studies. Recent studies in the elderly have shown the potential for significant improvements in strength and lean body mass with creatine ingestion (Tarnopolsky, 2008). It has been proposed that creatine supplementation augments the increase in satellite cells and mononuclei in skeletal muscle induced by strength training (Olsen *et al.*, 2006).

However, as with the studies on repeated bouts of high intensity exercise, there are a number of studies that reported no significant benefits of creatine on isometric strength (Rawson *et al.*, 1998), isotonic strength (Stout *et al.*, 1999) and isokinetic strength (Kreider *et al.*, 1996).

The reasons for discrepancies in these findings may be those expressed above, but in addition could include the level of resistance or weight training experienced by the subjects. The latter seems unlikely because studies showing positive effects have included experienced and novice subjects, as have those showing no significant effect. Again, on balance the evidence for a positive effect is greater than no effect.

18.4   Sodium bicarbonate

Intense bouts of activity invariably result in an increase in lactic acid production. The lactic acid dissociates into H^+ and La^- with a concomitant decrease in muscle pH from a value of 7.0 to around 6.4. It has been proposed that this increase in H^+ and decrease in pH may affect enzyme activity such as PFK (which thereby reduces glycolysis) and Ca-ATPase (which reduces Ca reuptake into the sarcoplasmic reticulum and subsequent release) as well as competitive inhibition of Ca^+ by H^+ (so reducing activation of cross-bridges). The overall effect is muscle fatigue, although other factors may also play important roles. For more detailed reviews on cellular factors and muscle fatigue, see Fitts (1994) and Allen et al. (2008). What is not in question is that lactic acid concentrations increase significantly in muscle and blood during and just after intense exercise, and also that muscle pH decreases.

Reduced pH has also been associated with an increased release of K^+ from muscle and a greater accumulation of K^+ in the muscle interstitium (Bangsbo et al., 1996). This increase in the extracellular K concentration is considered to depolarise the muscle membrane and result in excitation failure (Clausen, 2003). So, a further potential fatigue factor resulting from an increase in lactic acid production and reduction in intracellular pH is greater release of K^+ and excitation failure.

A primary buffer in blood is bicarbonate (HCO_3^-), which combines with H^+ to form H_2CO_3, which then immediately dissociates into CO_2 and H_2O. However, this buffer system is unable to prevent an increase in muscle acidosis following intense bouts of exercise but merely delays the inevitable.

Alkalinisers, such as sodium bicarbonate (and sodium citrate), have been ingested prior to intense exercise bouts in an attempt to slow down the decrease in muscle pH and so enhance performance (Nielsen et al., 2002). A typical dose of sodium bicarbonate ingested is 0.3 g/kg body weight, which for a 70-kg person amounts to 21 g. The effect is that blood pH increases from around pH 7.4 to pH 7.6 and bicarbonate concentration from 24 mM to around 30 mM. No changes are observed in muscle. The effects are extracellular, not intracellular.

How does elevating extracellular pH by the use of sodium bicarbonate promote performance? A proposed mechanism is the production of a pH gradient from muscle to blood, resulting in a faster efflux of H^+ and hence attenuation of the inevitable reduced intra-muscle pH (MacLaren, 1997). H^+, and lactate, transport across the sarcolemma is mediated by a monocarboxylate cotransporter (Juel, 1997), and this is supported by studies in which bicarbonate ingestion results in an accelerated release of lactate and H^+ from muscle (Nielsen et al., 2002). The consequences of maintenance of pH within the muscle (for even a short time) can be realised in higher lactic acid levels in blood, enhanced glycolysis and a reduction in K^+ efflux, thereby ensuring excitation-contraction coupling. Therefore, from a theoretical perspective, sodium bicarbonate ingestion prior to intense activity should result in improvements in performance or capacity.

Evidence from numerous studies supports the use of bicarbonate ingestion for various types of exercise performance (Matson and Tran, 1993; McNaughton et al., 2008). These include repeated sprint performance (Bishop et al., 2004; McNaughton, 1992), prolonged intermittent exercise (Bishop and Claudius, 2005), 400m running performance (Goldfinch et al., 1988), 800m running performance (Wilkes et al., 1983), 1500m running performance (Bird et al., 1995), running at an exercise intensity corresponding to 4mM lactate (George and MacLaren, 1988), swimming (Lindh et al., 2008), judo (Artioli et al., 2007), forearm exercise (Raymer et al., 2004) and muscle force (Verbitsky et al., 1997). More recently, a number of studies have examined the effects of chronic administration of sodium bicarbonate over days on performance with similar positive outcomes (Edge et al., 2006; McNaughton et al., 1999, 2000).

Sodium bicarbonate ingestion appears to have no significant effect on events lasting 30 seconds or less, quite possibly because glycolysis (and the ensuing reduction in muscle pH) is not a major process during such short durations.

A common problem with ingestion of sodium bicarbonate is that of diarrhoea. However, this can be reduced if the dose is partitioned and taken over the span of an hour with plenty of fluid rather than in a single consumption. The use of sodium citrate rather than bicarbonate was first employed by Parry-Billings and MacLaren (1986) in an attempt to resolve this potential issue. Results from subsequent studies have reported on the efficacy of "citrate loading" in a favourable manner similar to "bicarbonate loading", although a more recent publication favoured the use of bicarbonate in sprint running (Van Montfoort et al., 2004).

18.5   Beta-alanine

A relatively new ergogenic aid being investigated is that of beta-alanine. Beta-alanine is a non-proteogenic amino acid found mainly in meat and fish, and it is purported to be a limiting substrate in the synthesis of carnosine (beta-alanyl-L-histidine), which is a dipeptide present in high concentrations ($\sim$20 mM/kg dry muscle) in skeletal muscle. Greater amounts of carnosine are present in type IIx (fast twitch) fibres (Hill et al., 2007) where it acts as a buffer (Harris et al., 1990). It is a dipeptide synthesised in muscle from histidine and beta-alanine (Kendrick et al., 2008). The biochemical functions of carnosine, other than being a buffer, include a role as an antioxidant (Boldyrev, 1993), as a "suicide" peptide protecting the body against glycation (Hipkiss and Michaelis, 1995) and in Ca^{2+} sensitisation (Dukta and Lamb, 2004).

Carnosine levels in sprinters are significantly higher than in distance athletes or untrained subjects (Parkhouse et al., 1985). Furthermore, sprint training increases muscle carnosine, where a significant relationship has been established between muscle carnosine concentration and high intensity exercise performance (Suzuki et al., 2002).

Carnosine levels in muscle can be elevated by chronic ingestion (i.e. 2–10 weeks) of beta-alanine at doses between 4.0–6.4 g/day (Derave et al., 2007;

Harris *et al.*, 2006; Kendrick *et al.*, 2008). Furthermore, an increase in muscle carnosine has resulted in improved performance in anaerobic exercise capacity using cycling (Hill *et al.*, 2007), time to exhaustion during isometric strength of the knee extensors (Ponte *et al.*, 2007), and in sprint cycling following a simulated endurance race (Van Thienen *et al.*, 2009). However, not all studies have reported improvements in performance following beta-alanine supplementation in spite of enhanced levels of carnosine (Derave *et al.*, 2007; Kendrick *et al.*, 2008). In the study by Derave *et al.* (2007), improvements were observed in repeated knee extensor work but not in 400 m time using trained athletes.

Because the use of beta-alanine as a supplement is in its infancy, it may take a few more years before sufficient evidence is gleaned for the potential of using it as an ergogenic aid. However, the early findings are encouraging.

18.6   Conclusion

Fatigue associated with high intensity activities is a complex phenomenon, although factors relating to diminished levels of phosphocreatine and increasing concentrations of H^+ are important factors. Increasing total muscle creatine (and thereby the amount of PCr) by ingesting exogenous sources of creatine has been proven, and there is a substantial amount of evidence that subsequent improvements in repeated bouts of high intensity performance are observed in a range of sporting activities. The production of lactic acid as a consequence of intense exercise resulting in elevated concentrations within skeletal muscle is well established. The use of sodium bicarbonate (and sodium citrate) to induce alkalosis and thereby promote efflux of H^+ (and lactate) from the muscle to extracellular compartments has also been observed. More recently, induced alkalosis has been found to reduce K^+ in the interstitial spaces and result in enhanced muscle force generation. Sodium bicarbonate is a useful ergogenic aid for intense exercise lasting longer than 30 seconds. More recently, the use of beta-alanine to increase muscle carnosine levels has been established and has furthermore proved beneficial in some studies using intense exercise bouts. Research is still in its infancy (relatively speaking), although the signs are favourable.

18.7   References

Aaserud, R., Gramvik, P., Olsen, S.R. *et al.* (1998). Creatine supplementation delays onset of fatigue during repeated bouts of sprint running. *Scandinavian Journal of Medicine and Science in Sports* **8**, 247–251.

Allen, D.G., Lamb, G.D., and Westerblad, H. (2008). Skeletal muscle fatigue: Cellular mechanisms. *Physiological Reviews* **88**, 287–332.

Artioli, G.G., Gualano, B., Coelho, D.F. *et al.* (2007). Does sodium bicarbonate ingestion improve simulated judo performance? *International Journal of Sport Nutrition and Exercise Medicine* **17**, 206–217.

Balsom, P.D., Ekblom, B., Soderlund, K. *et al.* (1993). Creatine supplementation and dynamic high intensity intermittent exercise. *Scandinavian Journal of Medicine and Science in Sports* **3**, 143–149.

Balsom, P., Soderlund, K. and Ekblom, B. (1994). Creatine in humans with special reference to creatine supplementation. *Sports Medicine* **18**, 268–280.

Balsom, P.D., Soderlund, K., Sjodin, B. *et al.* (1995). Skeletal muscle metabolism during short duration high-intensity exercise. *Acta Physiologica Scandinavica* **154**, 303–310.

Bangsbo, J., Madsen, K., Kiens, B. *et al.* (1996). Effect of muscle acidity on muscle metabolism and fatigue during intense exercise in man. *Journal of Physiology* **495**, 587–596.

Barnett, C., Hinds, M. and Jenkins, D.G. (1996). Effects of oral creatine supplementation on multiple sprint cycle performance. *Australian Journal of Science and Medicine in Sports* **28**, 35–39.

Bemben, M.G. and Lamont, H.S. (2005). Creatine supplementation and exercise performance—Recent findings. *Sports Medicine* **35**, 107–125.

Bernus, G., Gonzale de Suso, J.M., Alonso, J. *et al.* (1993). ^{31}P-MRS of quadriceps reveals quantitative differences between sprinters and long-distance runners. *Medicine and Science in Sports and Exercise* **25**, 479–484.

Bird, S.R., Wiles, J. and Robbins, J. (1995). The effect of sodium bicarbonate ingestion on 1500-m racing time. *Journal of Sports Science* **13**, 399–403.

Bishop, D. and Claudius, B. (2005). Effects of induced metabolic alkalosis on prolonged intermittent sprint performance. *Medicine and Science in Sports and Exercise* **37**, 759–767.

Bishop, D., Edge, J., Davis, C. *et al.* (2004). Induced metabolic alkalosis affects muscle metabolism and repeated sprint ability. *Medicine and Science in Sports and Exercise* **36**, 807–813.

Boldyrev, A.A. (1993). Does carnosine possess direct antioxidant activity? *Journal of Biochemistry* **25**, 1101–1107.

Boobis, L.H. (1987). Metabolic aspects of fatigue during sprinting. In *Exercise: Benefits, limits and adaptations*, ed. D. Macleod, R. Maughan, M. Nimmo, T. Reilly and C. Williams, EandFN Spon, London. 116–143.

Bosco, C., Tihanyi, J., Pucspk, J. *et al.* (1997). Effect of oral creatine supplementation on jumping and running performance. *International Journal of Sports Medicine* **18**, 369–372.

Clausen, T. (2003). Na^+–K^+ pump regulation and skeletal contractility. *Physiological Reviews* **83**, 1269–1324.

Cooke, W.H., Grandjean, P.W. and Barnes, W.S. (1995). Effect of oral creatine supplementation on power output and fatigue during bicycle ergometry. *Journal of Applied Physiology* **78**, 670–673.

Delanghe, J., De Slypere, J.P., De Buyzere, M. *et al.* (1989). Normal reference values for creatine, creatinine, and carnitine are lower in vegetarians. *Clinical Chemistry* **35**, 1802–1803.

Deldicque, L. and Francaux, M. (2008). Functional food for exercise performance: Fact or foe? *Current Opinion in Clinical Nutrition and Metabolic Care* **11**, 774–781.

Derave, W., Ozdemir, M.S. and Harris, R.C. (2007). Beta-alanine supplementation augments muscle carnosine content and attenuates fatigue during repeated isokinetic contraction bouts in trained sprinters. *Journal of Applied Physiology* **103**, 1736–1743.

Dukta, T.L. and Lamb, G.D. (2004). Effects of carnosine on excitation-contraction coupling in mechanically-skinned rat skeletal muscle. *Journal of Muscle Research and Cell Motility* **25**, 201–213.

Earnest, C.P., Snell, P.G., Rodriguez, R. *et al.* (1995). The effect of creatine monohydrate ingestion on anaerobic power indices, muscular strength and body composition. *Acta Physiologica Scandinavica* **153**, 207–209.

Edge, J., Bishop, D. and Goodman, C. (2006). Effects of chronic NaHCO3 ingestion during interval training on changes to muscle buffer capacity, metabolism, and short-term endurance performance. *Journal of Applied Physiology* **101**, 918–925.

Fitts, R.H. (1994). Cellular mechanisms of muscle fatigue. *Physiological Reviews* **74**, 49–94.

Forsberg, A.M., Nilsson, E., Werneman, J. *et al.* (1991). Muscle composition in relation to age and sex. *Clinical Science* **81**, 249–256.

George, K.P. and MacLaren D.P.M. (1988). The effect of induced alkalosis and acidosis on endurance running at an intensity corresponding to 4mM blood lactate. *Ergonomics* **31**, 1639–1645.

Goldberg, P.G. and Bechtel, P.J. (1997). Effects of low dose creatine supplementation on strength, speed and power events by male athletes. *Medicine and Science in Sport and Exercise* **29**, S251.

Goldfinch, J., McNaughton, L. and Davies, P. (1988). Induced metabolic acidosis and its effects on 400-m racing time. *European Journal of Applied Physiology* **57**, 45–48.

Green, A.L., Hultman, E., MacDonald, I.A. *et al.* (1996). Carbohydrate ingestion augments skeletal muscle creatine accumulation during creatine supplementation in man. *American Journal of Physiology* **271**, E821–E826.

Greenhaff, P.L. (1997). The nutritional biochemistry of creatine. *Nutritional Biochemistry* **8**, 610–618.

Greenhaff, P.L., Casey, A., Short, A.H. *et al.* (1993). Influence of oral creatine supplementation of muscle torque during repeated bouts of maximal voluntary exercise in man. *Clinical Science* **84**, 565–571.

Harris, R.C., Martin, D.J., Dunnett, M. *et al.* (1990). Muscle buffering capacity and dipeptide content in the thoroughbred horse, greyhound and man. *Comparative Biochemistry and Physiology A—Physiology* **97**, 249–251.

Harris, R.C., Soderlund, K. and Hultman, E. (1992). Elevation of creatine in resting and exercised muscle of normal subjects by creatine supplementation. *Clinical Science* **83**, 367–374.

Harris, R.C., Tallon, M.J., Dunnett, M. *et al.* (2006). The absorption of orally supplied beta-alanine and its effects on muscle carnosine synthesis in human vastus lateralis. *Amino Acids* **30**, 279–289.

Hespel, P. and Derave, W. (2007). Ergogenic effects of creatine in sports and rehabilitation. *Subcellular Biochemistry* **46**, 245–259.

Hill, C.C., Harris, R.C., Kim, H.J. *et al.* (2007). Influence of β-alanine supplementation on skeletal muscle carnosine concentrations and high intensity cycling capacity. *Amino Acids* **32**, 225–233.

Hipkiss, A.R. and Michaelis, J. (1995). Non-enzymatic glycolysation of the dipeptide carnosine, a potential anti-protein, cross-linking agent. *FEBS Letters* **371**, 81–85.

Hultman, E., Soderlund, K., Timmons, J. *et al.* (1996). Muscle creatine loading in man. *Journal of Applied Physiology* **81**, 232–237.

Juel, C. (1997). Lactate-proton cotransport in skeletal muscle. *Physiological Reviews* **77**, 321–358.

Kendall, K.L., Smith, A.E., Graef, J.L. *et al.* (2009). Effects of four weeks of high-intensity interval training and creatine supplementation on critical power and anaerobic working capacity in college-aged men. *Journal of Strength and Conditioning Research* **23**, 1663–1669.

Kendrick, I.P., Harris, R.C., Kim, H.J. *et al.* (2008). The effects of 10 weeks of resistance training combined with beta-alanine supplementation on whole body strength, force production, muscular endurance and body composition. *Amino Acids* **34**, 547–554.

Kreider, R., Grindstaff, P., Wood, L. *et al.* (1996). Effects of ingesting a lean mass promoting supplement during resistance training on isokinetic performance. *Medicine and Science in Sports Exercise* **28**, S36.

Law, Y.L., Ong, W.S.G., Yap, T.L.L. *et al.* (2009). Effects of two and five days of creatine loading on muscular strength and anaerobic power in trained athletes. *Journal of Strength and Conditioning Research* **23**, 906–914.

Leenders, N., Sherman, W.M., Lamb, D.R. *et al.* (1999). Creatine supplementation and swimming performance. *International Journal of Sports Nutrition* **9**, 251–262.

Lindh, A.M., Peyrebrune, M.C., Ingham, S.A. *et al.* (2008). Sodium bicarbonate improves swimming performance. *International Journal of Sports Medicine* **29**, 519–523.

MacLaren, D.P.M. (1997). Alkalinizers: Influence of blood acid-base status on performance. In *The clinical pharmacology of sport and exercise*, ed. T. Reilly and M. Orme, Excerpta Medica, Amsterdam. 157–163.

Maganaris, C.N. and Maughan, R.J. (1998). Creatine supplementation enhances maximum voluntary isometric force and endurance capacity in resistance trained men. *Acta Physiologica Scandinavica* **163**, 279–287.

Matson, L.G. and Tran, Z.V. (1993). Effects of sodium bicarbonate ingestion on anaerobic performance: A meta-analytic review. *International Journal of Sports Nutrition* **3**, 2–28.

McNaughton, L.R. (1992). Sodium bicarbonate ingestion and its effects on anaerobic exercise of various durations. *Journal of Sports Sciences* **10**, 425–435.

McNaughton, L., Backx, K., Palmer, G. *et al.* (1999). Effects of chronic bicarbonate ingestion on the performance of high-intensity work. *European Journal of Applied Physiology and Occupational Physiology* **80**, 64–69.

McNaughton, L., Siegler, J. and Midgeley, A. (2008). Ergogenic effects of sodium bicarbonate. *Current Sports Medicine Reports* **7**, 230–236.

McNaughton, L., Strange, N. and Backx, K. (2000). The effects of chronic sodium bicarbonate ingestion on multiple bouts of anaerobic work and power output. *Journal of Human Movement Studies* **38**, 307–322.

Nevill, M.E., Boobis, L.H., Brooks, S. *et al.* (1989). Effect of training on muscle metabolism during treadmill sprinting. *Journal of Applied Physiolology* **67**, 2376–2382.

Nielsen, H.B., Hein, L., Svendsen, L.B. *et al.* (2002). Bicarbonate attenuates intracellular acidosis. *Acta Anaesthesiology Scandinavica* **46**, 579–584.

Noonan, D., Berg, K., Latin, R.W. *et al.* (1998). Effects of varying dosages of oral creatine relative to fat free mass on strength and body composition. *Journal of Strength and Conditioning Research* **12**, 104–108.

Olsen, S., Aagaard P., Kadi F. *et al.* (2006). Creatine supplementation augments the increase in satellite cell and myonuclei number in human skeletal muscle induced by strength training. *Journal of Physiology* **573**, 525–534.

Parkhouse, W.S., McKenzie, D.C., Hochachka, P.W. *et al.* (1985). Buffering capacity of deproteinised human vastus lateralis muscle. *Journal of applied Physiology* **58**, 14–17.

Parry-Billings M. and MacLaren, D.P.M. (1986). The effect of sodium bicarbonate and sodium citrate ingestion on anaerobic power during intermittent exercise. *European Journal of Applied Physiology* **55**, 524–529.

Peyrebrune, M.C., Nevill, M.E., Donaldson, F.J. *et al.* (1998). The effects of oral creatine supplementation in single and repeated swimming. *Journal of Sports Science* **16**, 271–279.

Ponte, J., Harris, R.C., Hill, C.A. *et al.* (2007). Effect of 14–28 days of beta-alanine supplementation on isometric endurance of the knee extensors. *Journal of Sports Sciences* **25**, 334.

Rawson, E.S., Clarkson, P.M. and Melanson, E.L. (1998). The effects of oral creatine supplementation on body mass, isometric strength, and isokinetic performance in older individuals. *Medicine and Science in Sports and Exercise* **30**, S140.

Raymer, G.H., Marsh, G.D., Kowalchuk, J.M. *et al.* (2004). Metabolic effects of induced alkalosis during progressive forearm exercise to fatigue. *Journal of Applied Physiology* **96**, 2050–2056.

Sahlin, K. (1998). Anaerobic metabolism, acid-base balance, and muscle fatigue during high intensity exercise. In *Oxford textbook of sports medicine*, ed. M. Harries, C. Williams, W.D. Stanish and L.J. Micheli, Oxford University Press, Oxford. 69–76.

Sharp, R.L., Costill, D.L., Fink, W.J. *et al.* (1986). Effects of eight weeks of bicycle ergometer sprint training on human muscle buffer capacity. *International Journal of Sports Medicine* **7**, 7–13.

Smart, N.A., McKenzie, S.G., Nix, L.M. *et al.* (1998). Creatine supplementation does not improve repeat sprint performance in soccer players. *Medicine and Science in Sports Exercise* **30**, S140.

Smith, S.A., Montain, S.J., Matott, R.P. *et al.* (1998). Creatine supplementation and age influence muscle metabolism during exercise. *Journal of Applied Physiology* **85**, 1349–1356.

Stout, J.R., Echerson, J., Noonan, D. *et al.* (1999). Effects of creatine supplementation on exercise performance and fat-free weight in football players during training. *Nutrition Research* **19**, 217–225.

Suzuki, Y., Ito, O. and Mukai, N. (2002). High level of skeletal muscle carnosine contributes to the latter half of exercise performance during 30-s maximal cycle ergometry sprinting. *Japanese Journal of Physiology* **52**, 199–205.

Tarnopolsky, M.A. (2008). Nutritional consideration in the aging athlete. *Clinical Journal of Sport Medicine* **18**, 531–538.

Vandenberghe, K., Goris, M., Van Hecke, P. *et al.* (1996). Prolonged creatine intake facilitates the effects of strength training on intermittent exercise capacity. *Insider* **4**, 1–2.

Van Montfoort, M.C., Van Dieren, L., Hopkins, W.G. *et al.* (2004). Effects of ingestion of sodium bicarbonate, citrate, lactate, and chloride on sprint running. *Medicine and Science in Sports and Exercise* **36**, 1239–1243.

Van Thienen, R., Van Proeyen, K., Eynde, B.V. *et al.* (2009). beta-Alanine improves sprint performance in endurance cycling. *Medicine and Science in Sports and Exercise* **41**, 898–903.

Verbitsky, O., Mizrah, J., Levin, M. *et al.* (1997). Effect of ingestion of sodium bicarbonate on muscle force, fatigue, and recovery. *Journal of Applied Physiology* **83**, 333–337.

Wilkes, D., Gledhill, N. and Smyth, R. (1983). Effect of acute induced metabolic alkalosis on 800 metre racing time. *Medicine and Science in Sports and Exercise* **15**, 277–280.

Wyss, M. and Kaddourah-Daouk, R. (2000). Creatine and creatinine metabolism. *Physiological Reviews* **80**, 1107–1213.

Chapter 19

Supplement use in sport

David R. Mottram

19.1 Introduction

Supplements used in sport include vitamins, minerals, carbohydrates, protein and various extracts, principally derived from plant sources. There is a commonly held view that "natural" products are, by definition, free of toxic side effects. This is clearly a misconception, particularly when it is remembered that in the early days of pharmacological science all drugs were derived from plant and animal sources and that many of these derivatives are amongst the most toxic chemicals known to man. Indeed, some nutritional supplements have the potential for harm (Beltz and Doering, 1993; Maughan *et al.*, 2004; Maughan, 2005).

19.2 Extent of supplement use

Taking substances to enhance athletic performance dates back to the Ancient Olympic Games. This behaviour persists today. Both recreational and competitive athletes use supplements. It has been suggested that between 40 per cent and 100 per cent of athletes use supplements, often as multiple regimes and at higher than normal doses (Baume *et al.*, 2007). Figures on the scope and extent of supplement use vary widely.

At a more recent Olympic Games, in Sydney in 2000, Corrigan and Kazlauskas (2003) recorded self-reported supplement use by the 2758 athletes who were tested at these Games. At least 17 different classes of supplements were reported, the most frequently cited being multivitamins (n = 1116), Vitamin C (810), creatine (316) and amino acids (190).

Sundgot-Borgen *et al.* (2003) investigated the use of selected supplements in Norwegian elite athletes compared with a control group. A similar percentage of female athletes (54 per cent) and controls (52 per cent) reported using one or more supplements, whereas more male athletes (51 per cent) than controls (32 per cent) used supplements. In the athlete group, the main supplements used were minerals (males 26 per cent, females 42 per cent), amino acids (males 12 per cent, females 3 per cent) and creatine (males 12 per cent, females 3 per cent).

A survey of high school athletes by Laure *et al.* (2004) in France showed that 4 per cent of respondents had used creatine and 41 per cent had used vitamins.

At the 2004 Olympic Games in Athens, 75.7 per cent of athletes declared a use of medication or supplements in the three days before testing. Of these, the most common were food supplements (45.3 per cent of respondents), vitamins (43.2 per cent) and proteins/amino acids (13.5 per cent) (Tsitsimpikou *et al.*, 2009).

Nieper (2005) found that 62 per cent of UK junior national track and field athletes were using supplements, with an average of 2.4 products per athlete and with males using ergogenic aids more often than females. Multivitamins and minerals were the most popular products used. The main reasons for using supplements were for health (45 per cent), to enhance the immune system (40 per cent) and to improve performance (25 per cent).

Erdman *et al.* (2006) surveyed Canadian high-performance athletes and found that 88.4 per cent reported using dietary supplements during the previous six months, with an average of 3.08 supplements per user. Sport drinks (22.4 per cent), sport bars (14.0 per cent), multivitamins and minerals (13.5 per cent), protein supplements (9.0 per cent) and Vitamin C (6.4 per cent) were most frequently reported. Protein supplements were significantly more likely to be used by athletes at the highest performance level.

19.3   Why supplements are used

There are considerable pressures placed on athletes to use supplements by their supporters and advisors and by the high-pressure advertising by companies that sell these products (Maughan *et al.*, 2007). In addition an athlete's lifestyle and/or training regime may not allow sufficient time to meet energy needs.

A number of reasons can therefore be identified to explain why athletes choose to use supplements so extensively (Baume *et al.*, 2007; Maughan *et al.*, 2004; Maughan *et al.*, 2007):

- to substitute for a poor quality diet;
- to provide additional nutrients to supplement an adequate or even a good diet;
- to prevent or aid the recovery from injury or ill-health;
- to facilitate recovery from training;
- to tailor nutritional support to provide ergogenic advantage in particular circumstances of higher level of physical activity.

The question that needs to be asked is whether supplements confer any advantage to the athlete. In a review by Deldicque and Francaux (2008), it was stated that several types of supplements have demonstrated improved sport performance at a higher level than that expected with a well-balanced diet. However, the evidence base for their effectiveness is not robust.

19.4   Types of supplements

There are several very useful reviews of the types of supplements available to athletes (Clarkson, 1996; Maughan, 1999; Maughan et al., 2004; UK Sport, 2006). In this section a brief synopsis is given of the more common supplements that have been cited as having potential benefits for athletes.

Classification

There is no single definition of what constitutes a dietary supplement (Maughan et al., 2007). Burke and Read (1993) proposed a classification based on dietary supplements and nutritional ergogenic aids. Dietary supplements include products such as sport drinks, carbohydrate and protein supplements, vitamins and minerals. Nutritional ergogenic aids include caffeine, bicarbonate, creatine, carnitine, ginseng and glycerol (Baume et al., 2007).

Vitamins

Vitamins are frequently taken by athletes on the supposition that they are experiencing a vitamin deficiency due to exercise and training regimes. However, Cotter (1988) has suggested that there is little evidence to suggest that exercise alone would necessitate vitamin supplementation.

In terms of using vitamin supplements as ergogenic aids, the B-complex vitamins have been taken because they are co-enzymes in the processes of red blood cell production and in the metabolism of fats and carbohydrates. Vitamin C is reputed to aid in the wound-healing process and vitamin E has been claimed to increase aerobic capacity. All these claims for ergogenic properties of vitamins have been discussed by Barone (1988) but, in general, there is little evidence available to substantiate such claims.

Vitamins are toxic when taken in excess. This applies particularly to the fat-soluble vitamins (A, D, E and K) that are stored in the body and can therefore accumulate. Even the water-soluble vitamins (B and C) can produce toxic effects when taken excessively (Hecker, 1987).

In general, a balanced diet will provide the necessary nutritional requirements of vitamins. Vitamin supplements are only of benefit where there is a clear deficiency, such as occurs with an exceptional nutritional intake (Wadler and Hainlain, 1989).

Proteins and amino acids

Protein and amino acid supplements are frequently used by athletes, often associated with training (Hawley et al., 2006). Protein is obviously an essential component of a balanced diet but there is no experimental evidence to show that protein supplementation enhances metabolic activity or leads to increased muscle mass (Wilmore and Freund, 1986; Hecker, 1987). However, protein supplements allow athletes the possibility of increasing protein intake without the unacceptable increase in fat intake that is associated with high protein foods (Maughan et al., 2007).

Excessive intake of protein can produce toxic effects, due to overproduction of urea with a concomitant loss of water. This can lead to dehydration with a risk to the competitor of muscle cramp and an impairment of body temperature regulation. Manipulation of diet, to induce metabolic acidosis by reducing carbohydrate intake or increasing fat and protein intake, have shown impaired performance (MacLaren, 1997).

Arginine and ornithine, which are amino acids, have been shown to stimulate the release of growth hormone (Bucci, 1989). Such an effect requires intravenous infusion of the amino acids. A similar effect, following oral administration of arginine or ornithine, has not been established. Furthermore, the literature does not support the idea that growth hormone releasers have an ergogenic effect (Beltz and Doering, 1993).

In general, it is considered that amino acids do not improve endurance performance (Wagenmakers, 1999) and that physically active individuals are advised to obtain necessary amino acids through consumption of natural, high-quality protein foods rather than through supplements (Williams, 1999).

Carbohydrates

Sports drinks, used to replace fluids, carbohydrates and electrolytes are widely used by athletes. During endurance exercise, suitable intake of such products has been shown to be beneficial for glycogen-depleted muscles and to enhance performance (Burke and Read, 1993).

Ginseng

Ginseng is a herbal preparation containing a complex mixture of glycosides, known as ginsenosides. There are many varieties of plant from which ginsenosides are extracted and multiple preparations within which they are presented. No two preparations will contain the same combination and dose of ginsenosides.

Ginseng has been used for thousands of years, particularly by the Chinese, and many claims have been made as to its therapeutic value. Few scientific experiments have been reported with regard to its performance-enhancing properties. Teves et al. (1983) failed to find any statistically significant difference in maximum aerobic capacity, heart rate or time to exhaustion during a comparative controlled trial on a small group of marathon runners.

Several disparate side effects have been described with long-term use of ginseng (Siegel, 1979).

Creatine

Creatine is one of the most widely used legal supplements available to athletes, with an estimated 30 per cent to 50 per cent of professional athletes using it on a regular basis (Puerini and Gorey, 2000). An extensive review of creatine is provided in Chapter 18.

L-Carnitine

L-Carnitine is synthesised in the kidneys and liver. It can be obtained through the diet from animal sources. L-Carnitine deficiency is extremely rare. It is required for the transport and oxidation of long-chain fatty acids into mitochondria for the production of energy. It is therefore postulated that ingesting more L-carnitine will lead to more fat being burned to supply energy. Athletes have used it to promote fat loss and to enhance aerobic and anaerobic capacity (Beltz and Doering, 1993). However, most placebo-controlled trials have failed to demonstrate any improvement in maximal oxygen uptake or in endurance performance in response to oral L-carnitine (Brown, 1993). A review by Cerretelli and Marconi (1990) was unable to show any beneficial effects on performance as a result of L-carnitine supplementation. At the dose ranges used, no reports of toxicity due to L-carnitine were described.

Caffeine

Caffeine was classified as a stimulant on the IOC prohibited list but was removed by WADA in 2004 and placed on a monitoring list. Since then, an increased interest in its use by athletes has been noted. An extensive review of caffeine is provided in Chapter 20.

Glucosamine

Glucosamine is promoted for its ability to stimulate the formation of proteoglycans within cartilage. There is some evidence from clinical trials that it can be beneficial to patients with osteoarthritis (Fillmore et al., 1999). There is little or no evidence for a beneficial use of glucosamine for athletes with joint pain (Maughan et al., 2007).

19.5   Availability of supplements

The supplements market is huge (Nieper, 2005). Many dietary supplements are produced by reputable international pharmaceutical companies and are available from pharmacies. Heavy advertising through magazines and the internet has allowed athletes unrestricted access to a wide range of supplements (Baume et al., 2007). Many prohormones, natural hormones and related steroids are available over the internet, despite attempts by government agencies to curtail this activity (Catlin *et al.*, 2008). Clearly, athletes intent on using supplements need to be vigilant with respect to the validity of the source of their products.

19.6   Problems associated with supplement use

WADA regulations

Most substances classified as supplements are not included on the WADA prohibited list. It is debatable whether WADA should revise its doping control regulations to include nutritional supplements (Williams, 1994; Mottram, 1999). Certainly, the fact that supplement use by athletes is so widespread and that many products are used solely in an attempt to improve ergogenic performance engenders a "doping attitude" in the sporting community (Baume *et al.*, 2007). This may encourage athletes to think beyond supplement use and to experiment with substances and methods from the prohibited list. It has also been suggested that supplement use by elite athletes encourages such use within the general population (Lippi *et al.*, 2008).

Even when athletes purchase supplements in good faith, there is an ever-present risk that the supplements may contain an unidentified substance from the WADA prohibited list. Under the strict liability rules of the World Anti-Doping Code, an adverse test result may lead to sanctions irrespective of the athlete's lack of knowledge that a prohibited substance was being taken. The WADA prohibited list is not definitive and does not therefore specify every single substance that is prohibited but includes specified classes of substances. Athletes must therefore guard against supplements that may contain new, untried and untested products.

Misleading advertising, inaccurate labelling and supplement contamination

Unlike therapeutic drugs, nutritional supplements are not required to have strong scientific and clinical proof that they are effective before they can be sold to the public (Clarkson, 1996). They are not subject to the same independent, scientific scrutiny as regulated medicines receive (Herbert, 1999; Maughan, 2005).

Manufacturers may make exaggerated claims regarding the ergogenic properties of their products (Beltz and Doering, 1993). Such claims are rarely substantiated by sound scientific data in peer-reviewed journals (Nieman and Pedersen, 1999). On the other hand, labelling of supplements may not correspond with the content of the product, which could contain prohibited substances.

In terms of contamination, studies have shown that between 10 per cent and 25 per cent of products were found to be contaminated (Baume *et al.*, 2007). Many of these contaminants are liable to result in an adverse finding during doping control testing. Two sources of contamination have been proposed

(Burke, 2004). One is cross-contamination due to poor practice on the part of the manufacturers; the other may be from undeclared additions of active ingredients to supplements that would otherwise be ineffective. Athletes should be aware that WADA-accredited laboratories can detect prohibited substances and their metabolites at much lower concentrations (parts per billion) than the levels detectable by the majority of supplement manufacturers (parts per million).

The main contaminants in supplements have been shown to be stimulants, such as ephedrine, anabolic steroids and precursors to anabolic steroids, often referred to as prohormones (Baume *et al.*, 2007). Nutritional supplements containing the plant *Ephedra sinica* (Ma-Huang) are marketed primarily as adjuvants in weight loss programmes (Yonamine *et al.*, 2004). Prohormones are legally available on the sports nutrition market and are aggressively marketed as having enormous potential to increase muscle growth and strength (Geyer *et al.*, 2008). The most common are the prohormones of testosterone and nandrolone. Such prohormones include 4-androstenedione, 4-androstenediol, 5-androstenediol (pre-cursors of testosterone), 19-norandrostenedione and 19-norandrostenediol (precursors of nortestosterone), as well as dehydroepiandrosterone (DHEA) (Yonamine *et al.*, 2004).

Geyer *et al.* (2008) have also identified prohibited stimulants such as ephedrines, methylenedioxymetamphetamine and sibutramine within supplements, despite their not being declared on the labels of the supplements tested.

Geyer *et al.* (2004) purchased 634 non-hormonal nutritional supplements from 13 countries, mostly from shops but including 52 samples from the internet. Analysis revealed that 94 (14.8 per cent) of the products contained anabolic androgenic steroids that had not been declared on the labels of the products. These were mainly prohormones of testosterone and nandrolone. The extent of contaminated supplements varied from country to country with the Netherlands (25.8 per cent), Austria (22.7 per cent), the UK (18.8 per cent) and the USA (18.8 per cent) having above average numbers.

A similar study was conducted on 103 dietary supplements bought on the internet (Baume *et al.*, 2006). The products were screened for the presence of stimulants, anabolic steroids and the precursors and metabolites of testosterone and nandrolone. Results showed that approximately one in five supplements were contaminated with products not declared on the label, all of which would have caused the athlete to test positive for prohibited substances.

Tribulus terrestris is an herbal nutritional supplement that has been promoted to produce gains in lean muscle mass and strength. Some of the manufacturers of this product claimed that it would not lead to positive drug tests whilst other manufacturers suggested it may increase the testosterone/epitestosterone ratio, the basis for determining if athletes have used exogenous testosterone. A study by Rogerson *et al.* (2007) showed that Tribulus terrestris did not alter T/E ratios but did not produce a large gain in strength or lean muscle mass either. Similarly, a study on two female athletes showed no impact of Tribulus terrestris on endogenous testosterone metabolites (Saudan *et al.*, 2008).

Accuracy and quality of advice on supplement use

Athletes often self-medicate with supplements but may seek advice from a variety of sources. Coaches were found to be the main advisors on supplement use for male (58 per cent) and female (52 per cent) elite Norwegian athletes (Sundgot-Borgen *et al.*, 2003). The authors were surprised that so many athletes were advised by non-medical members of the athletes' support teams, considering the lack of knowledge of nutrition by such supporters. Similar results were reported by Erdman *et al.* (2007), where family/friends (52.7 per cent of respondents), team mates (44.3 per cent) and coaches (40.7 per cent) were most often identified as sources of information on supplements.

In a survey by Nieper (2005), 72 per cent of respondents claimed to have access to a sports dietitian but tended to underutilise this resource. Subjects indicated that coaches (65 per cent) had the greatest influence on supplement use, with doctors (25 per cent) and sports dietitians (30 per cent) being less important.

Case studies involving supplements

There have been a number of high-profile cases involving athletes who have tested positive for the anabolic steroid nandrolone, where athletes had claimed that they had ingested the steroid in a "contaminated" nutritional supplement, an assertion that may be true (Ayotte, 1999).

Professional footballers in 2001

A number of professional footballers tested positive for nandrolone metabolites during 2001. Many of these cases were picked up by the IOC-accredited laboratory in Italy but the problem was not confined to this country. These cases involved players from many countries, including the Italians Christian Bucchi and Salvatore Monaco, Portugal's Fernando Couto, the Spaniard Josef Guardiola and the Dutch internationals Frank de Boer, Edgar Davids and Jaap Stam. In all these cases, the players received suspensions but it was widely acknowledged that the players had tested positive through using contaminated supplements.

Greg Rusedski, 2003

The tennis player Greg Rusedski tested positive for nandrolone in July 2003, and he claimed it was a result of taking "contaminated" electrolyte supplement pills that the Association of Tennis Professionals (ATP) had been giving out to tennis players through its trainers. A number of other tennis players similarly tested positive for nandrolone between September 2002 and May 2003. Many of these players were below the cut-off level that was in place for testing purposes and were therefore not sanctioned. Greg Rusedski and another six players were above the cut-off level but were exonerated by the ATP. The ATP anti-doping tribunal acknolwedged that it could not prosecute a case when it had created the situation itself by the action of its trainers distributing these "contaminated" supplements.

Subsequently, the ATP commissioned an anti-doping expert to investigate the source of the nandrolone but found no trace of nandrolone in around 500 pills tested. The expert's conclusion was ambiguous: "While the circumstantial evidence points to nandrolone-related contamination of the electrolyte-replacement products as the source . . . there is insufficient evidence to prove that the electrolytes were the cause of the test results. Similarly there is not sufficient evidence to prove they were not the cause".

19.7   Advice for athletes

Athletes have used supplements for centuries and will continue to do so, regardless of warnings. Therefore advice to avoid taking supplements is not helpful to athletes (Burke, 2004). Athletes have to be advised to consider the risk-benefit ratio of using supplements.

Are the benefits strong enough? Can nutritional support be achieved simply through a well-balanced diet? Does the taking of excess supplements, such as vitamins and minerals, confer any advantage or are they simply excreted because the body has specific nutritional limits for such products? Is there a strong evidence base to support the claims of ergogenic properties for some supplements? Some would say no (Deldicque and Francaux, 2008).

What is the potential cost of supplement use? Will the side effects outweigh any potential benefit? Can the source of the supplement be relied upon? What are the consequences of an adverse doping test result?

In the end, athletes must do their homework before making a rational, evidence-based decision. It is worth noting that, compared with other factors, the place of diet and supplements on performance is relatively small (Maughan *et al.*, 2007), although the margins for improvement that athletes seek over their fellow competitors are also often small.

The quality and accuracy of advice that athletes have sought in the past have been questioned (Sundgot-Borgen *et al.*, 2003). It is important for athletes to seek advice from qualified sport nutrition specialists or accredited sport dietitians (Maughan *et al.*, 2007) and to check information with their respective international federation, national anti-doping organisations (NADOs) or WADA.

No currently recognised analytical method is capable of distinguishing between a sample from an athlete deliberately taking a prohibited substance and one from an athlete who was passively exposed to a doping agent. Athletes and their advisors must be constantly alert to non-intentional doping as the WADA code applies strict liability rules (Yonamine *et al.*, 2004).

19.8   References

Ayotte, C. (1999). Nutritional supplements and doping controls. *New Studies in Athletics* **14**, 37–42.

Barone, S. (1988). Vitamins and athletes. In *Drugs, athletes and physical performance*, ed. J.A. Thomas, Plenum, New York. 1–9.

Baume, N., Hellemans, L. and Saugy, M. (2007). Guide to over-the-counter sports supplements for athletes. *International Sports Medicine Journal* **8(1)**, 2–10.

Baume, N., Mahler, N., Kamber, M. *et al.* (2006). Research of stimulants and anabolic steroids in dietary supplements. *Scandinavian Journal of Medical Science in Sports* **16**, 41–48.

Beltz, S.D. and Doering, P.L. (1993). Efficacy of nutritional supplements used by athletes. *Clinical Pharmacy* **12**, 900–908.

Brown M. (1993). Performance enhancement. *Coaching Focus* **23**, 5–6.

Bucci, L.R. (1989). Nutritional ergogenic aids. In *Nutrition in exercise and sport*, ed. I. Wolinsky and J.F. Hickson, CRC Press Boca Raton. 107–184.

Burke, L.M. (2004). Contamination of supplements: An interview with Professor Ron Maughan. *International Journal of Sport Nutrition and Exercise Metabolism* **14**, 493–496.

Burke, L.M. and Read, R.S.D. (1993). Dietary supplements in sport. *Sports Medicine* **15**, 43–65.

Catlin, D.H., Fitch, K.D. and Lungqvist, A. (2008). Medicine and science in the fight against doping in sport. *Journal of Internal Medicine* **264**, 99–114.

Cerretelli, P. and Marconi, C. (1990). L-Carnitine supplementation in humans: The effects on physical performance. *International Journal of Sports Medicine* **11**, 1–14.

Clarkson, P.M. (1996). Nutrition for improved sport performance: Current issues on ergogenic aids. *Sports Medicine* **21**, 393–401.

Corrigan, B. and Kazlauskas, R. (2003). Medication use in athletes selected for doping control at the Sydney Olympiad (2000). *Clinical Journal of Sports Medicine* **13**, 33–40.

Cotter, R. (1988). Nutrition, fluid balance and physical performance. In *Drugs, athletes and physical performance*, ed. J.A. Thomas, Plenum, New York. 31–40.

Deldicque, L. and Francaux, M. (2008). Functional food for exercise performance: Fact or foe? *Current Opinions in Clinical Nutrition and Metabolic Care* **11**, 774–781.

Erdman, K.A., Fung, T.S., Doyle-Baker, P.K. *et al.* (2007). Dietary supplementation of high performance Canadian athletes by age and gender. *Clinical Journal of Sports Medicine* **17**, 458–464.

Erdman, K.A., Fung, T.S. and Reimer, R.A. (2006). Influence of performance level on dietary supplementation in elite Canadian athletes. *Medicine and Science in Sports and Exercise* **38(2)**, 349–356.

Fillmore, C.M., Bartoli, L., Bach, R. *et al.* (1999). Nutrition and dietary supplements. *Physical Medicine and Rehabilitation Clinics of North America* **10**, 673–703.

Geyer, H., Parr, M.K., Koehler, K. *et al.* (2008). Nutritional supplements cross-contaminated and faked with doping substances. *Journal of Mass Spectrometry* **43**, 892–902.

Geyer, H., Parr, M.K., Mareck, U., *et al.* (2004). Analysis of non-hormonal nutritional supplements for anabolic androgenic steroids—Results of an international study. *International Journal of Sports Medicine* **25**, 124–129.

Hawley, J.A., Tipton, K.D. and Millard-Stafford, M.L. (2006). Promoting training adaptations through nutritional interventions. *Journal of Sports Sciences* **24**, 709–721.

Hecker, A.L. (1987). Nutrition and physical performance. In *Drugs and performance in sports*, ed. R.H.Strauss, Saunders, Philadelphia. 23–52.

Herbert, D.L. (1999). Recommending or selling nutritional supplements enhances potential legal liability for sports medicine practitioners. *Sports Medicine Alert* **5(11)**, 91–92.

Laure, P., Lecerf, T., Friser, A. *et al.* (2004). Drugs, recreational drug use and attitudes towards doping of high school athletes. *International Journal of Sports Medicine* **25**, 133–138.

Lippi, G., Franchini, M. and Guidi, G.C. (2008). Doping in competition or doping in sport? *British Medical Bulletin* **86**, 95–107.

MacLaren, D.P.M. (1997). *Alkalinizers: Influence of blood acid-base status on performance*. Esteve Foundation Symposium. Vol. 7. The clinical pharmacology of sport and exercise. Excerpta Medica, Amsterdam. 157–165.

Maughan, R.J. (1999). Nutritional ergogenic aids and exercise performance. *Nutritional Research Reviews* **12**, 255–280.

Maughan, R.J. (2005). Contamination of dietary supplements and positive drug tests in sport. *Journal of Sports Sciences* **23(9)**, 883–889.

Maughan, R.J., Depiesse, F. and Geyer, H. (2007). The use of dietary supplements by athletes. *Journal of Sports Sciences* **25(S1)**, S103–S113.

Maughan, R.J., King, D.S. and Lea, T. (2004). Dietary supplements. *Journal of Sports Sciences* **22**, 95–113.

Mottram, D.R. (1999). Banned drugs in sport. Does the International Olympic Committee (IOC) list need updating? *Sports Medicine* **27**, 1–10.

Nieman, D.C. and Pedersen, B.K. (1999). Exercise and immune function: Recent developments. *Sports Medicine* **27**, 73–80.

Nieper, A. (2005). Nutritional supplement practices in UK junior national track and field athletes. *British Journal of Sports Medicine* **39**, 645–649.

Puerini, A.J. and Gorey, K. (2000). Sports and drugs in primary care. *Medicine and Health* **83**, 169–172.

Rogerson, S., Riches, C.J., Jennings, C. *et al.* (2007). The effect of five weeks of Tribulus terrestris supplementation on muscle strength and body composition during preseason training in elite rugby league players. *Journal of Strength and Conditioning Research* **21(2)**, 348–353.

Saudan, C., Baume, N., Emery, C. *et al.* (2008). Short term impact of Tribulus terrestris intake on doping control analysis of endogenous steroids. *Forensic Science International* **178(1)**, e7–e10.

Siegel, R.K. (1979). Ginseng abuse syndrome: Problems with the panacea. *JAMA* **241**, 1614–1615.

Sundgot-Borgen, J., Berglund, B. and Torstveit, M.K. (2003). Nutritional supplements in Norwegian elite athletes—Impact of international ranking and advisors. *Scandinavian Journal of Medical Science in Sports* **13**, 138–144.

Teves, J.E., Wright, J.E. and Welch, M.J. (1983). Effects of ginseng on repeated bouts of exhaustive exercise. *Medicine and Science in Sports and Exercise* **15**, 162.

Tsitsimpikou, C., Tsiokanos, A., Tsarouhas, K. *et al.* (2009). Medication use by athletes at the Athens 2004 Summer Olympic Games. *Clinical Journal of Sports Medicine* **19(1)**, 33–38.

UK Sport. (2006). Sports supplements and the associated risk. Available at http//:www. uksport.gov.uk (accessed March 2009).

Wadler, G.I. and Hainlain, B. (1989). *Drugs and the athlete*. Davis, Philadelphia.

Wagenmakers, A.J.M. (1999). Amino acid supplements to improve athletic performance. *Current Opinion in Clinical Nutrition and Metabolic Care* **2**, 539–544.

Williams, M.H. (1994). The use of nutritional ergogenic aids in sports: Is it an ethical issue? *International Journal of Sports Nutrition* **4**, 120–131.

Williams, M.H. (1999). Facts and fallacies of purported ergogenic amino acid supplements. *Clinics in Sports Medicine* **18**, 633–649.

Wilmore, J.H. and Freund, B.J. (1986). Nutritional enhancement of athletic performance. In *Nutrition and exercise*, ed. M. Winick, Wiley, New York. 67–97.

Yonamine, M., Garcia, P.R. and de Moraes Moreau, R.L. (2004). Non-intentional doping in sports. *Sports Medicine* **34(1)**, 697–704.

Chapter 20

Caffeine

Neil Chester

20.1 Introduction

Caffeine is present in a variety of plant species widely distributed throughout the world, the most common sources being coffee, tea and cocoa. Because it is a constituent of a large number of commonly available beverages and foodstuffs (Table 20.1) and its use is generally unregulated and accepted throughout the world, caffeine is believed to be one of the most widely used drugs.

Caffeine has great appeal as an ergogenic aid with extensive scientific research supporting its performance-enhancing properties over a wide range of sporting activities. It is commonly employed amongst many individuals for its psychotropic properties, to increase wakefulness, alertness and concentration. However, despite the widespread use of caffeine as a performance-enhancing drug there remains conjecture regarding the exact mechanisms behind these properties.

As a consequence of caffeine's widespread consumption and limited side effects at low to moderate doses—together with the fact that it is extremely difficult, if not impossible to differentiate, via a drug test, between its consumption in a typical diet from that for the purpose of enhancing performance—WADA removed caffeine from its prohibited list in 2004. However, whilst caffeine is not prohibited it has been part of the WADA monitoring programme since its inception on January 1, 2004. The monitoring programme allowed WADA to examine the use of caffeine and other commonly available substances that were potential ergogenic aids and open to inadvertent doping offences. Evidence gathered from the programme would potentially support or oppose the reintroduction of a substance to the prohibited list.

There appears to have been an increase in caffeine consumption in recent years due to the growing popularity of café culture (Freedman, 2006). In sport the use of caffeine as an ergogenic aid appears to have increased following its removal from the prohibited list. Since 2004 there has been an expansion of the caffeinated drinks market and a concomitant rise in the sponsorship of various sports and sporting events by such drinks companies. In addition to being the most widely used social drug, caffeine's incorporation into various over-the-counter (OTC) medications implies that it has a useful therapeutic role. Indeed it is a key

Table 20.1 Caffeine content of selected beverages and OTC products

Beverage/OTC product	Caffeine content (mg)
Coffee	
Ground	105[*]
Instant	54[*]
De-caffeinated (instant)	2[*]
De-caffeinated (ground)	6[*]
Tea	
Black	40[*]
De-caffeinated	1[*]
Soft drinks	
Coca-Cola (355ml)	34.5[**]
Pepsi-Cola (355ml)	38[**]
Dr. Pepper (355ml)	41[**]
Sports drinks	
Lucozade Sport with caffeine boost (500ml)	80
Energy drinks	
Red Bull (250ml)	80
Relentless (500ml)	160
Red Bull Energy Shot (100ml)	133
Lucozade Alert (250ml)	80
OTC cold and flu medication	
Benylin Cold and Flu Max strength	25/capsule
Beechams Powders	50/sachet
Do-Do Chesteze[***]	50/tablet
Lemsip Max Cold and Flu	25/capsule
OTC pain relief medication	
Anadin extra	45/tablet
Askit Powders	110/sachet
Panadol extra	65/tablet
OTC products for the relief of tiredness	
Pro-Plus	50/tablet

[*] Average caffeine levels according to the Food Standards Agency (2004).
[**] Caffeine levels according to Reissig et al. (2009).
[***] Do-Do Chesteze also contains theophylline (100mg) and ephedrine (18.31mg).

constituent in numerous OTC medications for pain relief and the relief of upper respiratory tract conditions, including the common cold and influenza. (For further detail, refer to Chapter 21.) As a consequence of the general acceptance of caffeine use there remains almost an unwillingness to accept or appreciate its negative side effects and the ethical implications of its use as an ergogenic aid in organised sport.

20.2 Pharmacology

Chemically, caffeine is classified as a methylxanthine closely related to two other naturally occurring methylated xanthines, namely, theophylline and

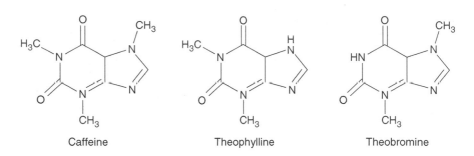

Figure 20.1 Chemical structure of naturally occurring methylxanthines.

theobromine (Figure 20.1). Caffeine (1,3,7-trimethylxanthine) is a tri-methylated xanthine whilst theophylline and theobromine are di-methylated xanthines. Pharmacologically, theophylline is considered to be the most potent of the naturally occurring methylxanthines; theobromine, a constituent of cocoa, is the least potent (Undem and Lichtenstein, 2001).

Following oral ingestion, caffeine is rapidly absorbed via the gastrointestinal tract and reaches peak plasma concentrations at 30 to 60 minutes (Sawynok and Yaksh, 1993). Due to its lipophilic properties, it is distributed widely around the body and easily crosses the blood-brain barrier and placenta. The half life of caffeine in healthy individuals is approximately four hours (Lelo *et al.*, 1986a) and it is metabolised extensively through demethylation into paraxanthine (80 per cent), theobromine (11 per cent) and theophylline (4 per cent) by chytochrome P450 enzymes in the liver (Lelo *et al.*, 1986b).

20.3   Mechanisms of action

Whilst it is accepted that caffeine has marked pharmacological, physiological and performance-enhancing effects there remains conjecture regarding the exact mechanisms involved. However, the principal mechanism by which caffeine exerts its effects is believed to be as an adenosine receptor antagonist. It is the only mechanism that is believed to occur at caffeine concentrations in the magnitude of those experienced following typical caffeine consumption (Fredholm, 1995).

Adenosine is a modulator of various physiological processes in both the CNS and the peripheral tissues via adenosine receptors. Adenosine receptors are located in most tissues, including the brain, heart, smooth muscle, adipocytes and skeletal muscle. The effects of adenosine are therefore widespread. Adenosine receptors, located on the cell membrane and coupled to G-proteins, can be divided into four subtypes: A_1, A_{2A}, A_{2B} and A_3. Stimulation of A_1 receptors typically initiates inhibitory responses through a reduction in cyclic AMP and stimulation of potassium channels. Inhibition of calcium flux is also believed to occur following A_1 receptor activation (Shimada and Suzuki, 2000). Activation also inhibits noradrenergic, dopaminergic, serotonergic and acetylcholinergic neurotransmission. The A_{2A} receptors are linked to dopaminergic neurons and stimulation of these receptors appears to be involved in the inhibition of dopaminergic neurotransmission. The A_{2B} receptors are believed to be low-affinity receptors serving a modulating role whilst A_3 receptors are believed to be sparsely distributed in the CNS (Graham, 1997).

Caffeine, which is similar in structure to adenosine, has the most affinity to the A_1 and A_{2A} receptors and its ability to cross the blood-brain barrier means that it readily affects the CNS. Because adenosine has largely an inhibitory effect, caffeine, as an adenosine receptor antagonist, therefore has a stimulatory effect. The complex nature of caffeine's actions relates to the ubiquitous nature of adenosine receptors and the fact that it is able to operate via the receptors in both direct or indirect ways.

Despite the importance of adenosine receptor antagonism in characterising the effects of caffeine, other related mechanisms are believed to play a role. Inhibition of cyclic nucleotide phosphodiesterase that leads to increased cyclic AMP and increased sensitivity of calcium translocation are both considered key mechanisms.

Caffeine's ability to inhibit cyclic nucleotide phosphodiesterase enzymes is significant because this increases intracellular levels of cyclic AMP and cyclic GMP. These molecules act as secondary messengers and enable signal response pathways to be enhanced. Cyclic AMP is involved in the signal response pathway that activates inactive hormone-sensitive lipase and stimulates lipolysis in adipose tissue. Increased sympathetic nervous system activity also results in enhanced intracellular cyclic AMP levels, leading to increased lipolysis. These mechanisms fit neatly with the positive effects of caffeine on endurance exercise performance and the proposed glycogen-sparing hypothesis. However, such mechanisms are not considered to account primarily for enhanced endurance following caffeine consumption. Indeed, research has found improvements without significant increases in circulating adrenaline and free fatty acids (FFAs) and reduction in the respiratory exchange ratio (RER) (Graham and Spriet, 1991, 1995).

The ability of caffeine to effect calcium translocation in the muscle may contribute directly to performance enhancement during physical exercise. Increases in intracellular calcium have been observed with caffeine. Caffeine seems to interfere with excitation-contraction coupling. Caffeine activates the release of calcium from the sarcoplasmic reticulum, which binds with troponin and activates the myofilaments leading to contraction. Whilst this has been demonstrated *in vitro*, using high caffeine doses, the ability to show similar effects using doses comparable with those taken by humans has proved difficult (Tarnopolsky, 2008).

Because the ability to combat fatigue may relate directly to the maintenance of electrolyte homeostasis, caffeine may impact potassium levels.

Lindinger *et al.* (1993) reported that plasma potassium increased to a lesser extent during exercise following caffeine administration. The significance of this finding is that fatigue is associated with suppression in resting membrane potential and therefore there would be less motor unit activation and force production. This may occur as a result of loss of potassium from the myocyte, thus increasing plasma potassium levels or less release of calcium from the sarcoplasmic reticulum. The lower plasma potassium levels observed following caffeine administration may be a consequence of increased plasma clearance or a lower efflux from the active muscle. It has been hypothesised that caffeine works directly or indirectly via adrenaline to stimulate muscle sodium/potassium ATPase and subsequent potassium uptake (Lindinger *et al.*, 1993, 1996)

20.4   Performance-enhancing properties

As an ergogenic aid, caffeine is used extensively across many sports to increase alertness and perception, mask the symptoms of fatigue, spare energy substrates and increase muscle force production and endurance. Whilst these effects following caffeine administration have not been demonstrated unequivocally, there is widespread support amongst the athletic and scientific communities.

The effects of caffeine administration on performance show a great interindividual variation. Individuals who display limited ergogenic effects following caffeine ingestion are often termed non-responders. The factors that are likely to contribute to this variation may relate to the source of caffeine ingestion, the dose and timing of ingestion and the individual characteristics relating to caffeine habituation and metabolism. The effects of caffeine have been most prominent amongst those who don't consume caffeine on a regular basis as opposed to those who consume it habitually (Bell and McLellan, 2002).

Whilst there is no evidence to support a dose-response relationship in terms of caffeine and performance, there appears to be an optimum dose above which adverse side effects may prevail and potentially be detrimental to performance. Positive improvements in performance have been shown following relatively low doses of caffeine (i.e. 2.1 mg.kg BW^{-1}) (Kovacs *et al.*, 1998). However, the optimum dose for performance enhancement is believed to be between 3 and 6 mg.kg BW^{-1} (Spriet, 2002). Higher doses of caffeine (i.e. 9 mg.kg BW^{-1}) have shown no further improvements in performance (Graham and Spriet, 1991; Pasman *et al.*, 1995).

Typically, caffeine is ingested one hour before competition. However, whilst caffeine is rapidly absorbed it is metabolised relatively slowly and remains at high concentrations in the circulation for several hours. There is a suggestion that its metabolic action (i.e. peak FFA levels) may peak at three hours post-exercise and may incur the greatest effect on endurance exercise performance (Nehlig and Debry, 1994). However, because caffeine-induced lipolysis is not deemed to be a central mechanism in improved endurance exercise, such a proposal is unlikely to significantly influence performance.

Interestingly, although coffee is considered the most widespread source of caffeine, its use as an ergogenic aid has been questioned. Whilst caffeine ingestion enhanced endurance performance, Graham *et al.* (1998) found no beneficial effect following coffee ingestion. It is suggested that some constituents of coffee may interfere with caffeine and its ergogenic properties (Graham, 2001). Further research is required to identify the compounds within coffee that may interact with caffeine and establish the mechanisms involved.

There has been limited research into the effects of other methylxanthines on sports performance. Theophylline is considered to be the most potent of the naturally occurring methylxanthines. However, Morton *et al.* (1989) found no effects on VO_{2max}, muscular performance (strength, power and endurance) and psychomotor performance following 10 to 13 mg.kg $BW^{-1}.day^{-1}$ administration of theophylline over a four-day period. Conversely, Greer and colleagues (2000) examined the effects of both caffeine and theophylline and found both enhanced endurance cycling performance.

Most research has tended to focus on the impact of acute caffeine supplementation on competitive events. Whilst there is a clear rationale for assessing the ergogenic effects of caffeine during competition it may be pertinent to examine the effects of caffeine supplementation during a training regimen. It is realistic to speculate that the use of caffeine as a training aid would have a significant impact on subsequent competitive performance.

Endurance exercise

Research by Costill and colleagues (1978) demonstrated significant increases in endurance cycling performance following moderate doses of caffeine. This research paved the way for the huge interest in caffeine as a performance-enhancing substance in endurance exercise. It was proposed that caffeine promoted FFA mobilisation through increased catecholamine release. Glycogen sparing was believed to occur as a consequence of greater FFA utilisation by the exercising muscles due to increased availability of circulating FFA. It is now understood that this is not the sole mechanism nor is it the most important. In most instances exercise performance is not limited by muscle glycogen. Whilst caffeine is clearly able to affect muscle fuel supply this mechanism does not account for the many ergogenic effects experienced during endurance and short-term exercise alike.

Nonetheless, the ergogenic effects of caffeine on endurance performance would appear to be unquestionable. Caffeine ingestion (3 to 13 mg.kg BW^{-1}) has been shown to improve time to exhaustion using exercise protocols at 80 to 85 per cent VO_{2max} (Graham and Spriet, 1995; Pasman *et al.*, 1995). Similarly, in more ecologically valid time trial protocols endurance performance lasting between 30 and 60 min has shown improvements following doses of caffeine between 3 and 4.5 mg.kg BW^{-1} (Kovacs *et al.*, 1998; Bridge and Jones, 2006). Performance of short-term endurance exercise has also shown improvements following caffeine ingestion. In rowing, caffeine ingestion (6 or 9 mg.kg BW^{-1}) significantly enhanced 2000 m time trial performance (Anderson *et al.*, 2000; Bruce *et al.*, 2000). In swimming, 1500 m time trial performance was enhanced following caffeine ingestion (6 mg.kg BW^{-1}) (MacIntosh and Wright, 1995).

Anaerobic exercise

Whilst the effects of caffeine on endurance exercise have been widely documented there has been less attention placed upon the effects of caffeine supplementation on short-term, high intensity exercise. The studies that have been conducted are not conclusive in their support for caffeine as an aid to anaerobic exercise performance.

Very few studies have examined the effects of caffeine on sport-specific sprinting performance. Collomp *et al.* (1992) assessed whether caffeine ingestion (250 mg) had any impact on 100 m freestyle swimming. When trained swimmers ingested caffeine, their swimming velocity significantly increased. As part of a protocol to simulate rugby action, Stuart *et al.* (2005) examined the effects of caffeine (6 mg.kg BW^{-1}) on 20 and 30 m sprints and found improvements in mean performance.

Maximal accumulated oxygen deficit (MAOD), an indirect measure of anaerobic capacity, has been employed to examine the effects of caffeine on anaerobic performance (Doherty, 1998; Bell *et al.*, 2001). Doherty (1998) found that caffeine ingestion (5 mg.kg BW^{-1}) improved time to exhaustion in a running protocol by 14 per cent whilst Bell and colleagues (2001) reported significant improvements in both time to exhaustion and MAOD using a cycling protocol under caffeine conditions (5 mg.kg BW^{-1}).

The Wingate test has also been used to assess potential improvements in anaerobic performance in response to caffeine supplementation (Collomp *et al.*, 1991; Kang *et al.*, 1998; Beck *et al.*, 2006; Greer *et al.*, 2006). However, only Kang and colleagues (1998) demonstrated enhanced performance. Following caffeine doses of 2.5 and 5 mg.kg BW^{-1}, significant improvements were reported in total, peak and mean power during a 30 s Wingate test.

If caffeine's effects are mediated by the CNS, any effects in competition may be masked by the heightened arousal experienced in competition (Davis and Green, 2009). Further research is required to establish the ergogenic value of caffeine on anaerobic performance.

Resistance exercise

In light of the reputed effects of caffeine on the contractile properties of muscle and on central mechanisms such as motivation it would seem extremely feasible that caffeine would have a positive impact upon resistance exercise. Despite several studies examining the ergogenic properties of caffeine on such exercise, there is no conclusive evidence to support its use.

Commonly used methods to assess muscular strength include the determination of one repetition maximum (1 RM), isokinetic peak torque or force produced during an isometric maximal voluntary contraction (MVC). Beck *et al.* (2006) reported a significant increase in bench-press 1 RM but no increase in leg-press 1 RM following caffeine ingestion. Astorino *et al.* (2008), however, found no increase in bench- or leg-press 1 RM following caffeine ingestion (6 mg.kg BW^{-1}). In a study by Bond *et al.* (1986) the effects of caffeine ingestion (5 mg.kg BW^{-1}) on isokinetic knee flexor and extensor strength were examined. There were no significant differences in peak torque across a range of speeds (30°, 150° and 300°.s^{-1}) between caffeine and placebo trials. In elite athletes Jacobson *et al.* (1992) reported greater peak torque for knee flexors at speeds of 30°.s^{-1}, 150°.s^{-1} and 300°.s^{-1} and for knee extensors at speeds of 30°.s^{-1} and 300°.s^{-1} following caffeine consumption (7 mg.kg BW^{-1}). Kalmar and Cafarelli (1999) reported a significant increase in MVC following caffeine administration (6mg.kg BW^{-1}), whilst Tarnopolsky and Cupido (2000) found no ergogenic value of caffeine in relation to MVC.

Several studies have examined muscular endurance using repetitions of exercises at a percentage of 1 RM until volitional fatigue. Beck *et al.* (2006) found no significant effect of caffeine on bench- and leg-press exercises (80 per cent 1 RM) to failure. Using a similar protocol (60 per cent 1 RM until failure), Astorino *et al.* (2008) reported non-significant increases in muscular endurance following caffeine ingestion in the order of 11 and 12 per cent for bench- and leg-press exercises, respectively. Muscular endurance has been assessed in other studies through sustained isometric contractions. Caffeine has shown positive effects on isometric knee extensions (50 per cent MVC) in doses of 6 mg.kg BW^{-1} (Kalmar and Cafarelli, 1999; Plaskett and Cafarelli, 2001; Meyers and Cafarelli, 2005).

Intermittent exercise

Team games such as football and rugby are characterised by aerobic exercise interspersed with repeated, intermittent bouts of high intensity anaerobic exercise. Assessing physiological performance has proved extremely difficult within these sports. Of those researchers who have attempted to assess intermittent exercise few have been successful in recreating the demands of a game. Paton *et al.* (2001) investigated the effects of caffeine ingestion (6 mg.kg BW^{-1}) on a repeated 20 m sprint protocol (10 × 20 m sprint with 10 s recovery following each sprint) and found no effect on performance or fatigue. Schneiker and colleagues (2006) examined the effect of caffeine supplementation (6 mg.kg BW^{-1}) on a repeated sprint protocol consisting of two 36-min halves (18 × 4 s sprints and 2-min active recovery between each sprint). Performance, with respect to total amount of sprint work and mean power output, was enhanced with caffeine use.

The difficulty in assessing physiological performance has led many researchers to focus on physiological function or skill performance. Stuart *et al.* (2005) examined the effects of caffeine (6 mg.kg BW^{-1}) in a battery of tests chosen to simulate the physical and skill demands of a rugby union match. Whilst improvements in most tests were evident, performance of tackle speed and reduction in fatigue in 30 m sprint speed were particularly enhanced by caffeine supplementation. Foskett *et al.* (2009) demonstrated improvements in passing accuracy and jump performance amongst football players participating in a simulated soccer-specific activity following caffeine ingestion (6mg.kg BW^{-1}). Such research clearly highlights the multi-faceted effects of caffeine and its ability to enhance not only physiological performance but also cognitive function and psychomotor performance.

Cognitive function

Caffeine is used extensively by the wider population to increase alertness in a variety of situations, such as in conditions of sleep deprivation, at night time, to avoid post-lunch fatigue and during periods of long hours of studying or driving. There is a large body of evidence to support the use of caffeine as a cognitive performance enhancer, especially in conditions of low arousal. It has been shown to increase cognitive function such as alertness and mood state (Penetar *et al.*, 1993) as well as vigilance, learning and memory (Lieberman *et al.*, 2002) under conditions of sleep deprivation.

Effects on mood and motor performance are believed to be related to caffeine's affinity to A$_{2A}$ receptors and stimulation of dopaminergic neurotransmission. The positive effect of caffeine on mood has been demonstrated via reports of lower anxiety and increased contentedness, self-confidence and motivation following ingestion (Lieberman *et al.*, 1987).

Decreased reaction time typically demonstrates improved selective attention and efficient information processing. The effect of caffeine on cognitive performance tasks has been demonstrated with reaction time (Smit and Rogers, 2000) and choice reaction time (Van Duinen *et al.*, 2005).

Most research has centred on the enhancement of generic behavioural characteristics following caffeine ingestion, and these are clearly transferable to sport. However, it may be difficult to assess the effects on more complex tasks within a sporting context because the heightened state of arousal that is typical of competition may mask any effects likely caused by caffeine ingestion.

20.5   Caffeine combinations

The co-administration of nutritional and pharmacological substances to enhance performance is common. Combinations of caffeine with additional supplements, including carbohydrates and sympathomimetic amines, may further enhance sports performance.

Many endurance athletes ingest carbohydrate supplements during exercise, and the introduction of caffeine as an ingredient of such supplements (i.e. in sports drinks, gels) is relatively new and has no doubt increased following caffeine's removal from the WADA prohibited list. A study examining the ingestion of a sports drink (carbohydrate-electrolyte solution) with added caffeine (2.1, 3.2 and 4.5 mg.kg BW^{-1}) during a one-hour cycling time trial led to an improvement in performance (Kovacs *et al.*, 1998). Similarly, Cox *et al.* (2002) reported improved time trial performance following two-hour steady state cycling amongst subjects that co-ingested carbohydrates and caffeine during exercise in the form of Coca-Cola (3 × ~1.5 mg.kg BW^{-1}). Caffeine in low doses (~1.5 to 3 mg.kg BW^{-1}) ingested with carbohydrates during exercise would therefore appear to have ergogenic benefits.

In recent work by Pederson *et al.* (2008) the co-ingestion of carbohydrates with high doses of caffeine (8 mg.kg BW^{-1}) after exhaustive exercise resulted in significantly greater muscle glycogen resynthesis during the four hours post-exercise when compared with carbohydrate ingestion alone. The rate of glycogen resynthesis (~60 mmol.kg dw^{-1}.h^{-1}) was deemed to be the highest that has been observed in humans under physiological conditions. Whilst further research is required, caffeine may play a key role in nutritional strategies designed to promote optimal recovery.

Caffeine in combination with sympathomimetic amines is often employed in weight-reduction therapy. Caffeine and ephedrine are usually combined for their thermogenic and anorectic properties. Boozer *et al.* (2001) found significant weight reduction in obese individuals following supplementation with natural sources of caffeine and ephedrine (Guarana and Ma Huang). Indeed, several products marketed as herbal weight-loss supplements typically contain caffeine from Guarana, a plant from South America whose seeds contain caffeine, theophylline and theobromine (Espinola *et al.*, 1997). These products also contain natural sources of sympathomimetics, such as ephedrine and synephrine, in the form of Ma Huang and Citrus Aurantium, respectively. Both caffeine and ephedrine are also commonly combined with acetylsalicylic acid (aspirin) for aspirin's weight-reduction properties (Astrup and Toubro, 1993). Whilst the mechanisms behind the weight-reducing effects of such drug combinations is not clearly understood, both caffeine and aspirin are believed to work synergistically with the thermogenic effects of ephedrine (Dulloo, 1993).

In addition to weight loss, research in recent years has supported the use of caffeine in combination with ephedrine or pseudoephedrine as a performance-enhancing aid (Bell *et al.*, 1998, 2002; Weatherby and Rogerson, 2002). Bell *et al.* (1998) demonstrated a significant improvement in time to exhaustion using a cycling protocol (85 per cent VO$_{2max}$), following caffeine (5 mg.kg BW^{-1}) and ephedrine (1 mg.kg BW^{-1}) supplementation over placebo and supplementation of caffeine alone. Ephedrine (0.8 mg.kg BW^{-1}) and caffeine (4 mg. kg BW^{-1}) in combination have also shown improvements in a 10-km run time trial whilst wearing fighting order weighing approximately 11 kg (Bell *et al.*, 2002). There is limited support for the combination of caffeine with pseudoephedrine; nevertheless, Weatherby and Rogerson (2002) reported an improvement in short-duration, supramaximal cycling exercise following the supplementation of 300 mg of caffeine with 120 mg of pseudoephedrine. Whilst the combination of caffeine with ephedrines appears to boast performance-enhancing properties further research is needed to elucidate the performance-enhancing mechanisms.

20.6   Therapeutic actions

Methylxanthines are used in many OTC medications as bronchodilators or analgesic adjuvants. Theophylline is largely incorporated into cold and flu preparation due to its role as a bronchodilator whilst caffeine is typically incorporated into pain relief medication as an adjuvant to aspirin or acetaminophen (paracetamol). When a peripheral acting analgesic such as acetaminophen is combined with caffeine the pain relief is similar to that experienced when combined with a centrally acting analgesic (Laska *et al.*, 1984). The significance of this is that the side effects of taking a centrally acting analgesic can be avoided and it precludes the need to take high doses of aspirin and paracetamol. Research has suggested that these effects are mediated by central amplification of cholinergic neurotransmission (Ghelardini *et al.*, 1997). However, the mechanisms behind these properties of caffeine are not clearly understood. Indeed, some studies have questioned the analgesic adjuvant properties of caffeine (Zhang and Li Wan Po, 1996, 1997).

20.7   Adverse side effects

Plasma caffeine concentrations above 15 µg/ml can cause toxic symptoms such as tachycardia, arrhythmia and tremor whilst concentrations greater than 80 µg/ml are considered fatal (Riesselmann *et al.*, 1999). Despite the widespread availability and consumption of products containing caffeine there are few reports of caffeine intoxication; nevertheless, two reports of fatal caffeine intoxication by Riesselmann *et al.* (1999) highlight blood caffeine concentrations of 260 and 180 µg/ml in the hearts of a young woman (19 years old) and an elderly woman (81 years old), respectively.

The safety of caffeine consumption in relation to the cardiovascular system has long been a contentious issue. Dietary caffeine intake has been linked with cardiovascular mortality and morbidity (James, 2004). Rosenberg *et al.* (1988) suggested that consumption of caffeinated coffee increased the risk of myocardial infarction. Also, research has shown a positive relationship between coffee consumption and elevations in systolic blood pressure (Jee *et al.*, 1999). However, there is a considerable body of evidence that opposes these conclusions. A large prospective study by Grobbee and colleagues (1990) found no connection between coffee consumption and increased risk of coronary heart disease or stroke. Indeed, low to moderate caffeine consumption in the form of coffee may even have cardio-protective effects attributed to the antioxidants present in coffee (Cornelis and El-Sohemy, 2007).

The most noticeable side effects from caffeine are those pertaining to the CNS. Whilst caffeine is ingested for its positive effects on cognitive function, excessive doses may cause insomnia, headaches, nervousness, restlessness, tremors and irritability. Chronic consumption of caffeine can lead to dependence and tolerance as the body up-regulates the number of adenosine receptors. Withdrawal symptoms are frequently experienced upon abrupt cessation of its consumption. According to Reeves *et al.* (1997) acute caffeine withdrawal can cause distress and symptoms of nausea, nervousness, tachycardia, arrhythmia, and insomnia. Interestingly the symptoms experienced during withdrawal are similar to those experienced after excessive caffeine consumption. Silverman *et al.* (1992) demonstrated that withdrawal symptoms, including a drop in mood, increased anxiety, fatigue and headache, can also be experienced in low to moderate caffeine consumers. Indeed, Evans and Griffiths (1999) confirmed that withdrawal and physical dependence can occur at low doses and following a short period of exposure (i.e. three consecutive days).

Frequent urination is common symptom of caffeine ingestion. Excessive fluid loss through urination may result in diuresis and a reduction in plasma volume. However, such concerns would appear to be unfounded. Whilst mild diuresis was demonstrated following administration of caffeinated drinks there were no significant changes in urine and plasma osmolarity, sweat rate or plasma volume (Wemple *et al.*, 1997).

Groups that are believed to be sensitive to caffeine include pregnant women, infants and children. Caffeine consumption is deemed to be particularly problematic due to the extended half-life of caffeine within pregnant women and infants and because of the high doses of caffeine, in relation to body weight, that can be consumed by children. The half-life of caffeine is extended during pregnancy approximately twofold when compared with non-pregnant women (Knutti *et al.*, 1981). This means that the time at which caffeine can exert its effects and increase the potential for toxicity is extended. Caffeine also freely crosses the placenta and passes into breast milk (Undem and Lichtenstein, 2001). Indeed further evidence has linked caffeine consumption in pregnant women with low birth weight (Cade, 2008).

Caffeine is often mistakenly associated with poor iron absorption. Whilst the consumption of tea and coffee has been shown to negatively affect dietary iron absorption (Morck *et al.*, 1983; Hurrell *et al.*, 1999), this has not been attributed to caffeine intake. Tea and coffee contain polyphenols that can bind to iron, making iron difficult to absorb. A recommendation to avoid such beverages at meal times is very important for people at risk of iron deficiency.

20.8   Caffeine use and WADA regulations

In 1984 caffeine was included in the IOC prohibited list and a urinary concentration threshold of 15 μg/ml was set in an attempt to combat inadvertent positive drug tests following "normal/acceptable" caffeine intake. In 1985 this threshold was reduced to 12 μg/ml and caffeine remained on the IOC list until 2004. In 2004 WADA produced its first prohibited list and specific stimulants such as caffeine, pseudoephedrine and phenylephrine were removed and included on the monitoring programme.

The monitoring programme examined specific substances with the aim of identifying potential misuse (WADA, 2009). This data may be used as evidence to support the reintroduction of substances back to the prohibited list (WADA, 2003). As a consequence the consumption of caffeine was allowed in sport without restriction. However, the motivation behind the removal of caffeine from the prohibited list remains unclear. According to the prohibited list committee, there was concern regarding whether caffeine levels in the urine were a good determinant of misuse due to the high degree of inter-subject variability in urine caffeine levels (WADA, 2003). It would appear that the premise behind the monitoring programme is to avoid the frustration and adverse publicity caused by an inadvertent positive drug test caused by legitimate use of therapeutic OTC medication or acceptable social consumption of caffeine. This would suggest that whilst caffeine has been removed from the prohibited list, WADA is not advocating its use as a performance-enhancing supplement. Unfortunately this message has not been clearly voiced.

With the advent of the monitoring programme there was the potential for caffeine use to increase markedly within sport. However, laboratory data do not support this (Van Thuyne and Delbeke, 2006). Analysis of urinary caffeine levels before and after the removal of caffeine from the list showed the overall percentage of positive samples remained the same. Surprisingly, overall urinary caffeine concentrations actually dropped after 2004. Following the examination of samples in relation to sport, only cycling showed an increase in positive samples. With a view to examining the motives of caffeine use before and after 2004, Chester and Wojek (2008) surveyed 480 track and field athletes and cyclists. It was revealed that use of caffeine for performance-enhancing purposes was high, especially amongst the elite and this had increased after 2004. Further work assessing the impact of the changes to the prohibited list in 2004 was carried out by Desbrow and Leveritt (2006). Almost 90 per cent of competitors questioned at the 2005 Ironman Triathlon World Championships intended to use caffeine prior to or during the competition.

The sports supplements market, even though considered a niche market, has attempted to profit from the re-classification of caffeine in elite sport. Caffeine has been added to numerous products in an attempt to increase their efficacy as ergogenic supplements. Evidence of their use amongst track and field athletes and cyclists is shown in Figure 20.2.

Central to the caffeinated sports supplements market is the caffeinated energy drinks market. This market has grown exponentially in recent years with UK sales believed to have risen by 75 per cent between the years 2000 and 2005 and sales figures for 2005 were believed to be over £1 billion, according to a market analysis report (Mintel International Group Limited, 2005). The primary consumers are thought to be males under 35 years of age.

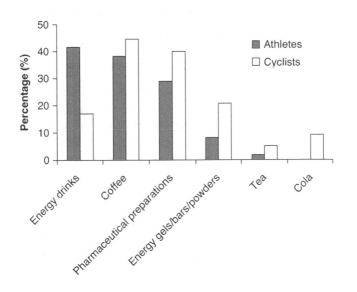

Figure 20.2 Caffeinated products used to enhance performance in cyclists (n = 172) and track and field athletes (n = 63) (Chester and Wojek, 2008).

An investigation into the consumption of caffeinated energy drinks amongst U.S. college students found that 51 per cent of participants regularly consume on average one energy drink per month (Malinauskas *et al.*, 2007). The reasons put forward for their consumption was to increase alertness following insufficient sleep (67 per cent), increase energy (65 per cent) and to consume with alcohol for social reasons (54 per cent). Side effects were regularly reported, such as headaches (22 per cent) and heart palpitations (19 per cent).

There is concern regarding the excessive use of caffeinated energy drinks and this has been compounded by reports of several deaths throughout Europe linked with such misuse (Dhar *et al.*, 2005). The sales of high-caffeine energy drinks are banned in a number of countries such as France and Denmark, which have imposed a statutory limit of 150 μg/ml of caffeine in soft drinks (Finnegan, 2003). Currently there is evidence that links consumption of caffeinated energy drinks with caffeine toxicity (Reissig *et al.*, 2009); however, further research is required to establish potential cardiotoxic effects from excessive use prior to exercise and in combination with alcohol.

Clearly only a small proportion of caffeinated energy drinks that are purchased are used in sport. Nevertheless, the expansion in the caffeinated energy drinks market coupled with the threefold increase in branded coffee retail outlets in the UK between 1997 and 2005 (Freedman, 2006) would suggest a significant increase in the consumption of caffeine across the population. Undoubtedly, a rise in general caffeine consumption is likely to impact on both the social use and ergogenic use of caffeine by those participating in sport.

20.9   Summary

Caffeine is arguably the most widely used performance-enhancing drug in the world, due to its wide-ranging effects and its appeal to athletes across a broad spectrum of sports. Because of caffeine's clear performance-enhancing properties, it still provokes great interest amongst the scientific community. Whilst significant improvements in numerous sporting activities have been shown following moderate dosing with caffeine, there remains some conjecture with respect to the mechanisms behind these effects. Although the use or consumption of caffeine is generally accepted, if not embraced within most cultures of the world, it still commands attention from health authorities. With the recent growth in coffee sales and the exponential growth in the caffeinated energy drinks market, particular attention should be paid to caffeine consumption by children. There should also be monitoring of the aggressive marketing techniques of such drinks companies and their effect on children. From a sporting perspective it may be difficult to accept anti-doping rules whilst caffeine, an established performance-enhancing drug, is condoned and even actively promoted within many sporting bodies.

20.10   References

Anderson, M.E., Bruce, C.R., Fraser, S.F. *et al.* (2000). Improved 2000 meter rowing performance in competitive oarswomen after caffeine ingestion. *International Journal of Sports Nutrition and Exercise Metabolism* 10, 464–475.

Astorino, T.A., Rohmann, R.L. and Firth, K. (2008). Effect of caffeine ingestion on one-repetition maximum muscular strength. *European Journal of Applied Physiology* 102, 127–132.

Astrup, A. and Toubro, S. (1993). Thermogenic, metabolic and cardiovascular responses to ephedrine and caffeine in man. *International Journal of Obesity* 17, S41–S43.

Beck, T.W., Housh, T.J., Schmidt, R.J. *et al.* (2006). The acute effects of caffeine-containing supplement on strength, muscle endurance and anaerobic capabilities. *Journal of Strength and Conditioning Research* 20, 506–510.

Bell, D.G., Jacobs, I. and Ellerington, K. (2001). Effect of caffeine and ephedrine on anaerobic exercise performance. *Medicine and Science in Sports and Exercise* 33, 1399–1403.

Bell, D.G., Jacobs, I. and Zamecnik, J. (1998). Effects of caffeine, ephedrine and their combination on time to exhaustion during high-intensity exercise. *European Journal of Applied Physiology and Occupational Physiology* 77, 427–433.

Bell, D.G. and McLellan, T.M. (2002). Exercise endurance 1, 3 and 6 h after caffeine ingestion in caffeine users and non-users. *Journal of Applied Physiology* 93, 1227–1234.

Bell, D.G., McLellan T.M. and Sabiston C.M. (2002). Effect of ingesting caffeine and ephedrine on 10-km run performance. *Medicine and Science in Sports and Exercise* 34, 344–349.

Bond, V., Gresham, K., McRae, J. *et al.* (1986). Caffeine ingestion and isokinetic strength. *British Journal of Sports Medicine* **20**, 135–137.

Boozer, C.N. Nasser, J.A., Heymsfield, S.B. *et al.* (2001). An herbal supplement containing Ma Huang-Guarana for weight loss: A randomised, double-blind trial. *International Journal of Obesity* **25**, 316–324.

Bridge, C.A. and Jones, M.A. (2006). The effect of caffeine on 8 km run performance in a field setting. *Journal of Sport Sciences* **24**, 433–439.

Bruce, C.R., Anderson, M.E., Fraser, S.F. *et al.* (2000). Enhancement of 2000 m rowing performance after caffeine ingestion. *Medicine and Science in Sports and Exercise* **32**, 1958–1963.

Cade, J. (2008). Maternal caffeine intake during pregnancy and risk of fetal growth restriction: A large prospective observational study. Available at http://www.foodbase.org.uk/results.php?f_category_id=&f_report_id=273 (accessed 20 November 2009).

Chester, N. and Wojek, N. (2008). Caffeine consumption amongst British athletes following changes to the 2004 WADA prohibited list. *International of Journal Sports Medicine* **29**, 524–528.

Collomp, K., Ahmaidi, S., Audran, M. *et al.* (1991). Effects of caffeine ingestion on performance and anaerobic metabolism during the Wingate test. *International Journal of Sports Medicine* **12**, 439–443.

Collomp, K., Ahmaidi, S., Chatard, J.C. *et al.* (1992). Benefits of caffeine ingestion on sprint performance in trained and untrained swimmers. *European Journal of Applied Physiology* **64**, 377–380.

Cornelis, M.C. and El-Sohemy, A. (2007). Coffee, caffeine and coronary heart disease. *Current Opinion in Clinical Nutrition and Metabolic Care* **10**, 745–751.

Costill, D.L., Dalsky, G.P., and Fink, W.J. (1978). Effects of caffeine ingestion on metabolism and exercise performance. *Medicine and Science in Sports* **10**, 155–158.

Cox, G.R., Desbrow, B., Montgomery, P.G. *et al.* (2002). Effect of different protocols of caffeine intake on metabolism and endurance performance. *Journal of Applied Physiology* **93**, 990–999.

Davis, J.K. and Green, J.M. (2009). Caffeine and anaerobic performance ergogenic value and mechanisms of action. *Sports Medicine* **39**, 813–832.

Desbrow, B. and Leveritt, M. (2006). Awareness and use of caffeine by athletes competing at the 2005 Ironman Triathlon World Championships. *International Journal of Sports Nutrition and Exercise Metabolism* **16**, 545–558.

Dhar, R., Stout, C.W., Link, M.S. *et al.* (2005). Cardiovascular toxicities of performance enhancing substances in sports. *Mayo Clinic Proceedings* **80**, 1307–1315.

Doherty, M. (1998). The effects of caffeine on the maximal accumulated oxygen deficit and short-term running performance. *International Journal of Sports Nutrition* **8**, 95–104.

Dulloo, A.G. (1993). Ephedrine, xanthines and prostaglandin-inhibitors: Actions and interactions in the stimulation of thermogenesis. *International Journal of Obesity* **17 (Suppl.)**, S35–S40.

Espinola, E.B., Dias, R.F., Mattei, R. *et al.* (1997). Pharmacological activity of Guarana (*Paullinia cupana* Mart.) in laboratory animals. *Journal of Ethnopharmacology* **55**, 223–229.

Evans, S.M. and Griffiths, R.R. (1999). Caffeine withdrawal: A parametric analysis of caffeine dosing conditions. *Journal of Pharmacology and Experimental Therapeutics* **289**, 285–294.

Finnegan, D. (2003). The health effects of stimulant drinks. *Nutrition Bulletin* **28**, 147–155.

Food Standards Agency (2004). Survey of caffeine levels in hot beverages. Available at http://www.food.gov.uk/science/surveillance/fsis2004branch/fsis5304 (accessed 25 November 2009).

Foskett, A., Ali, A. and Gant, N. (2009). Caffeine enhances cognitive function and skill during simulated soccer activity. *International Journal of Sports Nutrition and Exercise Metabolism* **19**, 410–423.

Fredholm, B.B. (1995). Adenosine, adenosine receptors and the actions of caffeine. *Pharmacology and Toxicology* **76**, 93–101.

Freedman, M. (2006). Café culture: A new tradition? Available at http://www.igd.com/index.asp?id=1&fid=1&sid=8&tid=16&cid=71 (accessed 20 November 2009).

Ghelardini, C., Galeotti, N. and Bartolini, A. (1997). Caffeine induces central cholinergic analgesia. *Naunyn Schmiedebergs Archives of Pharmacology* **356**, 590–595.

Graham, T.E. (1997). The possible actions of methylxanthines on various tissues. In *Proceedings of the Estelle Foundation symposium: The clinical pharmacology of sport and exercise*, ed. T. Reilly and M. Orme, vol. 7, Elsevier, Amsterdam. 257–270.

Graham, T.E. (2001). Caffeine and exercise: Metabolism, endurance and performance. *Sports Medicine* **31**, 785–807.

Graham, T.E., Hibbert, E. and Sathasivam, P. (1998). Metabolic and exercise endurance effects of coffee and caffeine ingestion. *Journal of Applied Physiology* **85**, 883–889.

Graham, T.E. and Spriet, L.L. (1991). Performance and metabolic responses to a high caffeine dose during prolonged exercise. *Journal of Applied Physiology* **71**, 2292–2298.

Graham, T.E. and Spriet, L.L. (1995). Metabolic, catecholamine and exercise performance responses to various doses of caffeine. *Journal of Applied Physiology* **78**, 867–874.

Greer, F., Friars, D. and Graham, T.E. (2000). Comparison of caffeine and theophylline ingestion: Exercise metabolism and endurance. *Journal of Applied Physiology* **89**, 1837–1844.

Greer, F., Morales, J. and Coles, M. (2006). Wingate performance and surface EMG frequency variables are not affected by caffeine ingestion. *Applied Physiology Nutrition and Metabolism* **31**, 597–603.

Grobbee, D.E., Rimm, E.B., Giovannucci, E. *et al.* (1990). Coffee, caffeine and cardiovascular disease in men. *New England Journal of Medicine* **324**, 991–992.

Hurrell, R.F., Reddy, M. and Cooke, J.D. (1999). Inhibition of non-haem iron absorption in man by polypenolic-containing beverages. *British Journal of Nutrition* **81**, 289–295.

Jacobson, B.H., Weber, M.D., Claypool, L. *et al.* (1992). Effects of caffeine on maximal strength and power in elite male athletes. *British Journal of Sports Medicine* **26**, 276–280.

James, J.E. (2004). Critical review of dietary caffeine and blood pressure: A relationship that should be taken more seriously. *Psychosomatic Medicine* **66**, 63–71.

Jee, S.H., He, J., Whelton, P.K. *et al.* (1999). The effect of chronic coffee drinking on blood pressure: A meta-analysis of controlled clinical trials. *Hypertension* **33**, 647–652.

Kalmar, J.M. and Cafarelli, E. (1999). Effects of caffeine on neuromuscular function. *Journal of Applied Physiology* **87**, 801–808.

Kang, H., Kim, H. and Kim, B. (1998). Acute effects of caffeine intake on maximal anaerobic power during the 30s Wingate cycling test. *Journal of Exercise Physiology Online* **1**. Available at http://faculty.css.edu/tboone2/asep/jan/3a.htm (accessed 5 August 2010).

Knutti, R., Rothweiler, H. and Schlatter, C. (1981). Effect of pregnancy on the pharmacokinetics of caffeine. *European Journal of Clinical Pharmacology* **21**, 121–126.

Kovacs, E.M.R., Stegen, J.H.C.H. and Brouns, F. (1998). Effects of caffeinated drinks on substrate metabolism, caffeine excretion and performance. *Journal of Applied Physiology* **85**, 709–715.

Laska, E.M., Sunshine, A., Mueller, F. *et al.* (1984). Caffeine as an analgesic adjuvant. *Journal of the American Medical Association* **251**, 1711–1718.

Lelo, A., Birkett, D.J., Robson, R.A. *et al.* (1986a). Comparative pharmacokinetics of caffeine and its primary demethylated metabolites paraxanthine, theobromine and theophylline in man. *British Journal of Clinical Pharmacology* **22**, 177–182.

Lelo, A., Miners, J.O, Robson, R.A. *et al.* (1986b). Quantitative assessment of caffeine partial clearances in man. *British Journal of Clinical Pharmacology* **22**, 183–186.

Lieberman, H.R., Tharion, W.J., Shukitt-Hale, B. *et al.* (2002). Effects of caffeine, sleep loss and stress on cognitive performance and mood during US Navy SEAL training. *Psychopharmacology* **164**, 250–261.

Lieberman, H.R., Wurtman, R.J., Emde, R.J. *et al.* (1987). The effects of low doses of caffeine on human performance and mood. *Psychopharmacology* **92**, 308–312.

Lindinger, M.I., Graham, T.E. and Spriet, L.L. (1993). Caffeine attenuates the exercise-induced increase in plasma [K^+] in humans. *Journal of Applied Physiology* **74**, 1149–1155.

Lindinger, M.I., Willmets, R.G. and Hawke, T.J. (1996). Stimulation of Na+, K+-pump activity in skeletal muscle by methylxanthines: Evidence and proposed mechanisms. *Acta Physiologica Scandinavica* **156**, 347–353.

MacIntosh, B.R. and Wright, B.M. (1995). Caffeine ingestion and performance of a 1,500-metre swim. *Canadian Journal of Applied Physiology* **20**, 168–177.

Malinauskas, B.M., Aeby, V.G., Overton, R.F. *et al.* (2007). A survey of energy drink consumption patterns amongst college students. *Nutrition Journal* **6**, 35.

Meyers, B.M. and Cafarelli, E. (2005). Caffeine increases time to fatigue by maintaining force and not by altering firing rates during submaximal isometric contractions. *Journal of Applied Physiology* **99**, 1056–1063.

Mintel International Group Limited. (2005). Energy and stimulant drinks—UK. Available at http://www.marketresearch.com/product/display.asp?productid=1130034&xs=r (accessed 20 November 2009).

Morck, T.A., Lynch, S.R. and Cook, J.D. (1983). Inhibition of food iron absorption by coffee. *American Journal of Clinical Nutrition* **37**, 416–420.

Morton, A.R., Scott, C.A. and Fitch, K.D. (1989). The effects of theophylline on the physical performance and work capacity of well-trained athletes. *Journal of Allergy and Clinical Immunology* **83**, 55–60.

Nehlig, A. and Debry, G. (1994). Caffeine and sports activity: A review. *International Journal of Sports Medicine* **15**, 215–223.

Pasman, W.J., van Baak, M.A., Jeukendrup, A.E. *et al.* (1995). The effect of different dosages of caffeine on endurance performance time. *International Journal of Sports Medicine* **16**, 225–230.

Paton, C.D., Hopkins, W.G. and Vollerbregt, L. (2001). Little effect of caffeine ingestion on repeated sprints in team-sport athletes. *Medicine and Science in Sports and Exercise* **33**, 822–825.

Pederson, D.J., Lessard, S.J., Coffey, V.G. *et al.* (2008). High rates of muscle glycogen resynthesis after exhaustive exercise when carbohydrate is coingested with caffeine. *Journal of Applied Physiology* **105**, 7–13.

Penetar, D., McCann, U., Thorne, D. *et al.* (1993). Caffeine reversal of sleep deprivation effects on alertness and mood. *Psychopharmacology* **112**, 359–365.

Plaskett, C.J. and Cafarelli, E. (2001). Caffeine increases endurance and attenuates force sensation during submaximal isometric contractions. *Journal of Applied Physiology* **91**, 1535–1544.

Reeves, R.R., Struve, F.A. and Patrick, G. (1997). Somatic dysfunction increase during caffeine withdrawal. *Journal of the American Osteopathic Association* **97**, 454–456.

Reissig, C.J., Strain, E.C. and Griffiths, R.R. (2009). Caffeinated energy drinks— A growing problem. *Drug and Alcohol Dependence* **99**, 1–10.

Riesselmann, B., Rosenbaum, F., Roscher, S. *et al.* (1999). Fatal caffeine intoxication. *Forensic Science International* **103**, S49–S52.

Rosenberg, L., Palmer, J.R., Kelly, J.P. *et al.* (1988). Coffee drinking and nonfatal myocardial infarction in men under 55 years of age. *American Journal of Epidemiology* **128**, 570–578.

Sawynok, J. and Yaksh, T.L. (1993). Caffeine as an analgesic adjuvant. A review of pharmacology and mechanisms of action. *Pharmacological Reviews* **45**, 43–85.

Schneiker, K.T., Bishop, D., Dawson, B. *et al.* (2006). Effects of caffeine on prolonged intermittent-sprint ability in team-sport athletes. *Medicine and Science in Sports and Exercise* **38**, 578–585.

Shimada, J. and Suzuki, F. (2000). Medicinal chemistry of adenosine receptors in brain and periphery. In *Adenosine receptors and Parkinson's disease*, ed. H. Kase *et al.*, Elsevier, Oxford. 31–48.

Silverman, K., Evans, S.M., Strain, E.C. *et al.* (1992). Withdrawal syndrome after the double-blind cessation of caffeine consumption. *New England Journal of Medicine* **327**, 1109–1114.

Smit, H.J. and Rogers, P.J. (2000). Effects of low doses of caffeine on cognitive performance, mood and thirst in low and higher caffeine consumers. *Psychopharmacology* **152**, 167–173.

Spriet, L.L. (2002). Caffeine. In *Performance-enhancing substances in sport and exercise*, ed. M.S. Bahrke and C.E. Yesalis, Human Kinetics, Champaign, IL. 267–278.

Stuart, G.R., Hopkins, W.G., Cook, C. *et al.* (2005). Multiple effects of caffeine on simulated high-intensity team sport performance. *Medicine and Science in Sports and Exercise* **37**, 1998–2005.

Tarnopolsky, M. (2008). Effect of caffeine on the neuromuscular system—Potential as an ergogenic aid. *Applied Physiology Nutrition and Metabolism* **33**, 1284–1289.

Tarnopolsky, M. and Cupido, C. (2000). Caffeine potentiates low frequency skeletal muscle force in habitual and nonhabitual caffeine consumers. *Journal of Applied Physiology* **89**, 1719–1724.

Undem, B.J. and Lichtenstein, L.M. (2001). Drugs used in the treatment of asthma. In *Goodman and Gilman's The pharmacological basis of therapeutics*, ed. J.G. Hardman *et al.*, 10th ed., McGraw-Hill, New York. 733–754.

Van Duinen, H., Lorist, M.M. and Zijdewind, I. (2005). The effect of caffeine on cognitive task performance and motor fatigue. *Psychopharmacology* **180**, 539–547.

Van Thuyne, W. and Delbeke, F.T. (2006). Distribution of caffeine levels in urine in different sports in relation to doping control before and after the removal of caffeine from the WADA doping list. *International Journal of sports Medicine* **27**, 745–750.

Weatherby, R.P. and Rogerson, S. (2002). Caffeine potentiation of the performance enhancing effects of pseudoephedrine. *Medicine and Science in Sports and Exercise* **35**, 110.

Wemple, R.D., Lamb, D.R. and McKeever, K.H. (1997). Caffeine vs. caffeine-free sports drinks: Effects on urine production at rest and during prolonged exercise. *International Journal of Sports Medicine* **18**, 40–46.

World Anti-Doping Agency (WADA). (2003). The Prohibited List and Therapeutic Use Exemptions. Available at http://www.wada-ama.org/Documents/Resources/PlayTrue_ Mag/PlayTrue_2003_3_Policy_Into_Practice_EN.pdf (accessed 20 November 2009).

World Anti-Doping Agency (WADA). (2009). World anti-doping code. Available at http:// www.wada-ama.org/Documents/World_Anti-Doping_Program/WADA_Anti-Doping_ CODE_2009_EN.pdf (accessed 20 November 2009).

Zhang W.Y. and Li Wan Po, A. (1996). Analgesic efficacy of paracetamol and its combination with codeine and caffeine in surgical pain—A meta-analysis. *Journal of Clinical Pharmacy and Therapeutics* **21**, 261–82.

Zhang W.Y. and Li Wan Po, A. (1997). Do codeine and caffeine enhance the analgesic effect of aspirin?—A systematic overview. *Journal of Clinical Pharmacy and Therapeutics* **22**, 79–97.

Chapter 21

Over-the-counter stimulants and herbal preparations

Neil Chester

21.1   Introduction

The term "over the counter" (OTC) in relation to pharmaceuticals refers to those products used primarily for the treatment of conditions that do not require direct medical attention. Over-the-counter drugs are non-prescription drugs that may be sold over the counter at pharmacies or be available for general sale off the shelf at various retail outlets including supermarkets. Over recent decades the classification of many drugs has changed as issues regarding their safety have been clarified. Some prescription drugs have been reclassified and are now sold over the counter and even off the shelf (e.g. the NSAID ibuprofen). Conversely, some OTC drugs have been withdrawn from the market in many countries following issues surrounding their safety (e.g. phenylpropanolamine).

Whilst there are countless drugs available over the counter, stimulants are typically deemed to be potential performance enhancers in sport. For this reason there are currently a number of OTC stimulants whose use is prohibited in sport (see Table 21.1). Many of these stimulants, known collectively as sympathomimetic amines, are contained in numerous OTC preparations for the treatment of symptoms associated with upper respiratory tract (URT) conditions, such as the common cold, sinusitis and seasonal rhinitis. In addition, methylxanthines, including caffeine and related substances, are stimulants commonly found in OTC preparations; however, their use is permitted in sport. Products designed specifically to increase alertness and combat drowsiness typically contain methylxanthines. Also, both sympathomimetic amines and methylxanthines are common constituents of products designed to promote weight loss.

In addition to being present within OTC pharmaceutical preparations, such stimulants are also commonly available in their naturally occurring botanical forms as herbal preparations. Whilst their use as herbal preparations has been common in traditional Chinese medicine for centuries, their recent use in the Western world has been limited. With the growth in the health food and supplements market it is clear that the popularity of alternative/complementary medicine is increasing, including the use of herbal preparations (Eisenberg *et al.*, 1998).

Table 21.1 Over-the-counter stimulants and their status in sport (January 2010) (WADA, 2009)

Stimulant	Permitted[*]	Prohibited in competition[**]
Sympathomimetic amines		
Ephedrine		✓
Norephedrine	✓	
Pseudoephedrine		✓
Norpseudoephedrine[***]		✓
Phenylephrine	✓	
Methylxanthines		
Caffeine	✓	
Theobromine	✓	
Theophylline	✓	

[*] Norephedrine (phenylpropanolamine), phenylephrine and caffeine are part of the WADA monitoring programme.
[**] Ephedrine, pseudoephedrine and norpseudoepedrine are prohibited when concentrations in urine are above 10, 150 and 5 µg/ml, respectively.
[***] Norpseudoephedrine is not available as an OTC stimulant but is commonly detected in urine as a metabolite of pseudoephedrine.

From an anti-doping perspective it would seem that the availability and general lack of control surrounding the use of OTC stimulants (in both their pharmaceutical and botanical forms) pose the most difficult problem in regulating their use.

21.2   Upper respiratory tract (URT) conditions and exercise

There is a causal link between intense exercise and the incidence of URT infection (Nieman *et al.*, 1990; Heath *et al.*, 1991). In the case of male endurance runners, there appears to be a dose-related effect of exercise training on the risk of URT infection (Heath *et al.*, 1991; Nieman *et al.*, 1990; Peters and Bateman, 1983). This relationship is highlighted by the "J" curve model proposed by Nieman *et al.* (1993), whereby the risk of URT infection is reduced below that of sedentary individuals when engaged in mild to moderate intensity exercise training and increased when engaged in high intensity, high-volume exercise training. However, a direct link between infection and disturbed immune function in athletes has not been fully established. There is evidence that there are important cofactors in the immune response to exercise including diet, lifestyle and stress (König *et al.*, 2000).

21.3   Treatment of URT conditions

Conditions that affect the URT, whose symptoms can be managed through the use of OTC preparations, include viral or bacterial infections, such as the common cold, influenza, pharyngitis, laryngitis, sinusitis and allergic reactions, such as seasonal allergic rhinitis. Symptoms are a consequence of an immune response to the infection or allergic reaction and at the very least are viewed as a nuisance. However, symptoms may be an important part of recovery from infection and whether symptomatic treatment using OTC preparations affects the recovery time course of URT infection is unclear (Eccles, 2005).

The number of OTC medications available for the treatment of symptoms associated with URT conditions is vast. There are 292 OTC cough, cold and flu preparations available in the UK with a market value of £453 million in 2008 (Proprietary Association of Great Britain, 2009a, 2009b). There are 27 OTC products available in the UK for the specific treatment of allergy and hay fever symptoms, totalling £84.6 million in 2008 (Proprietary Association of Great Britain, 2009a, 2009b).

The common cold and influenza

Both the common cold and influenza (flu) share similar symptoms and are caused by viral infections of the URT. Symptoms typical of cold and flu infections include pharyngitis, rhinorrhea, sneezing, nasal congestion and cough. In addition flu is characterised by fever, extreme lethargy and muscle and joint pain. Whilst the symptoms of the common cold gradually present themselves over the first three days after infection, the onset of flu symptoms is usually sudden. Both conditions normally last for approximately five to seven days. Both headache and sinusitis may also be symptoms.

Although effective vaccines are available to prevent flu they are generally limited to those who are at specific risk such as the elderly and infants or those working in environments where the risk of spread of infection is particularly high (e.g. health care professionals and those providing child care). Flu sufferers who have not been immunised or those with the common cold must rely on self-management involving the intake of additional fluids to combat the increased losses experienced from fever. Steam inhalations also help to hydrate the tissues of the URT and reduce congestion. In addition those who are ill may choose to use one of the many OTC preparations available to alleviate the symptoms. Cold and flu medications may contain the following drugs:

- sympathomimetic amines—to act as decongestants and bronchodilators;
- methylxanthines—to act as bronchodilators;
- analgesics—to relieve pain and provide centrally acting cough suppressants;
- antihistamines—as cough suppressants and to inhibit sneezing;
- expectorants—to loosen and increase bronchial secretions to enable removal via coughing.

Sinusitis

Sinusitis is an inflammatory condition typically caused by viral or bacterial infection of the mucosal lining of the paranasal sinuses. It typically presents itself following a URT infection and rhinitis, hence rhinosinusitis is now considered to be a more accurate name for the condition (Ryan, 2008). Rhinosinusitis may be classified as acute or chronic, depending on whether the condition lasts for less than or more than a period of 12 weeks.

A wide range of symptoms is typically experienced, including nasal congestion, nasal discharge, facial discomfort, headache and hyposmia (limited or no sense of smell). Decongestants, namely sympathomimetic amines, may be used to relieve a blocked nose and to ease breathing. Also, analgesics may be used to relieve headache and facial pain. However, as with other URT conditions the use of OTC medications simply help in alleviating the symptoms. Antibiotics may be prescribed if sinusitis is particularly troublesome and persistent.

Allergic rhinitis

Allergic rhinitis is a condition characterised by an allergic hypersensitivity reaction in the nasal mucosa caused by exposure to pollen or other allergens. Symptoms include rhinorrhea, sneezing, nasal congestion, nasal itching and watering and itching of the eyes. It affects over 20 percent of the UK population (Scadding *et al.*, 2008). When the trigger is pollen the condition is known as seasonal allergic rhinitis or hay fever. Grass pollen is the most common cause of hay fever with other major allergens including tree pollen, particularly birch and pollen from weeds such as plantains, mugwort and docks (Nathan, 2002). Allergens that may trigger allergic rhinitis other than plant pollen include fungal spores, fur from cats and dogs and the presence of cockroaches and house dust mites. Epidemiological data suggest that those suffering from asthma typically suffer from allergic rhinitis (Leynaert *et al.*, 1999) with both sharing similar triggers and pathophysiology. Allergic rhinitis is also a risk factor for the development of asthma (Scadding *et al.*, 2008). Management of co-existing asthma and allergic rhinitis should be as directed by a physician.

Allergic rhinitis occurs as a consequence of a type-I hypersensitive response whereby exposure to an allergen produces specific immunoglobulin E (IgE). The IgE then attaches to mast cells and basophils of the nasal mucosa and conjunctiva of the eye, resulting in sensitisation. Subsequent exposure to the allergen results in an antigen-antibody response that causes basophils and mast cell degranulation and releases inflammatory mediators such as histamine, cytokines, leukotrienes, interleukins and prostaglandins. Such mediators cause vasodilation and increased permeability of blood vessels, thus resulting in local oedema and irritation of nerve endings and leading to the characteristic eye and nasal itching.

The goals of treatment of allergic rhinitis include:

- unimpaired sleep;
- ability to undertake normal daily activities, including work and school attendance, without limitation or impairment and the ability to participate fully in sport and leisure activities;

- no troublesome symptoms;
- no or minimal side effects of treatment (Price *et al.*, 2006).

In addition to reducing the exposure to allergens, treatment includes the use of OTC oral and topical (intranasal and ocular) preparations, which include antihistamines and also sympathomimetics. Oral antihistamines are effective in treating rhinorrhea, sneezing, nasal itching and conjunctivitis. Antihistamines limit rhinitis by attaching themselves to the H_1 receptors and acting as antagonists, thus reducing capillary permeability and excessive mucus production. The overall decrease in mucus production complements the effects of sympathomimetics. Both oral and topical sympathomimetic amines, such as phenylephrine and oxymetazoline, may be useful in reducing nasal congestion. Nasal sprays are particularly useful in alleviating severe congestion; however, they should not be used for prolonged periods due to the risk of developing rhinitis medicamentosa (i.e. rebound congestion and possible mucosal damage; Graf, 1997).

21.4   Weight loss

Whilst weight-loss products may be useful to the athlete by increasing lean body mass, they are often the domain of those interested in image enhancement such as the body builder. However, with levels of obesity increasing and increased attention on image enhancement there is a growing market for weight-loss products amongst the general public.

Whilst their efficacy is questionable, current OTC weight-loss products typically contain herbal extracts that contain a number of active ingredients including sympathomimetic amines, methylxanthines and acetylsalicylic acid (aspirin). Such products may act directly via adrenergic receptors to produce thermogenic or lypolytic effects or indirectly via serotonergic pathways in the hypothalamus to bring about appetite suppression (anorectics). The popularity of combining ephedrine, caffeine and aspirin (ECA stack) in weight management would appear to be related to the purported synergistic effects of these three substances. The dampening of the thermogenic effects of sympathomimetics caused by the negative feedback mechanisms is said to be reduced by both methylxanthines and aspirin (Dulloo, 1993).

21.5   Relief from fatigue and drowsiness

Fatigue and drowsiness are common conditions experienced in response to poor sleep hygiene, and poor work–rest balance. However, chronic fatigue may be symptomatic of a more serious underlying problem (e.g. depression, diabetes mellitus, hypothyroidism, heart disease or cancer) and requires medical attention. Whilst there are numerous pharmacological treatments for fatigue it is important to assess and address the root cause of the symptoms.

Nevertheless the treatment of acute fatigue and drowsiness can be successfully managed in the short term through the use of one of numerous OTC products available. Such products generally contain methylxanthines, typically caffeine. Some products have herbal ingredients that contain natural sources of both methylxanthines and sympathomimetic amines. Ingredients are intended to increase alertness and combat drowsiness by activating the release of central neurotransmitters, such as dopamine (sympathomimetic amines), and affecting dopamine transmission by displacement of adenosine at A1 and A2 receptors (methylxanthines).

They are often marketed as energy supplements because they combat symptoms of fatigue and contain high quantities of caffeine. Energy drinks are extremely popular amongst both adults and children alike and are a central component of the supplements market designed to combat drowsiness. However, there are serious concerns regarding the regulation of these products and consequently the level of caffeine in these drinks and the aggressive marketing campaigns targeted largely at young adults. This has led to significant use of these high-caffeine drinks amongst adolescents and children and increasing numbers of reports of caffeine intoxication following the consumption of such drinks (Reissig *et al.*, 2009).

21.6 Sympathomimetic amines

Drugs that mimic the effects of the endogenous mediators of the sympathetic nervous system (i.e. adrenaline and noradrenaline) are referred to as sympathomimetic amines. Sympathomimetic amines work by direct activation of adrenoceptors or indirect activation via the stimulation of release of endogenous catecholamines. The response of any cell or organ to sympathomimetic amines is directly related to the density and proportion of α- and β-adrenoceptors present.

According to Hoffman (2001) the actions of sympathomimetic amines can be classified into the following types: (1) peripheral stimulatory action on vascular smooth muscle in blood vessels supplying the skin, kidneys and mucous membranes and glandular smooth muscle in salivary and sweat glands; (2) peripheral inhibitory action on the smooth muscle of the gut wall, the bronchioles and the blood vessels supplying the skeletal muscles; (3) cardiac excitatory action, inducing increased heart rate and force of contraction; (4) metabolic actions, including increased rate of glycogenolysis in the liver and muscles and mobilisation of free fatty acids from adipose tissue; (5) endocrine actions, including regulation of the secretion of insulin, renin and pituitary hormones; (6) CNS actions, including respiratory stimulation, increased wakefulness, psychomotor activity and reduction in appetite; and (7) presynaptic actions resulting in the inhibition or facilitation of release of neurotransmitters, such as acetylcholine and noradrenaline. Not all sympathomimetic amines display all of the actions mentioned to a similar extent.

The profile of effects of each sympathomimetic amine is determined by its relative affinity for the subgroups of adrenoceptors and forms the basis for their classification. Beta$_2$-receptors are located on airway smooth muscle and cause bronchodilation when stimulated. Alpha$_1$-receptors are located on arterial smooth muscle and cause vasoconstriction when stimulated. Consequently, β_2-agonists (e.g. salbutamol) are used as bronchodilators to treat asthma whilst α_1-agonists (e.g. phenylephrine) are used as vasoconstrictors to treat symptoms of the common cold and associated URT conditions. The primary role of sympathomimetic amines in the treatment of URT conditions is to act as decongestants. When the mucus membranes lining the nose and paranasal sinuses are irritated by infection or allergy, the blood vessels supplying the membranes become enlarged. This leads to fluid accumulation in the surrounding tissue and encourages the production of larger than normal amounts of mucus. Alpha$_1$-agonists constrict the blood vessels, reducing the swelling in the lining of the nose and sinuses and acting as decongestants. The most widely available α_1-agonists present in OTC medications include ephedrine, its stereoisomer pseudoephedrine and phenylephrine. These sympathomimetics pose several potential problems for the sportsperson. First, they can cause significant side effects and second, both ephedrine and pseudoephedrine are prohibited in competition according to the 2010 WADA prohibited list (Table 21.1).

Potential side effects of sympathomimetic amines

Decongestants, although widely available in OTC preparations, are potent vasoconstrictors. In the UK, ephedrine is licensed for the treatment of hypotension caused by spinal or epidural anaesthesia and phenylephrine is licensed for the treatment of acute hypotension. Ephedrine, phenylephrine and pseudoephedrine use is contra-indicated in hypertensive patients.

The use of ephedrine has been linked to cardiomyopathy (To et al., 1980) and stroke (Bruno et al., 1993) whilst pseudoephedrine use has also been linked to stroke (Cantu et al., 2003) and temporal coronary artery spasm and myocardial infarction (Weiner et al., 1990). Until recent years phenylpropanolamine (PPA) was a common ingredient of OTC decongestant preparations. However, its use has been linked with hypertensive reactions, cerebral haemorrhage and psychosis (Gibson and Warrell, 1972; Norvenius et al., 1979; Berstein and Diskant, 1982; Johnson et al., 1983; Kernan et al., 2000; Cantu et al., 2003). A fairly recent study has demonstrated an odds ratio for association between haemorrhagic stroke and the use of PPA of 1.23 for cough and cold preparations and 15.92 for appetite suppressants (Horwitz et al., 2000). According to the United States Food and Drug Administration (FDA) Non-prescription Drugs Advisory Committee, the use of PPA in OTC medications is deemed unsafe (FDA, 2009). Thus PPA has been removed from all OTC medications in the USA. However, in the UK the Committee on Safety of Medicines, the expert group of the Medicines and Healthcare Products Regulatory Agency (MHRA), has not recommended a ban on PPA. It considers the evidence of the link between PPA use and haemorrhagic stroke to be weak and largely related to its use as an appetite suppressant, an application not licensed in the UK. Also, in the UK the recommended maximum dose for PPA contained in OTC products is lower than in the USA (100 mg compared to 150 mg) (MHRA, 2000). Nevertheless, OTC products containing PPA have tended to be reformulated or withdrawn from the market in the UK (Arroll, 2008).

It is clear, therefore, from clinical data that, when taken orally, α_1-agonist sympathomimetic amines can evoke profound systemic cardiovascular side effects. Moreover, these effects are both drug-specific and dose-dependent. The current recommended oral doses for common decongestants are shown in Table 21.2.

There have been numerous reports of the effects upon cardiovascular parameters of sympathomimetic amines contained in OTC medicines. Ephedrine administration (0.8 mg^{-1}. kg^{-1} BW) was found to increase systolic blood pressure significantly before exercise (Jacobs *et al.*, 2003). Doses equivalent to more than three to four times the recommended therapeutic dose of pseudoephedrine raised diastolic blood pressure above 90 mm Hg (Drew *et al.*, 1978). These results were in accord with two other studies. Bye *et al.* (1974) reported significant increases in heart rate and systolic blood pressure following relatively high doses of ephedrine (50 mg) and pseudoephedrine (120 mg and 180 mg). Empey *et al.* (1980) found doses of 120 mg and 180 mg produced statistically significant increases in both pulse and systolic blood pressure. However, the increases were deemed to be clinically unimportant because they were considerably less than might be expected to occur in response to either emotion or mild exercise.

Whilst several studies have reported increased cardiovascular stimulation following ingestion of OTC sympathomimetics, it is evident that doses used were at least twice the recommended therapeutic dose. Reports of the effects following the ingestion of sympathomimetics in therapeutic doses have been conflicting. Bye *et al.* (1974) found that a single dose of ephedrine (25 mg) significantly elevated both heart rate and systolic blood pressure. In the same study, a single therapeutic dose of pseudoephedrine (60 mg) significantly elevated only systolic arterial blood pressure, whilst Bright *et al.* (1981) found only a nonsignificant rise in resting heart rate following a single therapeutic dose. Empey *et al.* (1980) reported that ingestion of pseudoephedrine in a therapeutic dose of 60 mg provided maximal nasal decongestion without any cardiovascular or other side effects.

Few researchers have examined the effects of multiple dosing regimes on cardiovascular parameters. Chester (2000) found significant increases in blood pressure following a multiple therapeutic dosing regimen for pseudoephedrine (i.e. six 60-mg doses over a 36-hour period). Bye *et al.* (1975) reported significant increases in heart rate but not systolic blood pressure after three different dose

Table 21.2 Recommended maximal therapeutic doses of common sympathomimetic amines in OTC decongestant preparations

Sympathomimetic	Single dose (mg/4–6 h)	Daily dose (mg)
Ephedrine	25	100
Phenylephrine	10	40
Pseudoephedrine	60	240

regimes, one involving two different sustained-release formulations. Prolonged administration of a sustained-release formulation of pseudoephedrine (180 mg twice daily for two weeks) increased heart rate and decreased systolic blood pressure.

The bronchodilator effects of OTC sympathomimetics have been less well documented than the cardiovascular effects as might be expected from their receptor affinities. The OTC sympathomimetics exert their effect principally on the α_1-receptors on vascular smooth muscle with minimal effect on β_2-receptors in the bronchial smooth muscle. However, some brochodilation has been claimed following administration of supratherapeutic doses of ephedrine (60 mg) and pseudoephedrine (210 mg) (Drew et al., 1978).

In terms of action on the CNS, most evidence suggests that OTC sympatho-mimetics have no stimulatory effect in the relatively low doses used (Bye et al., 1975; Kuitunen et al., 1984). Bye et al. (1974) found that whilst pseudoephedrine lacked any stimulatory effect even at supratherapeutic doses (180 mg), ephedrine possessed a stimulatory effect at therapeutic doses. According to Wadler and Hainline (1989), OTC sympathomimetic amines exhibit less central stimulatory effects than amphetamines because they are less lipid-soluble. Differences in central stimulation are related to differences of lipid solubility within the bio-logical membranes and hence penetration of the blood-brain barrier determines the ease with which these compounds gain access to central receptors (Lanciault and Wolf, 1965).

Danger during endurance exercise has been associated with impaired thermoregulation as a result of the use of sympathomimetic amines. Clearly the use of stimulants to mask the symptoms of fatigue may enable an individual to continue exercising in a hyperthermic state. Indeed, the deaths of several cyclists during major competition, most notably that of Tom Simpson on Mont Ventoux in the 1967 Tour de France, have been attributed to hyperthermia related to the use of amphetamines (Williams, 1974). More recently the death of Steve Bechler, a Major League Baseball player, in 2003, as a result of heat-stroke was attributed to the use of excessive ephedrine, contained in a weight-reduction supplement (Charatan, 2003). It is likely that hyperthermia is a consequence of increased motor activity and impaired thermoregulation. Although published studies have identified increased thermogenesis (Dulloo and Miller, 1986) and a reduction in the drop in core temperature during exposure to low temperature (Vallerand, 1993) following administration of ephedrine, no studies have assessed body tem-perature at comfortable ambient temperatures following the administration of ephedrines.

Reputed ergogenic effects

The sympathetic response involves a myriad of reactions that heighten the capacity of the body to respond to stressful situations. These actions enable an individual to perform physical activity and relate to an increased potential in terms of sports performance.

Amphetamines are structurally related to the OTC sympathomimetics and are possibly the most well-known stimulants prohibited by WADA. Enhanced performance following amphetamine administration may be explained by the fact that amphetamines appear to mask the body's symptoms of fatigue. Both ephedrine and pseudoephedrine are classified as prohibited substances because of their chemical similarity to amphetamines. Therefore, it is assumed that they, like amphetamines, have similar ergogenic properties. However, the literature regarding the effects of common OTC sympathomimetics on sports performance is limited.

Few studies have examined the effects of OTC stimulants on steady-state exercise. Bright et al. (1981) investigated the effects of pseudoephedrine on submaximal treadmill exercise. They concluded that pseudoephedrine in single or double therapeutic doses failed to cause significant cardiovascular and metabolic adjustments in healthy subjects during submaximal exercise. It was likely that any sympathoadrenergic effects that occurred as a result of drug administration were masked during exercise.

Most research that has attempted to elucidate the effects of such drugs on exercise has focused on exercise performance parameters. One of the most appropriate physiological indicators of physical endurance capacity is maximal oxygen consumption (VO_{2max}). An increase in this parameter following drug administration may indicate increased aerobic power and the potential to enhance aerobic exercise performance. However, Sidney and Lefcoe (1977) found no effect of a therapeutic dose of ephedrine on VO_{2max}. Similarly, Swain et al. (1997) reported no effect from pseudoephedrine and phenylpropanolamine on maximal aerobic capacity following the administration of single or double the therapeutic dose. Clemons and Crosby (1993) examined the effect of a single therapeutic dose of pseudoephedrine prior to performance of a graded exercise test and found no difference in total exercise time to exhaustion.

In relation to time trial performance Gillies et al. (1996) found no improvement in 40-km cycling following administration of double the therapeutic dose of pseudoephedrine. Similarly Chester et al. (2003a) found no improvement in 5-km running performance following a multiple, therapeutic dosing regimen of pseudoephedrine (i.e. six 60-mg doses over a 36-hour period). Whilst data pertaining to endurance exercise suggest that pseudoephedrine has limited ergogenic effect, exercise of shorter duration has shown positive results. In a study by Hodges et al. (2006) it was concluded that pseudoephedrine administration in greater than the therapeutic dose (i.e. 2.5 mg per kg body weight) significantly improves 1500 m run performance. Using comparable doses of pseudoephedrine (i.e. 180 mg) Gill et al. (2000) found a significant increase in peak power output during a 30-s sprint cycle test and maximum torque produced in an isometric knee extension exercise. From the available data it would appear that pseudoephedrine administration in high doses (i.e. greater than the therapeutic dose) has the potential to augment high intensity exercise performance. However, further research in this area is necessary to confirm this.

Recent work has found that, when combined with caffeine, pseudoephedrine (Weatherby and Rogerson, 2002) and ephedrine (Bell *et al.*, 1998, 2002) significantly improve exercise performance. Bell and colleagues (1998) investigated the time to exhaustion during high intensity cycling exercise following ingestion of such a combination of drugs (5 mg.kg BW^{-1} caffeine and 1 mg.kg BW^{-1} ephedrine). Results showed a significant increase in time to exhaustion when compared with trials following placebo ingestion and ingestion of caffeine and ephedrine alone. These results were attributed to increased central nervous system stimulation. There is, however, a paucity of research that assesses the effect of combining caffeine with pseudoephedrine and thus this requires further examination.

Whilst there are limited data to support the ergogenic effects of OTC sympathomimetic amines upon complex exercise performance, it is possible that effects may be evident upon less complex athletic parameters such as isometric muscle strength and reaction time. However, Sidney and Lefcoe (1977) found no effect of a single therapeutic dose of ephedrine on grip strength or endurance, muscle power, anaerobic capacity or reaction time. Following multiple therapeutic doses of pseudoephedrine (i.e. six 60-mg doses over a 36-hour period) Chester (2000) found no effect on isometric grip, leg and back strength or reaction time.

There has been considerable interest in the use of sympathomimetic drugs to promote weight loss by increasing energy expenditure and reducing food intake through appetite suppression. In an animal study performed by Ramsey *et al.* (1998), it was reported that energy expenditure was increased and, in some animals, food intake was reduced following the administration of ephedrine and caffeine. Consequently it was concluded that ephedrine and caffeine treatment could promote weight loss through its action as a thermogenic and anorectic. It appears that ephedrine is effective in increasing thermogenesis and has the potential for body weight loss in obese individuals (Bukowiecki *et al.*, 1982) especially when combined with caffeine or aspirin (Astrup and Toubro, 1993). Boozer *et al.* (2001) found significant short-term reduction in weight amongst overweight and obese subjects following supplementation of natural sources of ephedrine and caffeine (Ma Huang and Guarana). However, there have been no studies that have focused on sympathomimetic drug use and non obese, athletic populations to promote leanness.

Sympathomimetic amine use and WADA regulations

The use of specific sympathomimetic amines, namely ephedrine, pseudoephedrine and cathine, is restricted by WADA. However, the detection of these substances in urine only constitutes an adverse analytical finding when their concentration is above a specific threshold (Table 21.3).

Prior to 2004, Chester *et al.* (2003b) found that athletes participating at high levels tended to avoid OTC medicines because they contained prohibited substances. Nevertheless, in April 2002–2003 UK Sport reported that out of the

Table 21.3 Urinary concentration thresholds for specific sympathomimetic amines above which constitutes an adverse analytical finding (January 2010) (WADA, 2009)

Prohibited substance	Urinary concentration ($\mu g.ml^{-1}$)
Cathine/norpseudoephedrine	5
Ephedrine	10
Pseudoephedrine	150

100 anti-doping results that required further investigation, 49 were for stimulants. Almost half of these were due to the stimulants phenylpropanolamine, ephedrine, pseudoephedrine and phenylephrine (UK Sport, 2003). Recent data from Chester *et al.* (2006) suggest that whilst use of OTC products amongst elite athletes is common their use is primarily for therapeutic purposes. However, elite athletes appear to have limited knowledge in terms of OTC medication in relation to anti-doping legislation (Mottram *et al.*, 2008). Nevertheless, recent studies have reported that athletes frequently use products containing pseudoephedrine and ephedrine (Bents *et al.*, 2004; Bents and Marsh, 2006) with the intention of improving performance.

Data from UK Sport's testing programme over the last 5 years (2004 to 2009) reveal a total of 231 anti-doping rule violations, of which a third were related to the use of stimulants (Figure 21.1). Further analysis shows that OTC stimulants such as ephedrine made up a significant proportion of these positive drug tests (Figure 21.2). It is interesting to note that whilst there were 18 cases of cathine detected in athlete samples, following investigation the outcome in all cases was that there was "no case to answer". It is likely that pseudoephedrine was also present in all samples and therefore the presence of cathine was deemed to be a result of its metabolism.

Since the introduction of the IOC prohibited list and drug testing, there have been numerous instances of positive tests for OTC sympathomimetic amines. In the 1972 Munich Olympics Rick DeMont lost his gold medal in the 400m free-style after testing positive for ephedrine. He claimed that he had inadvertently taken ephedrine contained in asthma medication. In 1988, a number of US athletes including the multi-Olympic champion Carl Lewis tested positive for ephedrine prior to the Seoul Olympics. They were excused, having claimed that the drug had been taken inadvertently. In 1994, Diego Maradona was banished from the World Cup after testing positive for a cocktail of ephedrine and ephedrine-related substances. In 2000, the Russian synchronised swimmer Maria Kisseleva was stripped of her European duet title after testing positive for ephedrine. She claimed that it had been given to her by a team doctor to help her lose weight. She was only given a one-month ban and subsequently won gold in Sydney. Most recently Paddy Kenny, an Irish International and Sheffield United footballer, received a nine-month ban following a positive test for ephedrine, believed to be

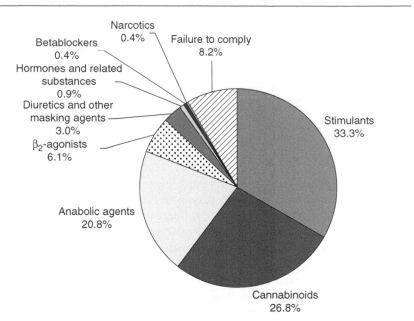

Figure 21.1 Anti-doping rule violations between 2004 and 2009 from the UK Sport's testing programme (UK Sport, 2009).

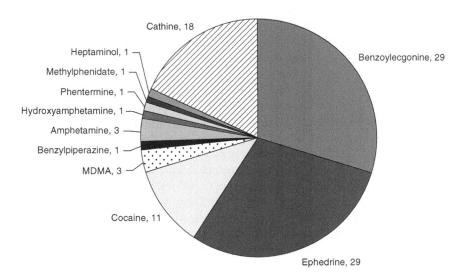

Figure 21.2 Anti-doping rule violations between 2004 and 2009 from the UK Sport's testing programme relating to the detection of prohibited stimulants (UK Sport, 2009).

as a consequence of using an OTC cold preparation containing ephedrine. There have also been high-profile cases that have involved positive tests for pseudoephedrine. In 1988 at the Seoul Olympics, a UK and subsequent Olympic 100m champion, Linford Christie, tested positive for pseudoephedrine. He was exonerated as he was believed to have taken the drug unknowingly as an ingredient of the Chinese health supplement ginseng. At the 2000 Sydney Olympics the IOC demonstrated rather less leniency when Andreea Răducan, a Romanian gymnast, was stripped of her individual gold medal after testing positive for pseudoephedrine, which was contained in cold medication prescribed by the team doctor. Whilst there was an unsuccessful appeal by Răducan, she did not receive a ban; however, the team doctor was banned from the next two Olympiads.

In an attempt to reduce the number of positive cases especially by those athletes using sympathomimetics for legitimate therapeutic reasons, the IOC introduced quantitative levels below which drug detection would not be deemed to be a positive result. In recent years these threshold levels have been revised in an attempt to differentiate between therapeutic use and misuse (see Table 21.3). Between the years 2004 and 2010 pseudoephedrine was not classified as a prohibited substance but it was part of WADA's monitoring programme. The monitoring programme (introduced in 2004) enabled WADA to assess the use of particular substances that are open to accidental use due to their presence in numerous OTC preparations. Evidence from the programme together with support of its performance-enhancing effects from several scientific studies (Gill *et al.*, 2000; Hodges *et al.*, 2006) led to the re-introduction of pseudoephedrine on the prohibited list. In an attempt to address the extreme inter-subject variability in the pharmacokinetics of OTC stimulants as demonstrated in studies by Lefebvre *et al.* (1992), Chester *et al.* (2004) and Strano-Rossi *et al.* (2009), WADA has set the threshold of pseudoephedrine at 150 µg/ml. Further research is needed regarding the pharmacokinetics of OTC stimulants if doping control is to successfully differentiate between therapeutic use and misuse.

21.7 Methylxanthines

Caffeine, theophylline and theobromine are methylxanthines. In the UK, both caffeine and theophylline are common constituents of preparations for the treatment of symptoms associated with URT conditions. In addition caffeine is typically the primary constituent of products designed to relieve fatigue and tiredness and many OTC weight-loss preparations.

There are several commonly accepted mechanisms thought to account for the pharmacological and ergogenic effects of methylxanthines. These mechanisms include the inhibition of cyclic nucleotide phosphodiesterase enzymes, which break down cyclic AMP and cyclic GMP; increased sensitivity of intracellular Ca translocation; and antagonism of adenosine receptors. It is generally accepted that adenosine receptor antagonism is the most important mechanism. The adenosine receptors mediate inhibitory signals, resulting in effects such as suppressed neurotransmission, sedation, pain relief, bronchoconstriction, sodium retention, beta receptor antagonist. As antagonists, methylxanthines block these signals and therefore in effect lead to a stimulatory response. The effectiveness of methylxanthines is directly related to their affinity to the adenosine receptors of which theophylline and paraxanthine are considered to be the most potent. The significance of these methylxanthines in relation to caffeine is that following ingestion it is converted to theobromine, theophylline and paraxanthine through demethylation in the liver.

Pharmacologically, methylxanthines (typically theophylline) are used for their bronchodilatory effects through adenosine antagonism and inhibition of phosphodiesterase enzymes. Also, their CNS stimulatory properties are widely exploited, especially in products designed to combat fatigue. Clearly this effect has been used extensively in sport and underpins much of the use of caffeine as an ergogenic aid. Other uses of caffeine relate to its positive result on endurance activity due to its reputed effects on the mobilisation of fatty acids, subsequent fat oxidation and glycogen sparing. Also, these effects in addition to its reputed ability to suppress appetite make caffeine and other methylxanthines ideal ingredients in weight-reduction supplements.

Interest in the effects of caffeine on sports performance has been widespread. The ingestion of moderate doses of caffeine (3–6 mg.kg^{-1} BW) 60 minutes prior to exercise is associated with the enhancement of performance during prolonged, submaximal exercise (Graham and Spriet, 1995; Pasman *et al.*, 1995) and during high intensity exercise of short (Jackman *et al.*, 1996; Bruce *et al.*, 2000) and moderate duration (MacIntosh and Wright; 1995; Bruce *et al.*, 2000). Evidence suggesting such an effect on high-power output and sprint performance is inconclusive (Collomp *et al.*, 1992; Greer *et al.*, 1998; Paton *et al.*, 2001; Doherty *et al.*, 2004). Research into the ergogenic effects of methylxanthines, other than caffeine, has been limited. However, Greer *et al.* (2000) examined the effects of both caffeine and theophylline on a time to exhaustion cycling protocol and concluded that both were ergogenic.

As discussed previously, caffeine is commonly supplemented with sympathomimetic amines (typically ephedrine) in an attempt to heighten its effect on exercise performance. However, whilst the combination of caffeine with ephedrine appears to augment its ergogenic effect the mechanisms are not completely understood. It is likely that both substances have a complementary effect rather than an additive one.

The attractiveness of caffeine as an ergogenic aid lies not only in the fact that it has been shown to be performance enhancing over a wide range of sporting disciplines but also because it is relatively safe and readily available. The effects of caffeine on sports performance have been shown to occur following an optimum dose (Graham and Spriet, 1995) and this dose is considered to be relatively safe. Nevertheless, as with all drugs there are side effects and safety issues concerning individuals sensitive to caffeine and those who consume caffeine in large quantities. Side effects may include nausea, insomnia, tachycardia, arrhythmia and tremor. Further in-depth discussion regarding the use of caffeine in sport and its side effects can be found in Chapter 20.

Whilst caffeine is not classified as a prohibited substance, it remains in the monitoring programme to enable WADA to monitor its use. Whilst caffeine remains a common constituent of an individual's diet it is clear that its use as a performance-enhancing drug is increasing. Recent studies have found athletes using products containing caffeine (Chester and Wojek, 2008; Desbrow and Leveritt, 2006) with the intention of improving performance. The rise in the energy drinks market and the sponsorship of various sports by such drinks companies clearly promote this practice.

21.8   OTC herbal stimulants

There are many products available for reducing weight, combating drowsiness, relieving fatigue and enhancing sports performance, and all contain a variety of herbal stimulants. Herbal stimulants are from plants or plant extracts that may be categorised according to the agents that they contain. Typically, they contain caffeine and related methylxanthines; the most common herbal stimulants are coffee and tea. Herbal stimulants may also contain ephedrine and related sympatho-mimetics. Herbs may, however, contain many active ingredients and the exact quantities and contents are seldom labelled. Whilst herbal products contain active ingredients they are classified as food supplements rather than as drugs and they undergo less stringent quality control procedures prior to sale. Most herbal supplements have not been subject to extensive scientific scrutiny and rigorous clinical trials. This poses a significant problem in terms of the safety of herbal supplement use. The major risks of taking herbal supplements include the purity of the ingredients and the possibility of contamination, and possible interactions between the ingredients and between other supplements consumed simultaneously. Athletes should therefore exercise extreme caution when contemplating the use of natural/ herbal supplements.

Guarana

Guarana is a South American plant whose seeds contain caffeine (2.5 to 5 per cent) and theophylline and theobromine in small amounts and large amounts of tannins (Carlini, 2003). Guarana is widely available as a constituent of numerous OTC supplements designed to suppress appetite, relieve tiredness and enhance sports performance. The effects of guarana are mediated largely through its active ingredients—caffeine and theophylline—via the mechanisms outlined previously for caffeine. There has been limited research into the efficacy of guarana supplementation in humans. Research examining the effects of herbal supplements containing guarana and Ma Huang has shown significant fat reduction and weight loss in humans (Boozer et al., 2001). Research using animal models has shown that guarana reduced fatigue in mice in forced swimming and increased memory in rats (Espinola et al., 1997). Supplementation of doses of caffeine equivalent to that contained in the guarana extract did not show any improvement in performance. It has been suggested that the content of guarana (i.e. tannins), other than methylxanthines, may be responsible for the improvements in performance observed (Espinola *et al.*, 1997).

Ephedra sinica/Ma Huang

In Chinese medicine Ma Huang is the name given to the plant species Ephedra sinica. Ephedra sinica is a natural source of ephedrine, pseudoephedrine, norephedrine and norpseudoephedrine. Ephedra sinica is typically an ingredient in weight-loss preparations because of ephedrine's thermogenic and anorectic properties. Ma Huang typically contains up to 24 mg of ephedrine and related sympathomimetics per unit dose (Bucci, 2000). Limited research has examined the use of Ma Huang as an ergogenic aid and whilst it is likely that it offers the same ergogenic benefits as its isolated constituents, further work is necessary to elucidate the effects of consuming combined sympathomimetics in herbal form.

Citrus aurantium

Weight-loss products often marketed as "ephedra free" typically contain Citrus aurantium (Seville orange or bitter orange extract) as a substitute for ephedra. The peel of bitter orange is known as Zhi shi in traditional Chinese medicine and is used in the treatment of gastrointestinal complaints, such as indigestion and constipation. The principal active ingredients of Citrus aurantium include the sympathomimetics synephrine (~6 per cent) and octopamine (Haller *et al.*, 2005).

Synephrine acts at the α_1-adrenergic receptors and causes vasoconstriction and increased blood pressure (Bui *et al.*, 2006). Evidence from animal models suggests that octopamine activates lipolysis via the β_3-adrenoreceptors of adipocytes, thus accounting for Citrus aurantium's purported thermogenic effect in humans (Carpene *et al.*, 1999). However, β_3-adrenoreceptor agonists are less active in human adipocytes (Fugh-Berman and Myers, 2004) and therefore it is likely that any positive effect on weight loss may be attributed to the effects on appetite suppression. However, "ephedra-free" weight-loss products not only contain Citrus aurantium but also other herbs such as guarana and green tea, all rich in methylxanthines. It is this combination of sympathomimetics and methylxanthines that is thought to produce marked effects in weight loss.

Whilst "ephedra-free" products are deemed to be safer than their ephedra counterparts, there has been limited research examining their safety. It is possible that the combined effects of synephrine and caffeine may be similar to the reported effects from ephedrine and caffeine, including hypertension, myocardial infarction and stroke. Haller and colleagues (2005) demonstrated significant cardiovascular stimulation following the administration of a supplement containing synephrine, octopamine and caffeine. However no effect on blood pressure was found following administration of a supplement containing only synephrine (46.9 mg). Bui *et al.* (2006) found increases in heart rate and systolic and diastolic blood pressure in young, healthy adults following a single 900-mg dose of a Citrus aurantium (6 per cent synephrine) supplement. It is also ironic that the term "ephedra free" is used to highlight the fact that the supplement does not contain ephedrine, which is a prohibited substance, and yet Citrus aurantium is a source of octopamine, which is also a prohibited substance (WADA, 2009).

21.9 Summary

Sympathomimetic amines and methylxanthines contained in OTC medications have clear therapeutic roles in alleviating the symptoms of URT conditions. In therapeutic doses these sympathomimetics are typically devoid of adverse side effects and performance-enhancing properties. Even in supratherapeutic doses research has found it difficult to elucidate the performance-enhancement properties of these drugs. However, pseudoephedrine and ephedrine (both commonly available OTC stimulants) are prohibited in competition. As a consequence of the principle of strict liability there is a huge responsibility for ensuring that athletes are aware of these stimulants and the products that contain them. This responsibility lies with the athletes and their support personnel. These issues are even more pertinent when the use of herbal preparations is considered. Due to the limited research into the efficacy of these products and the general lack of regulations surrounding their quality and therefore their safety, it is advisable that athletes are warned against using such products.

21.10 References

Arroll, B. (2008). Common cold. *British Medical Journal, Clinical Evidence* 6, 1510.

Astrup, A. and Toubro, S. (1993). Thermogenic, metabolic and cardiovascular responses to ephedrine and caffeine in man. *International Journal of Obesity* 17, S41–S43.

Bell, D.G., Jacobs, I. and Zamecnik, J. (1998). Effects of caffeine, ephedrine and their combination on time to exhaustion during high-intensity exercise. *European Journal of Applied Physiology and Occupational Physiology* 77, 427–433.

Bell, D.G., McLellan T.M. and Sabiston, C.M. (2002). Effect of ingesting caffeine and ephedrine on 10-km run performance. *Medical Science in Sports and Exercise* 34, 344–349.

Bents, R.T., Tokish, J.M. and Goldberg, L. (2004). Ephedrine, pseudoephedrine and amphetamine prevalence in college hockey players. *Physician and Sports Medicine* 32, 30–34.

Bents, R.T. and Marsh, E. (2006). Patterns of ephedra and other stimulant use in collegiate hockey athletes. *International Journal of Sport Nutrition and Exercise Metabolism* 16, 636–643.

Berstein, E. and Diskant, B.M. (1982). Phenylpropanolamine: A potentially hazardous drug. *Annals of Emergency Medicine* 11, 311–315.

Boozer, C.N. Nasser, J.A., Heymsfield, S.B. *et al.* (2001). An herbal supplement containing Ma Huang-Guarana for weight loss: A randomised, double-blind trial. *International Journal of Obesity* 25, 316–324.

Bright, T.P., Sandage, B.W. and Fletcher, H.P. (1981). Selected cardiac and metabolic responses to pseudoephedrine with exercise. *Journal of Clinical Pharmacology* **21**, 488–492.

Bruce, C.R., Anderson, M.E., Fraser, S.F. *et al.* (2000). Enhancement of 2000-m rowing performance after caffeine ingestion. *Medicine and Science in Sports and Exercise* **32**, 1958–1963.

Bruno, A., Nolte, K.B. and Chapin, J. (1993). Stroke associated with ephedrine use. *Neurology* **43**, 1313–1316.

Bucci, L.R. (2000). Selected herbals and human exercise performance. *American Journal of Clinical Nutrition* **72(Suppl.)**, 624S–636S.

Bui, L.T., Nguyen, D.T. and Ambrose, P.J. (2006). Blood pressure and heart rate effects following a single dose of bitter orange. *Annals of Pharmacotherapy* **40**, 53–57.

Bukowiecki, L., Jahjah, L. and Follea, N. (1982). Ephedrine, a potential slimming drug, directly stimulates thermogenesis in brown adipocytes via β-adrenoreceptors. *International Journal of Obesity* **6**, 343–350.

Bye, C. Dewsbury, D. and Peck, A.W. (1974). Effects on the human central nervous system of two isomers of ephedrine and triprolidine and their interaction. *British Journal of Clinical Pharmacology* **1**, 71–78.

Bye, C., Hill, H.M., Hughes, D.T.D. *et al.* (1975). A comparison of plasma levels of L(+) pseudoephedrine following different formulations, and their relation to cardiovascular and subjective effects in man. *European Journal of Clinical Pharmacology* **8**, 47–53.

Cantu, C., Arauz, A., Murillo-Bonilla, L.M. *et al.* (2003). Stroke associated with sympathomimetics contained in over-the-counter cough and cold drugs. *Stroke* **34**, 1667–1672.

Carlini, E.A. (2003). Plants and the central nervous system. *Pharmacology and Biochemistry and Behaviour* **75**, 501–512.

Carpene, C., Galitzky, J., Fontana, E. *et al.* (1999). Selective activation of β_3-adrenoceptors by octopamine: Comparative studies in mammalian fat cells. *Naunyn-Schmiedeberg's Archives of Pharmacology* **359**, 310–321.

Charatan, F. (2003). Ephedra supplement may have contributed to sportsman's death. *British Medical Journal* **326**, 464.

Chester, N. (2000). The use of exogenous sympathomimetic amines in sport and exercise. Unpublished PhD thesis.

Chester, N., Mottram, D., Atkinson, G. *et al.* (2006). The impact of changes to the prohibited list on the use of OTC medication by athletes. Unpublished report.

Chester, N., Mottram, D.R., Reilly, T. *et al.* (2004). Elimination of ephedrines in urine following multiple dosing and the consequences for athletes, regarding doping control. *British Journal of Clinical Pharmacology* **57**, 62–67.

Chester, N., Reilly T., and Mottram D.R. (2003a). Physiological, subjective and performance effects of pseudoephedrine and phenylpropanolamine during endurance running exercise. *International Journal of Sports Medicine* **24**, 3–8.

Chester, N., Reilly T., and Mottram D.R. (2003b). Over-the-counter drug use amongst athletes and non-athletes. *Journal of Sports Medicine and Physical Fitness* **43**, 111–118.

Chester, N. and Wojek, N. (2008). Caffeine consumption amongst UK cyclist and track and field athletes. *International Journal of Sports Medicine* **29**, 524–528.

Clemons, J.M. and Crosby S.L. (1993). Cardiopulmonary and subjective effects of a 60mg dose of pseudoephedrine on graded treadmill exercise. *Journal of Sports Medicine and Physical Fitness* **33**, 405–412.

Collomp, K., Ahmaidi, S., Chatard, J.C. *et al.* (1992). Benefits of caffeine ingestion on sprint performance in trained and untrained swimmers. *European Journal of Applied Physiology* **64**, 377–380.

Desbrow, B. and Leveritt, M. (2006). Awareness and use of caffeine by athletes competing at the 2005 Ironman Triathlon World Championships. *International Journal of Sport Nutrition and Exercise Metabolism* 16, 545–558.

Doherty, M., Smith, P.M., Hughes, M.G. *et al.* (2004). Caffeine lowers perceptual response and increases power output during high-intensity cycling. *Journal of Sports Science* **22**, 637–643.

Drew, C.D.M., Knight, G.T., Hughes, D.T.D. *et al.* (1978). Comparison of the effects of D-(−)-ephedrine and L-(+)-pseudoephedrine on the cardiovascular and respiratory systems in man. *British Journal of Clinical Pharmacology* 6, 221–225.

Dulloo, A.G. (1993). Ephedrine, xanthines and prostaglandin-inhibitors: Actions and interactions in the stimulation of thermogenesis. *International Journal of Obesity* **17(Suppl.)**, S35–S40.

Dulloo, A.G. and Miller, D.S. (1986). The thermogenic properties of ephedrine methylxanthine mixtures—Human studies. *International Journal of Obesity* 10, 467–481.

Eccles, R. (2005). Understanding the symptoms of the common cold and influenza. *Lancet* 5, 718–725.

Eisenberg, D.M., Davis, R.B., Ettner S.L. *et al.* (1998). Trends in alternative medicine use in the United States 1990–1997: Results of a follow-up national survey. *JAMA* **287**, 337–344.

Empey, D.W., Young G.A., Letley E. *et al.* (1980). Dose-response of the nasal decongestant and cardiovascular effects of pseudoephedrine. *British Journal of Clinical Pharmacology* **9**, 351–358.

Espinola, E.B., Dias, R.F., Mattei, R. *et al.* (1997). Pharmacological activity of Guarana (Paullinia cupana Mart.) in laboratory animals. *Journal of Ethnopharmacology* **55**, 223–229.

Federal Food and Drug Administration (FDA). (2009). Phenylpropanolamine (PPA) information page. Available at http://www.fda.gov/Drugs/DrugSafety/Informationby DrugClass/ucm150738.htm (accessed 5 November 2009).

Fugh-Bernam, A. and Myers, A. (2004). Citrus aurantium, an ingredient of dietary supplements marketed for weight loss: Current status of clinical and basic research. *Experimental Biology and Medicine* **229**, 698–704.

Gibson, G.J. and Warrell, D.A. (1972). Hypertensive crisis and phenylpropanolamine. *Lancet* **2**, 492.

Gill, N.D., Shield, A., Blazevich, A.J. *et al.* (2000). Muscular and cardiorespiratory effects of pseudoephedrine in human athletes. *British Journal of Clinical Pharmacology* **50**, 205–213.

Gillies, H., Derman, W.E., Noakes, T.D. *et al.* (1996). Pseudoephedrine is without ergogenic effects during prolonged exercise. *Journal of Applied Physiology* 81, 2611–2617.

Graf, P. (1997). Rhinitis medicamentosa: Aspects of pathophysiology and treatment. *Allergy* **52**, 28–34.

Graham, T.E, and Spriet, L.L. (1995). Metabolic, catecholamine and exercise performance responses to varying doses of caffeine. *Journal of Applied Physiology* **78**, 867–874.

Greer, F., Friars, D. and Graham, T.E. (2000). Comparison of caffeine and theophylline ingestion: Exercise metabolism and endurance. *Journal of Applied Physiology* **89**, 1837–1844.

Greer, F., McLean, C. and Graham, T.E. (1998). Caffeine, performance, and metabolism during repeated Wingate exercise tests. *Journal of Applied Physiology* **85**, 1502–1508.

Haller, C.A., Benowitz, N.L. and Jacob, P. (2005). Hemodynamic effects of ephedra-free weight-loss supplements in humans. *American Journal of Medicine* **118**, 998–1003.

Heath, G.W., Ford, E.S., Craven, T.E. *et al.* (1991). Exercise and the incidence of upper respiratory tract infections. *Medicine and Science in Sports Exercise* **23**, 152–157.

Hodges, K., Hancock, S., Currell, K. *et al.* (2006). Pseudoephedrine enhances performance in 1500-m runners. *Medicine and Science in Sports Exercise* **38**, 329–333.

Hoffman, B.B. (2001). Catecholamines, sympathomimetic drugs, and adrenergic receptor antagonists. In *Goodman and Gilman's The Pharmacological Basis of Therapeutics*, ed. J.G. Hardman, L.E. Limbird, and A.G. Gilman, 10th ed., McGraw-Hill, New York. 215–268.

Horwitz, R.I., Brass, L.M., Kernan, W.M. *et al.* (2000). Phenylpropanolamine and risk of hemorrhagic stroke: Final report of the Yale Hemorrhagic Stroke Project.

Jackman, M., Wendling, P., Friars, D. *et al.* (1996). Metabolic, catecholamine and endurance responses to caffeine during intense exercise. *Journal of Applied Physiology* **81**, 1658–1663.

Jacobs, I., Pasternak, H. and Bell, D.G. (2003). Effects of ephedrine, caffeine and their combination on muscular endurance. *Medicine and Science in Sports and Exercise* **35**, 987–994.

Johnson, D.A., Etter, H.S. and Reeves, D.M. (1983). Stroke and phenylpropanolamine use. *Lancet* **970**, 1983.

Kernan, W.N., Viscoli, C.M., Brass, L.M. *et al.* (2000). Phenylpropanolamine and the risk of hemorrhagic stroke. *New England Journal of Medicine* **343**, 1826–1832.

König, D, Grathwohl, D., Weinstock, C. *et al.* (2000). Upper respiratory tract infection in athletes: Influence of lifestyle, type of sport, training effort and immunostimulant intake. *Exercise Immunology Review* **6**, 102–120.

Kuitunen, T., Karkkainen, S. and Ylitalo, P. (1984). Comparison of the acute physical and mental effects of ephedrine, fenfluramine, phentermine and prolitane. *Methods & Findings in Experimental and Clinical Pharmacology* **6**, 265–270.

Lanciault, G. and Wolf, H.H. (1965). Some neuropharmacological properties of the ephedrine isomers. *Journal of Pharmaceutical Sciences* **54**, 841–844.

Lefebvre R.A., Surmont F., Bouckaert J. *et al.* (1992). Urinary excretion of ephedrine after nasal application in healthy volunteers. *Journal of Pharmacy and Pharmacology* **44**, 672–675.

Leynaert, B., Bousquet, J., Neukirch, C. *et al.* (1999). Perennial rhinitis: An independent risk factor for asthma in nonatopic subjects. Results from the European Community Respiratory Health Survey. *Journal of Allergy Clinical Immunology* **104**, 301–304.

MacIntosh, B.R. and Wright, B.M. (1995). Caffeine ingestion and performance of a 1,500-metre swim. *Canadian Journal of Applied Physiology* **20**, 168–177.

Medicines and Healthcare Products Regulatory Agency (MHRA). (2000). Phenyl-propanolamine and haemorrhagic stroke—Update. Available at http://www.mhra.gov.uk/Safetyinformation/Safetywarningsalertsandrecalls/Safetywarningsandmessagesformedicines/CON019551 (accessed 5 November 2009).

Mottram, D.R., Chester, N., Atkinson, G. *et al.* (2008). Athletes' knowledge and views on over-the-counter medication. *International Journal of Sports Medicine* **29**, 851–855.

Nathan, A. (2002). How to treat hay fever and associated allergic conditions in the pharmacy. *Pharmaceutical Journal* **268**, 575–578.

Nieman, D.C., Henson, D.A. and Gusewitch, G. (1993). Physical activity and immune function in elderly women. *Medicine and Science in Sports and Exercise* **25**, 823–831.

Nieman, D.C., Johanssen, L.M., Lee, J.W. *et al.* (1990). Infectious episodes in runners before and after the Los Angeles Marathon. *Journal of Sports Medicine and Physical Fitness* **30**, 316–328.

Norvenius, G., Widerlov, E. and Lönnerhölm, G. (1979). Phenylpropanolamine and mental disturbance. *Lancet* **2**, 1367–1368.

Pasman, W.J., van Baak, M.A., Jeukendrup, A.E. *et al.* (1995). The effect of different dosages of caffeine on endurance performance time. *International Journal of Sports Medicine* **16**, 225–230.

Paton, C.D., Hopkins, W.G. and Vollebregt, L. (2001). Little effect of caffeine ingestion on repeated sprints in team-sport athletes. *Medicine and Science in Sports and Exercise* **33**, 822–825.

Peters, E.M. and Bateman, E.D. (1983). Ultramarathon running and upper respiratory tract infections. *South African Medical Journal* **64**, 582–584.

Price, D., Bond, C., Bouchard, J. *et al.* (2006). International Primary Care Respiratory Group (IPCRG) guidelines: Management of allergic rhinitis. *Primary Care Respiratory Journal* **15**, 58–70.

Proprietary Association of Great Britain. (2009a). OTC directory 2009/10: Treatments for common ailments. Available at http://www.medicinechestonline.com/ (accessed 19 October 2009).

Proprietary Association of Great Britain. (2009b). 2009 PAGB annual review. Available at http://www.pagb.co.uk/publications/PDFs/annualreview2009.pdf (accessed 19 October 2009).

Ramsey, J.J., Colman, R.J., Swick, A.G. *et al.* (1998). Energy expenditure, body composition and glucose metabolism in lean and obese rhesus monkeys treated with ephedrine and caffeine. *American Journal of Clinical Nutrition* **68**, 42–51.

Reissig, C.J., Strain, E.C. and Griffiths, R.R. (2009). Caffeinated energy drinks—A growing problem. *Drug and Alcohol Dependence* **99**, 1–10.

Ryan, D. (2008). Management of acute rhinosinusitis in primary care: Changing paradigms and the emerging role of intranasal corticosteroids. *Primary Care Respiratory Journal* **17(3)**, 148–155.

Scadding, G.K., Durham, S.R., Mirakian, R. *et al.* (2008). BSACI guidelines for the management of allergic and non-allergic rhinitis. *Clinical and Experimental Allergy* **38(1)**, 19–42.

Sidney, K.H. and Lefcoe N.M. (1977). The effects of ephedrine on the physiological and psychological responses to submaximal and maximal exercise in man. *Medicine and Science in Sports and Exercise* **9**, 95–99.

Strano-Rossi, S., Leone, D., de la Torre, X. *et al.* (2009). The relevance of the urinary concentration of ephedrines in anti-doping analysis: Determination of pseudoephedrine, cathine, and ephedrine after administration of over-the-counter medications. *Therapeutic Drug Monitoring* **31**, 520–526.

Swain, R.A., Harsha, D.M., Baenziger, J. *et al.* (1997). Do pseudoephedrine or phenylpropanolamine improve maximum oxygen uptake and time to exhaustion? *Clinical Journal of Sport Medicine* **7**, 168–173.

To, L.B., Sangster, J.F., Rampling, D. *et al.* (1980). Ephedrine-induced cardiomyopathy. *Medical Journal of Australia* **2**, 35–36.

UK Sport. (2003). The UK anti-doping programme results: Quarter 4 and full year figures 2002/03. Available at http://www.uksport.gov.uk/pages/historical_results/ (accessed 11 November 2009).

UK Sport. (2009). Drugs results database. Available at http://www.uksport.gov.uk/drugs/ (accessed 11 November 2009).

Vallerand, A.L. (1993). Effects of ephedrine/xanthines on thermogenesis and cold tolerance. *International Journal of Obesity* **17**, S53–S56.

Wadler, G.I. and Hainline, B. (1989). *Drugs and the athlete.* F.A. Davis Company, Philadelphia.

Weatherby, R.P. and Rogerson, S. (2002). Caffeine potentiation of the performance enhancing effects of pseudoephedrine. In *Conference proceedings: Sixth IOC World Congress on Sport Sciences.* St Louis. Abstract, p.110.

Weiner, I., Tilkian, A.G. and Palazzolo, M. (1990). Coronary artery spasm and myocardial infarction in a patient with normal coronary arteries: Temporal relationship to pseudoephedrine ingestion. *Catheterization and Cardiovascular Diagnostics* **20**, 51–53.

Williams, M.H. (1974). Drugs and athletic performance. Charles C. Thomas, Springfield, Illinois.

World Anti-Doping Agency (WADA). (2009). The 2010 prohibited list international standard. Available at http://www.wada-ama.org/Documents/World_Anti-Doping_Program/WADP-Prohibited-list/WADA_Prohibited_List_2010_EN.pdf (accessed 10 November 2009).

Chapter 22

Non-steroidal anti-inflammatory drugs

Peter N. Elliott

22.1 Introduction

All sports have developed from the natural capabilities of the human mind and body and so, when partaken at modest levels, few sports involve great risk of physical injury. This situation changes dramatically when sporting pursuits are undertaken at higher competitive levels. As it becomes necessary to push the body further, in an effort to achieve greater performance, a point may well be reached where the stresses and strains exerted on the structural framework of the body may exceed that which the body is capable of withstanding, resulting in connective tissues being torn or joints being dislocated. Many sports carry their own peculiar additional risks of injury to the body; the boxer may suffer repeated blows to the face, causing extensive bruising and laceration and the footballer may receive kicks to the legs, resulting in bruising or even bone fracture.

Any traumatic injury to a competitor will result in a reduced level of performance capability and may require the abstention from sport for a period of recuperation. As well as the pain and personal discomfort associated with injury the individual's performance is likely to deteriorate during a period of inactivity. Muscle bulk may be lost and an extended training period will inevitably be required to regain peak fitness.

In a sport where a career may be of limited duration and where there is a short season of competition the result of even minor trauma may be devastating. To the keen amateur, years of training may be wasted by an inability to participate competitively in a once-in-a-lifetime event. To a top international professional, a day on the bench may represent the loss of vast sums of money.

Whatever the cause or nature of the injury, one of its inevitable features will be the occurrence of an inflammatory reaction at the damaged site. If we are to appreciate the potential to treat sports injuries we must understand the inflammatory response.

22.2 The inflammatory response

The term "inflammation" is derived from the Latin *inflammare*, which means to set on fire. It is a term widely employed to describe the pathological process that occurs at the site of tissue damage. A precise definition of the condition is difficult as its nature can vary quite significantly. If we accept that it is a process that is aimed at maintaining the integrity of the tissues and that the bloodstream carries a huge range of cells and chemicals that have protected the body, then it is feasible to construct a useful, descriptive definition.

Inflammation enables the body's defensive and regenerative resources to concentrate on tissues that have suffered damage or are contaminated with abnormal material (such as invading micro-organisms). It aims to limit the damaging effects of any contaminating material, to cleanse and remove any foreign particles and damaged tissue debris, and to allow healing processes to restore the tissues to some kind of normality. Inflammation is fundamentally important for survival.

Inflammation is a phenomenon that was well known to ancient civilisations. Examples of inflammatory conditions can be identified in early writings of Chinese, Egyptian, Greek and Roman origin. Hieroglyphic symbols, which can be translated as representing inflammation, can be identified in an Egyptian manuscript about 4000 years old. The classical description of inflammation was undoubtedly given by Celsus in the first century AD. In his *De re medicinia* he states that "the signs of inflammation are four, redness and swelling with heat and pain". To these four signs was added a fifth, loss of function, by Virchow (1858), the founding researcher of modern cellular pathology. Loss of function is a consequence of the swelling and pain associated with inflammation and is clearly an indication that affected tissues require rest for rapid rehabilitation.

Inflammation is a dynamic process, and this process may, on occasion, be capable of causing more harm to the organism than the initiating stimulus itself would. Clearly, not all inflammatory reactions are useful. There is, for example, no obvious reason why the inflammatory reactions that occur in diseases such as rheumatoid arthritis benefit individuals. What is abundantly clear is that the combined effect of the components of the body's defensive mechanism may often be excessive. A study of inflammation tends to leave one with the distinct impression that the body generally overreacts to stimuli. If this is the case, then we may be drawn to the view that inhibiting inflammatory reactions may in some circumstances be beneficial. Could it be that suppressing the inflammatory reactions associated with traumatic sports injuries falls into such a category?

Whilst there are many and varied kinds of inflammation it is possible to consider that the basic components of the inflammatory reaction result from the combined effects of changes in the microcirculation, alteration of permeability of the blood vessel walls to protein and immigration of leucocytes and leucocyte-derived cells, which exhibit activities such as phagocytosis.

Changes in microcirculation during the inflammatory response

The immediate reaction of tissues to a physical trauma is to increase the blood supply to the area. In superficial tissues this may be seen as an increased redness and the affected area may feel warmer than the surrounding, unaffected areas (two of the cardinal signs of inflammation).

Another of the cardinal signs, swelling, is also the consequence of a change in the vascular system. In this case it is a change in the permeability of the blood vessel wall to protein. Normally the fluid found outside the blood system, in the tissues, is composed of water with some low molecular weight solutes such as oxygen, sodium ions, chloride ions and glucose. The protein content of this fluid is very low whilst the protein content of blood is relatively high. This state of affairs is maintained by virtue of the fact that the blood vessel wall is permeable only to water and salts. Proteins cannot normally move from the blood vessel through the vessel wall into the surrounding tissues.

Water is forced out of small blood vessels at the arteriolar end of capillary beds due to the pressure under which blood is maintained by the heart's activity. The colloid osmotic pressure exerted by the protein present in the blood counterbalances this force, causing water to be drawn back into the blood system. Without the presence of the plasma protein, blood volume would very rapidly diminish due to the net movement of water from the blood to the tissues.

During an inflammatory reaction the fluid equilibrium is altered. The permeability of small blood vessels changes to allow plasma protein to leak out of the vessel into the surrounding tissue. This change in distribution of protein is followed by a net movement of water from the blood into the tissues, giving rise to oedema, which may ultimately be seen as swelling. Electron microscopic examination of blood vessels to which vasoactive substances were applied revealed the production of gaps 0.1µm to 0.4µm in diameter between adjacent endothelial cells. These gaps are temporary and there is no apparent damage caused to the endothelium of the leaking vessel.

Another consequence of oedema formation is the development of pain. Pain is, at least in part, due to the increased pressure on sensory nerves caused by the accumulation of the oedematous fluid in an enclosed space. There is, however, some evidence that pain may also be due to the release of pain-inducing chemicals at the site of the reaction. The local generation of peptides such as bradykinin can give rise to pain and the effect of such pain-producing substances may be enhanced by the action of prostaglandins.

A loss of function, the fifth cardinal sign, is perhaps the most significant issue associated with inflammation in the injured sportsman or sportswoman. It results, largely, as a consequence of the swelling that accrues in the reaction. The swelling of an articular joint inhibits normal movement and promotes pain. This pain is particularly evident when the sufferer attempts to use the affected limb.

Leucocytes in inflammation

Acute inflammatory reactions to minor trauma may well be restricted to changes in the microcirculation as described above. Such reactions may resolve quite quickly.

More persistent inflammatory reactions of the type common to sports injuries, however, involve another major physiological change, which is the influx of leucocytes. One of the most significant leucocytes in the normal reaction to traumatic injury is the polymorphonuclear leucocyte. There are several different kinds of these polymorphs but the most abundant can be identified in a blood smear by virtue of their affinity to take up a neutral pH stain. These cells are sometimes referred to as neutrophils.

Normal tissues contain few extravascular polymorphs but in an inflammatory reaction these cells may pass from the microcirculation into the damaged tissue site. Following an injury, blood polymorphs stick momentarily to the endothelium; they roll along the inside surface of the vessel wall, adhering briefly until they re-enter the circulation. After a few minutes, more and more cells adhere, and eventually these are not dislodged by the blood flow. In this way the endothelium comes to be lined with leucocytes, a process known as margination. Other leucocytes, platelets, and red cells may also stick. Margination is promoted by the rapid deployment of cell adhesion molecules (CAMs) on the surfaces of the endothelial cells, which can attach to the leucocytes.

The marginated polymorphs leave the intravascular site by a process, which starts with a pseudopodium insinuating itself between two adjacent endothelial cells that form the blood vessel wall by attachment to the platelet/endothelium CAM or PECAM exhibited on the surface of the ends of endothelial cells . The bulk of the polymorph, including the nucleus, then passes between the endothelial cells and comes to lie outside the endothelial cell but within the basement membrane. The cell then passes through the basement membrane.

These cells provide an important contribution to the inflammatory process. Polymorphonuclear leucocytes are the first inflammatory cells to accumulate in large numbers in an injured area. These cells are phagocytic and play a protective role by ingesting and subsequently digesting invading micro-organisms or tissue debris in the affected area. Polymorphs do not survive for more than a few hours outside blood vessels and when they die they release their contents (which include a whole host of very destructive lysosomal enzymes) into the surrounding area. The release of these enzymes may help to clear the affected area of damaged tissue fragments prior to the laying down of new tissue. These highly destructive enzymes may also be responsible for additional damage occurring to the tissues and may help to sustain an inflammatory reaction.

Besides the influx of polymorphonuclear cells from the blood there is also a movement of mononuclear cells. Monocytes begin to move into the affected site at the same time as the polymorphs but they arrive more slowly and are, therefore, generally outnumbered by polymorphonuclear cells at the start of a reaction. Mononuclear cells are, however, much more enduring than the poly-morphs and in many reactions begin to predominate after a day or so. Outside the circulation, monocytes go through a maturation phase to become macrophages, which, as the name implies, are large phagocytic cells. These cells can undergo cell division, which also contributes to the large numbers of mononuclear cells that accumulate at the inflamed site. Mononuclear cells such as macrophages do have a number of other significant roles. They are capable of secreting many different chemicals that affect defensive activities and they have a key role in determining whether the body mounts an antibody response to a challenge.

The contributions of the leucocytes to the inflammatory reactions are various. The presence of cells capable of phagocytosis at an injured site is an advantage. The removal of damaged tissues and any foreign material such as micro-organisms is of obvious importance. The local increase in leucocyte numbers at the site of inflammation results in a general increase in the concentration of proteolytic enzymes, because the lysosomes of the leucocytes contain cathepsins, hydrolases and other catabolic enzymes. Release of these enzymes may be an important factor in the maintenance of inflammation by the production of altered tissue proteins and by the nonspecific activation of thrombin, kinin and plasmin systems. Polymorphs also provide a source of enzymes with more specific activities for maintaining the inflammatory reaction.

Acute and chronic inflammation

The initial reaction to most types of sport injuries is an acute inflammatory response exhibiting the prominent feature of increased vascular permeability. This reaction will normally resolve in time, and, if actual tissue necrosis is slight, no identifiable trace of the reaction will be left. In a more severe situation repair is effected by the synthesis of connective tissue to form a scar.

In some circumstances, however, inflammation may persist. The characteristic feature of chronic inflammation is the presence of leucocytes at the site of reaction. Some acute inflammatory reactions may proceed without migration of phagocytic cells into the tissues, but chronic inflammation is invariably associated with large numbers of extravascular white cells. Chronic inflammation is also characterised by concurrent tissue destruction and resultant inflammation. The death of invading polymorphs at an inflamed site with the resultant release of all their intercellular enzymes can give rise to a suppurative lesion. A suppurative lesion may continue at the site of some foreign material but the necrotic area may become surrounded by a deposition of fibrous material and white cells to give rise to an abscess. A separation of degenerative and synthetic processes as in the case of an abscess is not always seen, with the two processes often occurring simultaneously at the same site. Such a chronic inflammatory mass is called a granuloma.

Chronic inflammation can occur, however, without passing through an acute or suppurative phase. Histological examination of chronic inflammatory lesions reveals the presence of a variety of different types of white cells. In rheumatoid synovial fluids, large numbers of white cells, principally polymorphs, can be found. These have extremely short half lives on the order of only three to four hours and the variety of damaging agents that can be released from these cells has already been outlined. Polymorphs are also actively phagocytic but this function may not be important in chronic inflammatory situations because their short life span will frequently result in the release of any ingested material on the death of the cell.

Most chronic inflammatory reactions are characterised by large numbers of mononuclear cells. Those mononuclear cells may be derived either by emigration or division and the persistence of these cells may be due to their great longevity. Macrophages, like polymorphs, are phagocytic and this would seem to be an important function, the removal of foreign material and tissue debris being a prerequisite for the resolution of an injury.

Within an area of chronic inflammation macrophages may be transformed into two other cell types: epithelioid cells and foreign body giant cells. Epithelioid cells are a common feature of granulomatous inflammation and can be transformed into epithelial cells by natural maturation if they live long enough and do not have undigested phagocytosed material within the cell. Giant cells are multinucleate and have been shown to be produced by cell fusion, although this fusion may be followed by nuclear division without cytoplasmic fission. These cells are found in large numbers around foreign bodies that are too large for macrophages to engulf. Other cells present in chronic inflammatory reactions are fibroblasts, which are probably derived from local connective tissue fibroblasts and are responsible for collagen deposition, and lymphocytes and plasma cells, which are responsible for the production of antibodies to facilitate the elimination of micro-organisms.

Our knowledge of inflammatory processes has largely been derived from observations made in humans with chronic inflammatory disease and in laboratory experiments with animals. The contribution that any of the factors described above may make in the inflammatory sequel to a sporting injury cannot be specified but undoubtedly there will be several predictable phenomena:

1   an influx of blood giving rise to the characteristic heat and redness;
2   a movement of plasma protein and associated water into the tissue, causing swelling;
3   an influx of phagocytic cells that have the potential to cause tissue destruction;
4   pain, perhaps due to pressure on the nerve endings caused by the swelling or to the effect of chemical mediators of pain being released; and
5   finally, and perhaps most importantly for the sportsman, there will be a loss of function: Virchow's fifth cardinal sign.

The persistence of the problem depends on many factors but certainly the influx of leucocytes and the release of their enzyme-rich content may compound the damage already caused and may prolong the duration of the reaction. Given that no further aggravation occurs and that there are no complications, resolution should occur within days or weeks and at worst months.

A pertinent question to ask at this point is whether the inflammation that follows a traumatic injury is necessary. Clearly, the body automatically takes what it deems to be the safest course of action when injured. It directs its defensive systems to the area to make sure that no microbial invasion occurs and that all the necessary resources are made available to repair the damage. It is evident, however, that the body has a tendency to overreact. The response in many cases may be more serious than the stimulus.

22.3   The treatment of sporting injuries

The acronym RICE will be familiar to those with experience in treating sports injuries. Rest, ice, compression and elevation are all of value. Rest enables healing and limits adding to the damage already sustained. Applying pressure to an affected area and the elevation of a limb above the level of the heart can influence the intravascular/extravascular fluid balance equilibrium with a resultant inhibition of oedema development.

Cooling a traumatised part of the body is also effective. The use of aerosol sprays that contain volatile compounds that evaporate on the skin surface, causing rapid chilling of the area, is quite common. The practice of cooling an injured area whether by volatile spray, cold compress or ice-packs, etc., if applied rapidly, may well reduce the immediate response to minor trauma by inhibiting the active processes that initiate an inflammatory reaction. Problems have arisen because of the abuse of these solvent-based products for "sniffing". Nevertheless, cooling will undoubtedly reduce the immediate reaction to a traumatic stimulus. Given that the body does seem to have a natural inclination to overreact, inducing a delay in the response produced by cooling may well prevent, or at least limit, any subsequent inflammation.

Other nonspecific topical applications that can be used successfully for the treatment of injured tissues include liniments. These preparations are rubefacients and are thought to act by counterirritation. This is a phenomenon where mild or moderate pain can be relieved by irritating the skin. Counterirritation is effective in providing relief from painful lesions of muscles, tendons and joints. There is, however, little evidence that the topical application of preparations containing adrenaline or aspirin is of value in the relief of pain.

A number of more specific anti-inflammatory treatments are available to deal with sporting injuries. The reduction of pain and inflammation represents an obvious therapeutic target. It is clear, however, that great care must be taken in judging the severity of an injury. Pain is the cue that intimates the severity of a problem. There are many drugs that can reduce our appreciation of pain, but a reduction of pain sensation may lead to the induction of further damage to an injury due to the failure to respond to the natural inclination to rest. Anti-inflammatory drugs may, nevertheless, be of value.

The use of non-steroidal anti-inflammatory drugs to treat inflammatory conditions

Although the treatment of inflammation with anti-inflammatory agents was practised by Hippocrates, who recommended the chewing of willow bark for a variety of ailments, such sensible practices were largely forgotten during subsequent centuries. It was not until 1876 that a physician named MacLagan revolutionised the treatment of rheumatic fever (and, indeed, other inflammatory conditions) by the re-introduction of an extract of willow bark called salicin. MacLagan had been unimpressed with the treatments that were routinely used to treat rheumatic fever (a condition characterised by extensive inflammatory lesions) such as bloodletting. A synthetic analogue of salicin, a glycoside, was soon produced and in 1899 a German pharmaceutical company, Bayer, introduced a more palatable derivative, acetylsalicylic acid, under the trade name Aspirine. Over 100 years later we still have aspirin readily available as a simple, cheap and effective remedy for a wide variety of ailments. It has been the subject of innumerable clinical trials in many diverse areas of medicine ranging from the treatment of food intolerance to the prevention of heart attacks. Without doubt, the bulk of the tens of thousands of tons of aspirin consumed each year is taken for the alleviation of pain, inflammation and fever.

Since the introduction of aspirin, many other drugs with similar therapeutic profiles have been developed and there are now about 20 aspirin-like drugs available for clinical use in the UK, some of which are available for general purchase. These aspirin-like drugs, generally referred to collectively as non-steroidal anti-inflammatory drugs, or NSAIDs, all have proven anti-inflammatory activity in the treatment of chronic inflammatory conditions such as rheumatoid arthritis. Countless clinical trials have demonstrated the efficacy of these agents in alleviating both objective and subjective symptoms of inflammatory disease. Whilst some of these agents are more popular than others, there is no overwhelming evidence that any particular member of this group is the most effective. Indeed, it is difficult to find convincing proof that any of the newer drugs in this class is more effective than aspirin. The assessment of activity of this type of drug is, however, fraught with difficulties. It is not easy to find large numbers of patients with similar disease states who are prepared to be subjected to the withdrawal of their effective therapies so that they may be used as controls in such trials. It is also very difficult to quantify a reduction in inflammation.

Given that these difficulties exist when testing drugs on common chronic conditions, it is not hard to appreciate that the difficulties involved in testing anti-inflammatory agents in acute sporting injuries, which may affect any part of the body, are considerably greater. A traumatic sporting injury should progressively heal over a fairly limited period without intervention. How then can you measure the efficacy of an anti-inflammatory drug superimposed on a naturally regressing inflammatory condition? The simple answer is, with great difficulty!

The majority of clinical trials published on the efficacy of NSAIDs in sports injury are organised with two groups of injured subjects. One group is treated with one example of an NSAID whilst the other group is treated with a different NSAID. The usual result of these trials is that no significant difference is established between the two drugs under test. Clinical trials using this protocol have usually been used to establish that a new NSAID is effective. The trial protocol makes the assumption that the older, perhaps more established, drug is itself effective. This is not good science.

Whilst NSAIDs are clearly effective in treating chronic disease, evidence that they do have a role to play in acute traumatic injury treatment is much more limited. To establish definitively that drugs can effectively treat a sports injury a number of criteria have to be met. First, suitable injuries, preferably all of a certain type, are needed in reasonable numbers. Second, some measure of meaningful effectiveness is required. Third, a comparison would have to be made with a group of similar patients receiving no active treatment, that is, a control group. Because many individuals are responsive to suggestion, subjects in the control group would have to receive what appears to be the same treatment as the test group but, of course, without the active drug. In other words one group would be given tablets containing the drug whilst the other group would be given identical looking nondrug tablets, so-called placebos.

Experience in treating sports injuries has increased profoundly as specialised clinics have increased in numbers. This has improved the standard of clinical trials quite profoundly as large numbers of subjects with similar injuries are now much more readily available for assessment. A measurement of the period of time following injury until the injured person is fit for competition or full training again could serve as the key to assess effectiveness. If this time is reduced in the drug-treated group then it could be concluded that the drug is a successful therapy.

As soon as it is evident that a therapy is effective a substantial ethical and moral problem becomes evident. If a drug works or even if it is thought to work, it is difficult to justify the withholding of that treatment for the purpose of a trial since this action might unnecessarily prolong the period of absence from the sport. In many professional clubs such an action would be unacceptable (Boyne and Medhurst, 1967).

There is a widely held view that NSAIDs exert their anti-inflammatory effects by inhibiting the synthesis of prostaglandins. Prostaglandins are long-chain, poly-unsaturated fatty acid derivatives formed by the action of cyclo-oxygenase enzymes. Prostaglandins exhibit many properties that may contribute to inflammatory reactions.

The use of NSAIDs in the treatment of chronic inflammatory disease is well established and their efficacy is beyond question. Similarly in the treatment of acute traumatic injury their use has become commonplace and although far too many clinical trials have failed to furnish proof of their efficacy, clear evidence that these drugs are of benefit in sports injury has been produced. These drugs represent a simple and relatively safe means of reducing the inflammatory response to an injury. They may also help to return an injured sports participant to competitive fitness more rapidly. Many clinical trials compare the use of two different anti-inflammatory drugs but the most common finding is that there is no significant difference between the two. Where differences are reported they are not consistent. It would therefore be difficult to indicate a rank order of efficacy for these drugs.

Sprains (rupture of ligaments, which may be partial), strains (partial tearing of muscles) and bruises are all painful examples of sports injuries. Commonly they may warrant the use of painkilling (analgesic) drugs such as paracetamol or even, in severe cases, a narcotic analgesic compound such as dihydrocodeine. Since, however, these conditions are generally associated with an inflammatory component the use of an analgesic drug with anti-inflammatory activity would seem to be a more logical choice.

Given that the injured athlete is an otherwise normal, healthy adult, the major problem liable to be encountered following the use of aspirin (or indeed, for that matter, any of the NSAIDs) is gastric irritation, which may be experienced as a form of dyspepsia. The most common approach to minimising this problem is to avoid the use of these drugs when the stomach is empty. If the drugs are taken following a meal then any increased acid production that ensues can be utilised in the digestive process and would not be free to attack the lining of the stomach.

NSAIDs, which are selective inhibitors of cyclo-oxygenase-2 enzyme, were introduced in an attempt to reduce inflammation (by inhibiting synthesis of pro-inflammatory prostaglandin synthesis by COX-2 at the inflammatory site) without interfering with the synthesis of gastro-protective prostaglandins in the stomach (by cyclo-oxygenase-1). These drugs may offer some advantage to subjects who do not tolerate nonselective NSAIDs well but such drugs are associated with an increased risk of thrombotic events. NSAIDs are not currently licensed for the treatment of acute musculoskeletal disorders.

In the United Kingdom, about 20 different non-steroidal anti-inflammatory drugs are available to treat sports injuries and some details are given here of a small selection of them.

Aspirin

Aspirin is a very effective analgesic drug at a dose of 2–3 g per day. (In the UK, aspirin tablets generally contain 300 mg.) At higher doses, that is, in excess of 4 g per day, aspirin will reduce the swelling of an inflamed joint, a property not shown at the lower, analgesic level. Whilst anti-inflammatory activity is seen only at higher doses it is inadvisable to exceed the normal recommended doses without qualified medical supervision. Despite the antiquity of this preparation unequivocal evidence that any of the newer NSAIDs offers an all-round superior performance is lacking. The general availability and low cost of aspirin make it an ideal candidate for self-treatment following sports injury. Aspirin use is, however, not devoid of side effects, although the risks involved with the use of the drug are probably generally overstated.

In 1984 Anderson and Gotzsche compared the use of aspirin and naproxen, another NSAID, in patients with sports injuries. Perhaps, not surprisingly, they found no significant differences between the two drugs. Whilst this type of trial is common and the finding typical, the authors did highlight a phenomenon very relevant to the treatment of this type of traumatic injury. They demonstrated that significantly better results were obtained when the interval between injury and the start of treatment was shorter. This effect is widely appreciated now and is exactly what would be predicted from experimental inflammation studies in animals. In laboratory tests of the type used to screen for anti-inflammatory activity of new drugs for arthritis, it can be shown clearly that NSAIDs are much more effective against developing inflammation than they are against established inflammation.

The implications of this are clear. If it is deemed necessary to use an anti-inflammatory drug to treat a sports injury it should be given as early as possible after the damage is sustained and certainly before the inflammation becomes established. The principle reason for this probably lies in the realm of the intra-vascular/extravascular fluid equilibrium. The role of permeability changes has already been highlighted. Protein moves through the blood vessel wall during the development of the inflammatory reaction and draws water with it, resulting in the oedematous swelling. Once this oedema is formed, its resolution is dependent on the removal of the extravascular protein. NSAIDs do not appear to have any effect on the extravascular protein. It is an inevitable conclusion, therefore, that preventing oedema development is easier than resolving established oedema as there is no mechanism for the rapid removal of this protein the resolution of an established reaction.

Naproxen

Naproxen is one of the mainstays of treatment for chronic inflammatory conditions. Its efficacy and safety record are excellent and it is one of the most frequently prescribed drugs for the treatment of arthritis. Since its introduction in the early 1970s naproxen has been the subject of a large number of trials in the treatment of soft tissue injuries. Whilst many of these compare naproxen to another non-steroidal anti-inflammatory drug and find no difference in activity, several trials have shown naproxen to be better than the other drug in some respects and naproxen has been shown to be superior to placebo. In view of the popularity of this drug and the generally good reports of its efficacy in the literature, naproxen must rank high amongst the most suitable drugs for the treatment of sporting injuries. The drug is given at a dose of 0.75–1.25 g per day in three or four divided doses. Initially a high loading dose of 500mg may be given to aid the rapid attainment of suitable plasma levels of the drug (750 μg/ml). The drug may be taken at meal times to help combat any gastric discomfort, although in the presence of food the drug is absorbed more slowly. More rapid absorption occurs with the use of naproxen sodium. A 500 mg naproxen suppository preparation is available, principally for use at night.

Ibuprofen

Ibuprofen is another non-steroid anti-inflammatory drug with a similar structure to naproxen. It is the oldest propionic acid derivative anti-inflammatory agent in use and considerable experience has, therefore, been obtained with it. This drug is also one of the few drugs of this class available in the UK without prescription. It has a reputation for being well tolerated. In other words, it is widely felt that this particular anti-inflammatory agent does not induce the same degree of dyspepsia as many of its rivals.

Ibuprofen has always been perceived to be a well-tolerated drug. It is possible, however, that much of its reputation is based on early experiences with the drug when it was used at relatively low dose levels. To improve the often disappointing activity of ibuprofen the doses used have been increased and, whilst the drug is still generally well tolerated, it is certainly not without gastric irritant activity at these higher levels. Trials using ibuprofen at doses as low as 1200 mg per day have been shown to reduce pain and recovery time of soft-tissue sports injuries. Trials have, however, tended to use higher doses than this. Hutson (1986) found no significant differences between the activity of ibuprofen given at doses of 1800 mg or 2400 mg daily amongst 46 patients with knee injuries. The normal recommended dose range for ibuprofen for musculoskeletal disorders is 1.2–1.8 g daily in three to four divided doses, preferably after food. This may be increased if necessary to the maximum recommended daily dose of 2.4 g.

Indomethacin

Indomethacin has been used for treating inflammatory conditions since the mid-1960s and remains a very frequently prescribed drug. Whilst being an effective anti-inflammatory drug it does suffer, apart from the gastric irritant activity somewhat typical of this type of drug, from a number of central nervous system side effects such as headaches, dizziness and lightheadedness. Generally, indomethacin is found to be of similar efficacy to other non-steroidal anti-inflammatory drugs, such as naproxen, in the treatment of soft-tissue sports injuries. As might be expected, the drop-out rate due to side effects of this drug is generally higher than for other NSAIDs with normal therapeutic doses of indomethacin (50–200 mg daily). The drug is normally initiated at 25 mg two or three times daily and gradually increased if necessary. Edwards et al. (1984) found it necessary to withdraw only one patient from a group of 53 who were receiving 75 mg indomethacin daily for acute soft-tissue sports injuries. It is possible that at this low starting dose toxicity is less of a problem.

Indomethacin is also available in 100-mg suppositories for nighttime use and these may be of benefit in some individuals. It should be remembered that the combined rectal and oral doses should not amount to more than 200 mg in a 24-hour period.

Piroxicam

Piroxicam appears to be comparable to indomethacin or naproxen in treating acute musculoskeletal injuries and it is generally well tolerated. One particular advantage of piroxicam is that it has a long half-life, which permits its use as a single daily dose, usually of 20 mg. An initial, loading dose of 40 mg on each of the first two days of treatment, reducing to 20 mg for subsequent days, may be used for acute musculoskeletal disorders. In a large study of acute sports injuries in Norway the authors concluded that piroxicam at 40 mg daily for the first two days and 20 mg daily for a further five days resulted in significant improvements in mobility and reductions in pain when compared to placebo (Lereim and Gabor, 1988). This treatment gave a marginally superior response when compared to naproxen at 500 mg twice daily, and both drugs were well tolerated.

Piroxicam may also be given as a deep intramuscular injection for the initial dose. Effective concentrations of drugs are usually achieved earlier in this way than when they are administered orally.

Diclofenac

Available in both 75-mg and 100-mg tablets, diclofenac is another useful drug. Daily doses of either 75 mg or 150 mg are recommended. In a trial involving subjects with severe sprained ankles, diclofenac, at 150 mg daily, was shown to be superior to both placebo and piroxicam at 20 mg daily (Bahamonde and Saavedra, 1990). Both drugs were well tolerated. One possible advantage of this drug is that it is available in a slow-release form that is administered once daily, although this may be less of an advantage in an acute situation. In general, therapeutic levels are not achieved as rapidly with drugs that have a long half-life. Drugs with a short duration of action will normally give therapeutic levels in a very short period of time.

Phenylbutazone

Phenylbutazone was introduced into clinical medicine in 1949 to take its place alongside the salicylates for the treatment of arthritic conditions. It is a powerful anti-inflammatory drug and is capable of treating acute exacerbations of rheumatoid arthritis and severe ankylosing spondylitis (an inflammatory condition of the spine). Compared to the many, newer anti-inflammatory agents now available, phenylbutazone is subject to a large number of toxic side effects, some of which have led to fatal outcomes. It is no longer available in clinical medicine in the UK. Its inclusion in this chapter is because of its historical use in sports injuries and its use in equestrian sport. In the past it has been somewhat abused, particularly in the United States. A report by Marshall (1979) indicates that in the National Football League, for example, an average of 24-40 unit doses of phenylbutazone was used per player per season.

Equestrian sport

Whatever the role of phenylbutazone in injuries in sportsmen and sportswomen in the past, there is no doubt that it has been used with considerable success in the field of equestrian sports. In show jumping the horses' feet are subjected to constant concussion. By the age of 10 many show-jumping horses suffer pathological changes in their feet but, in many cases still be at their peak. Similarly, three-day event horses are subject to considerable physical stress with the strain of a tendon or the suspensory ligament being common injuries. Even without jumping-related competition, regular galloping activity, as in, for example, flat racing or polo, may result in substantial changes in horses' bones, joints and ligaments. When pushed too hard or for too long, lameness may develop due to pain and inflammation. The time-honoured remedy for reducing the pain and inflammation of these injuries in horses is to administer an anti-inflammatory drug; the most frequently used example is phenylbutazone.

Horses generally tolerate phenylbutazone very well and may be treated with the drug to improve their comfort. Whilst there are many indications for the use of phenylbutazone in horses, dilemmas do arise as to whether their use may mask an injury and lead to a complete breakdown of an affected limb. The governing bodies of equestrian sports generally recognise the usefulness of this drug but exclude its use on, or immediately before, competition days so that no unfair advantage may be gained by improving performance and so that unfit horses are protected from being used competitively.

Duration of NSAID treatment

There are obvious advantages to the early treatment of inflammatory responses to injury. How long treatment should continue is less clear. Studies of NSAID treatment of soft-tissue injuries in animals have generally demonstrated the advantage of treatment in the early, post-injury stage. The effectiveness of treatment over longer periods is less apparent. Some sports-injury studies have also reported no differences between treated and untreated groups at later stages of the inflammatory and healing processes.

In self-limiting injuries, healing generally occurs without treatment. It is perhaps inevitable that differences between treated and nontreated groups will diminish with time. Whilst treatment may result in an earlier return to normality untreated subjects are likely to "catch up". There is, however, an alternative interpretation, which is that NSAIDs may actually slow down the healing process. Inhibiting the influx of inflammatory cells, particularly polymophonuclear leucocytes, may limit the amount of local tissue injury that occurs following injury. It is possible that this may lead to the slower removal of damaged tissue and a consequent delay in the injury's resolution. The production of scar tissue may be impaired if fibroblast activity is reduced and this could, indeed, reduce the speed in which fully functional tissues are reformed (see Almekinders, 1999).

There is no consistent evidence that NSAIDs delay healing and, in consequence, explanations of possible mechanisms are largely speculative. Whilst sports injuries studies with NSAIDs do not universally demonstrate their efficacy the majority do. It would, therefore, seem to be a reasonable approach to treat acute traumatic sporting injuries immediately with NSAIDs but to discontinue treatment as soon as it is apparent that the acute inflammatory problem is resolving.

The use of NSAIDs to enhance performance in endurance sports

Given that NSAIDs are able to reduce the reaction to minor trauma it has been hypothesised that these drugs may be useful as prophylactic treatment to limit the body's reaction to endurance activities. From the few studies conducted, particularly using ibuprofen, there is no convincing evidence that an enhanced performance can be achieved (Nieman *et al.*, 2006). Concerns have been raised that masking pain may lead to even greater levels of tissue damage.

Topical NSAIDs in sports injury

Several pharmaceutical companies produce topical preparations of non-steroidal anti-inflammatory drugs for the relief of musculoskeletal pain. Topical preparations of piroxicam, ibuprofen, ketoprofen, felbinac (the active metabolite of fenbufen) and diclofenac are currently available in the UK (Table 22.1).

The concept of applying a non-steroidal anti-inflammatory drug locally in an effort to maximise the level of the drug at the site of injury whilst minimising the systemic level of the drug is an interesting one. In theory this technique may achieve a good therapeutic effect without the troublesome gastrointestinal side effects sometimes encountered with systemic therapy. There is good evidence that these preparations afford good penetration of the drug through the skin and that high levels of the active drug are achieved in the underlying tissues. Clinical trials with these preparations generally demonstrate that active drug formulations are more effective than placebo but the differences are generally slight. In one celebrated double-blind study, patients suffering bilateral inflammatory knee joint effusions were treated with diclofenac gel to one knee and a placebo gel to the other (Radermacher *et al.*, 1991). It was found that there were small reductions in swelling in both knees and no significant difference between the drug-treated and placebo-treated knees could be detected. In other words it did not seem to matter which knee the NSAID was applied to!

The massage of an affected area with a gel or cream may in itself be beneficial irrespective of the presence of a non-steroidal anti-inflammatory drug.

Table 22.1 Topical NSAID preparations commonly available in the UK

Diclofenac	Pennsaid, Voltarol Emulgel, Voltarol Gel Patch
Felbinac	Traxam
Ibuprofen	Fenbid Forte Gel, Ibugel Forte
Ketoprofen	Oruvail, Powergel
Piroxicam	Feldene

A significant point that should be considered here is whether these compounds actually exert their anti-inflammatory action at the inflamed site or elsewhere. If, for example, the reality of the situation is that the drugs reduce inflammation by interacting in some way with components in the bloodstream, then the concept of local application would be flawed. The statement found in the British National Formulary (2008) that these preparations "may provide some slight relief of pain in musculoskeletal conditions" would seem to be a reasonable conclusion to this section.

22.4   References

Almekinders, L.C. (1999). Anti-inflammatory treatment of muscular injuries in sport. An update of recent studies. *Sports Medicine* **28**, 383–388.

Anderson, L.A. and Gotzsche, P.C. (1984). Naproxen and aspirin in acute musculo-skeletal disorders: A double-blind, parallel study in patients with sports injuries. *Pharmacotherapeutica* **3**, 531–537.

Bahamonde, L.A. and Saavedra, C. (1990). Comparison of the analgesic and anti-inflammatory effects of diclofenac potassium versus piroxicam versus placebo in ankle sprain patients. *Journal of International Medical Research* **18**, 104–111.

Boyne, P.S. and Medhurst, H. (1967). Oral anti-inflammatory enzyme therapy in injuries in professional footballers. *The Practitioner* **198**, 543–546.

British National Formulary. (2008). British Medical Association and Royal Pharmaceutical Society of Great Britain.

Celsus. *De re medicinia*. Available at http://penelope.uchicago.edu/Thayer/E/Roman/Texts/Celsus/home.html.

Edwards, V., Wilson, A.A., Harwood, H.F. *et al.* (1984). A multicentre comparison of piroxicam and indomethacin in acute soft tissue sports injuries. *Journal of International Medical Research* **12**, 46–50.

Hutson, M.A. (1986). A double-blind study comparing ibuprofen 1800mg or 2400mg daily and placebo in sports injuries. *Journal of International Medical Research* **4**, 142–147.

Lereim, P. and Gabor, I. (1988). Piroxicam and naproxen in acute sports injuries. *American Journal of Medicine* **84 (Suppl. 5A)**, 45–49.

Marshall, E. (1979). Drugging of football players curbed by central monitoring plan, NFL claims. *Science* **203**, 626–628.

Nieman, D.C., Henson, D.A., Dumke, C.L. *et al.* (2006). Ibuprofen use, endotoxemia, inflammation, and plasma cytokines during ultramarathon competition. *Brain, Behaviour and Immunity* **20**, 578–584.

Radermacher, J., Jentsch, D., Scholl, M.A. *et al.* (1991). Diclofenac concentrations in synovial fluid and plasma after cutaneous application in inflammatory and degenerative joint disease. *British Journal of Clinical Pharmacology* **31**, 537–541.

Virchow, R. (1858) *Cellular pathology.*

Chapter 23

Melatonin and related substances

Thomas Reilly and Jim Waterhouse

23.1 Background

Melatonin is a hormone secreted by the pineal gland located deep within the brain. It is synthesised from the amino acid tryptophan by the enzymes N-acetyltransferase and 5-hydroxyindole-O-methyltransferase (HIOMT). It is itself a substrate for serotonin or 5-hydroxytryptamine, a neurotransmitter engaged in regulating sleep (see Table 23.1).

Melatonin has a relatively short half-life of 35–50 min, poor bioavailability and numerous nonspecific as well as specific actions. It is synthesised in practically all living organisms and in plants such as rice. Occurring naturally in the body, melatonin can also be obtained over-the-counter in some countries in supra-physiological doses. The original commercial products contained extracts from cow pineal gland, now replaced with purer forms due to the risk of carrying infections, or with synthetic analogues. Ingested melatonin is capable of crossing the blood-brain barrier and binding to receptor sites in the brain. It can be purchased as a dietary supplement in the USA, since 1993, but is accessible only by prescription throughout the European Union. Its consumer acceptance in the USA, Singapore and elsewhere is linked to expectations of health benefits due to nonspecific effects. Highly specific effects are noted in the role of naturally occurring melatonin in regulating human circadian rhythms.

Melatonin levels peak at night at about 60 ng with values during daytime being 30 times lower. There is a pronounced rhythm in the activity of N-acetyltransferase, nocturnal values exceeding daytime figures a thousand fold. Inhibition of melatonin by light is due to the suppression of another enzyme engaged in its synthesis, hydroxyl-O-methyltransferase. Suppression during daylight hours is caused by noradrenaline released from the sympathetic nervous system.

The main neural pathway for registering information about light is the retino-hypothalamic tract, which connects the eyes to the suprachiasmatic nuclei cells of the hypothalamus. These pairs of grouped cells are the site of the body clock that regulates human circadian rhythms. Melanopsin is selectively sensitive to light at short wavelengths (460–480 nm) and this opsin in specialised ganglion

Table 23.1 Steps in metabolism of melatonin

Metabolism starts with uptake of tryptophan from the circulation into the pineal gland.
Tryptophan is converted to 5-hydrohytrypophian by the enzyme tryptophan
  5-monooxygenase.
Further conversion is to serotonin (5 hydroxytryptamine, or 5-HT) by the enzyme
  5-hydroxy-tryptophan decarboxylase.
Serotonin is converted to melatonin (N-acetyl-methoxytryptamine) by a two-step
  process:

  1. N-acetylation of serotonin by arylalkylaline N-acetyl-transferase to give
     N-acetylserotonin;
  2. Methylation of the 5-hydroxy group by hydroxyindole-O- methyltransferase
     (HIOMT).

cells in the retina rather than the rods and cones of the visual system relays photoreception to the suprachiasmatic nuclei. Many blind people display circadian rhythms that run freely, into and out of phase with the 24-hour rhythm of the solar day. Another neural link through the intergeniculate leaflet carries information about general excitement to the suprachiasmatic nuclei. The nuclei cells and the pineal gland are connected via the superior cervical ganglion.

Two principal membrane receptors for melatonin (MT1 and MT2) are found in the central nervous system and in peripheral tissues. The suprachiasmatic nuclei possess melatonin receptors, being the anatomical site of the body clock. These cells are situated close to the areas where body temperature, the autonomic nervous system, hormone secretion, feeding cycles and the sleep-wakefulness cycle are regulated. The existence of melatonin receptors in the periphery illustrates how ubiquitous circadian rhythms are in the body, integrated into an overall 24-hour oscillating system. Their entrainment by the time-keeping cells of the suprachiasmatic nuclei indicates how the central body clock affects peripheral tissues via core temperature and output from the endocrine and central nervous systems.

The body clock regulates rhythms in physiological functions over a 24-hour period. These fluctuations constitute circadian rhythms and contain endogenous and exogenous components. Endogenous rhythms are determined by activity of the body clock in conjunction with pineal function. Various clock genes have been linked to circadian rhythms, whose generation is a consequence of a series of negative feedback loops involving clock gene expression. The natural length of the endogenous rhythm has been estimated to be 24.3 hours (Middleton *et al.*, 1996; hence, *circa diem*). Exogenous factors that lock the free-running rhythm into an exact 24-hour cycle coinciding with the light-darkness cycle include, mainly, the light-dark cycle itself but also rhythms of ambient temperature, habitual activity, meal times and social exchanges. In nycthemeral conditions, whole-body rhythms have endogenous and exogenous components in different proportions. For example, body temperature is largely an endogenous rhythm whereas digestive functions are mainly exogenous.

The circadian rhythm in melatonin is closely linked to that of core body temperature, which generally peaks at about 17:00 hours and reaches a nadir in mid-sleep (Reilly and Brooks, 1986). The classical cosine function of the rhythm in core temperature reflects the switches from heat gain to heat loss, which in turn lead to changes in other physiological functions. Melatonin induces subjective changes and the combination of increased drowsiness and cutaneous heat loss and decreased metabolic rate prepares the body for its night time sleep. These changes illustrate the soporific effects and vasodilatory properties of melatonin, and form the basis of its use in treating certain sleep disorders. It has also been used to entrain the free-running circadian rhythm in blind people (Lewy *et al.*, 2005).

Humans display a phase-response curve for melatonin, effects of the hormone on characteristics of circadian rhythms depending on the time of day. A melatonin stimulus in the morning moves the acrophase or peak time to the right, a direction associated with a phase delay. Increased melatonin concentrations in the evening shift the acrophase to the left, representing a phase advance. Light opposes the effects of melatonin and has a phase-response curve that is the reverse, the respective peaks being a half-cycle apart. The interplay of light and melatonin in concert with alternations between daytime and darkness constitutes the basis of timing of circadian rhythms. Changes in day length and hours of darkness due to seasonal variations are likely to affect melatonin levels in humans and other species. In the lizard, for example, the pineal gland was known as the "third eye".

23.2   Melatonin and biological rhythms

Melatonin is not only the hormone associated with circadian rhythms but also is engaged in rhythms of greater lengths. These rhythms include the human menstrual cycle (circamensal), associated with fluctuations in female reproductive hormones, and the annual cycle of seasons (circannual). There may be interactions between these different rhythms: the increases in body temperature and catecholamine activity that are induced by changes in ovarian hormones across the menstrual cycle could interact with circadian variations in these variables to influence physiological responses to exercise.

The menstrual cycle is controlled by an axis formed by the pituitary gland, the hypothalamus and the ovaries. It is characterised by systematic rises and falls in the reproductive hormones oestrogen and progesterone. Typically, the cycle length is about 28 days, the count commencing on the first day of menses. The new ovarian follicle develops after four to five days of menses, stimulated by FSH (follicle-stimulating hormone) and ovulation is triggered by a surge in LH (luteinizing hormone), marked by a rise in core temperature of about 0.5 °C. The follicular phase is dominated by oestrogen whereas progesterone dominates the luteal cycle, although oestrogen is produced by the corpus luteum that emerges from the ovarian follicle. Unless conception has occurred at ovulation, levels of oestrogen and progesterone fall pre-menses, which ends the luteal phase of the cycle. Oestradiol, one of the oestrogens, can increase lipolysis and inhibit glycolysis and glycogenolysis, in effect sparing glycogen stores and altering the preferred substrate as fuel for exercise. Forsyth and Reilly (2005) reported lower levels of blood lactate in the luteal compared to the follicular phase in response to exercise on a rowing ergometer. This difference had consequences when the lactate threshold was determined. The exercise intensity, heart rate, VO_2 corresponding to a fixed blood lactate concentration (VO_2- 4 mM) were higher in mid-luteal than in mid-follicular phase, irrespective of time of day.

In many species melatonin regulates mating behaviour. Its seasonal variations allow some animals to tolerate changes in environmental conditions between summer and winter. Melatonin has been linked to the growth and shedding of pelage in ponies, to provide insulation against cold conditions in winter and facilitate heat loss in summer. The thickness of covering is related to latitude. Shetland ponies have less covering than their Icelandic counterparts further north but more than Connemara ponies further south. Humans living in Arctic regions may have disrupted circadian rhythms in winter due to the long hours of darkness. Seasonal affective disorder (SAD) is a clinical condition linked to circadian disturbances, and treatment of the condition entails morning bright light or evening exogenous melatonin administration (Peiser, 2009). Such treatment might be acting via clock adjustment (and the relevant phase response curve) but this is not certain.

The increased duration of melatonin synthesis and secretion from summer to winter acts as a biological signal for seasonal functions that depend on day length. Besides reproduction and coat growth, these functions include in some instances camouflage colouring and habitual activity. In seasonal breeders that mate in daylight hours, melatonin controls variables related to sexual activity. It can inhibit the anterior pituitary hormones LH and FSH in animals with a breeding season during daylight hours when days are long. In contrast, melatonin is stimulated in short-day breeders. In humans there is a seasonal variation in melatonin related to the length of day, but this cannot explain seasonal patterns of reproductive behaviour. Similarly, variations in fitness measures are affected more by training variables and activity patterns that are influenced by weather and climatic conditions than by internal circannual cycles (Reilly and Peiser, 2006).

23.3   Other properties of melatonin

Melatonin is an antioxidant that helps in protecting nuclear and mitochondrial DNA. It does not undergo redox cycling, which allows other antioxidants like vitamin C to regain their antioxidant properties. Once it is oxidised, melatonin cannot be reduced to its former state and is therefore known as a terminal antioxidant. A molecule of the main metabolite in the antioxidant pathway can neutralise up to 10 reactive oxygen species. Melatonin's antioxidant activity is thought to decrease damage due to certain types of Parkinson's disease, prevent cardiac arrhythmias and increase longevity. Hence it is used on the assumption that it counters ageing effects (Bartsch *et al.*, 2009).

Melatonin is thought to interact with the immune system. Positive effects are attributed to its action on MT1 and MT2 receptors expressed in immunocompetent cells. Cytokine production may be enhanced, thereby compensating for acquired immunodeficiencies. Hence, melatonin may help in fighting viral and bacterial infections (Maestroni, 2001). Small quantities of melatonin are synthesised in human lymph cells and the hormone is therefore thought to be involved in clonal expression of antigen-stimulated T-lymphocytes. Taken in conjunction with calcium, melatonin acts as an immunostimulant. Its production is elevated in patients with rheumatoid arthritis compared to age-matched healthy controls (Cutolo and Maestroni, 2005). Its reduction in nocturnal shift workers has been linked to various disorders including cancer and cardiovascular disease (Schernhammer *et al.*, 2003).

Melatonin has demonstrated positive effects in the treatment of certain insomnias. It is the standard treatment for "delayed sleep phase syndrome" and has been used for reducing subjective symptoms of seasonal affective disorder, a depressive condition linked to the long hours of winter darkness. Its primary use as a dietary supplement is for improving the quality of sleep from which incidental benefits to health and well-being may accumulate. As sleep disruption suppresses the immune system, melatonin is also taken by advocates due to its stimulation of immune function. Typically, supplements are sold as 3-mg or 5-mg pills although a smaller dose of 0.3 mg has been reported to be equally effective and large doses of around 20 mg may be counterproductive (Lewy *et al.*, 2002).

23.4 Exercise and the melatonin rhythm

Since noradrenaline suppresses the synthesis of melatonin, the same effect might be associated with exercise. The lowering effect on melatonin was reported by Montelone *et al.* (1990) when exercise was conducted at 22:40 to 23:00 hours and its difference from control values lasted three hours post-exercise. Later, the same group (Montelone *et al.*, 1992a) reported an implied role for cortisol secretion with increases in plasma levels of this hormone preceding a night time blunting of melatonin secretion. Further, night time melatonin concentrations were unaffected when earlier depressed by bright light (Montelone *et al.*, 1992b). These findings conflict with reported increases in melatonin when exercise was conducted during the day. Carr (1981) found an increase of 100–200 per cent in melatonin levels for exercise performed between 13:00 and 18:00 hours for 60 min. Values were restored to baseline 30 min post-exercise. Similar phenomena were reported for males exercising between 09:00 and 13:00 hours (Theron *et al.*, 1984) and the increase due to exercise was accentuated when activity was conducted in a room darkened to 54 lux. These conflicting results have been attributed to confounding effects of various factors that include light, exercise intensity, habitual activity, age and sex (Atkinson *et al.*, 2003).

The exercise intensity may itself be important. Low levels of exercise for three hours at 40–60 per cent VO_{2max} had no effect whereas intense exercise at 75 per cent VO_{2max} acutely increased melatonin concentrations. Whatever the conflicting findings on the normal circadian rhythm in melatonin, the transient nature of the effect is consistent across studies. What is less clear is whether there are long-term effects as a result of training repeatedly at a particular time of day. Considering the Tour of Spain cycling race that lasts more than three weeks, Lucia *et al.* (2001) reported a progressive decline in circulating 6-sulphatoxymelatonin, a metabolite of melatonin, but an increase in the evening compared to baseline pre-tour values.

23.5   Melatonin and thermoregulation

Apart from its widespread effects in the body, the main consequences of administering exogenous melatonin are on the nervous, thermoregulatory and circadian systems. The effects are manifested in increased sleepiness, hypothermia and correction of circadian disturbances. These areas have a potential impact on exercise performance, the first two of which are covered in this section. The role of melatonin as a chronobiotic is covered separately.

Melatonin induces drowsiness for about two to four hours after ingestion. Following daytime ingestion of melatonin capsules, individuals are advised against driving a car, operating machinery or performing other tasks that would place themselves or others at risk. Subjective fatigue increases and so melatonin is not recommended during the daytime before strenuous exercise or competitive sport. If ingested late in the evening to aid sleep, there are no hangover effects the next morning. Atkinson *et al.* (2001) found no impairment in psychomotor tasks at 08:00 hours the morning after subjects took a 3-mg melatonin tablet prior to retiring to sleep at midnight.

The soporific effects of melatonin are evident in short-term performance as well as subjective states. Impairments have included slowed reaction time (Lieberman *et al.*, 1984), decreased alertness and increased errors in a vigilance task (Dollins *et al.*, 1993) and reduced cognitive performance (Slotten and Krekling, 1997). Fraschini *et al.* (1999) reported that balance and proprioception were adversely affected after administration of 10 mg of melatonin. Similarly, ingestion of 5 mg of melatonin at 11:45 hours caused impairments in performance tests when administered between 13:00 and again at 17:00 hours (Atkinson *et al.*, 2003). These measures included subjective alertness, choice reaction time, short-term memory and decreased heart rate responses to a 4-km cycling time trial, with a trend towards a decrement in pace over the 4 km. Elsewhere, Rogers *et al.* (1997) found that a deleterious effect of melatonin on reaction time was restricted to visual but not auditory stimuli. This finding may be linked with other reports of no effect of the hormone on short-term memory, possibly due to the acoustical coding inherent in memory tasks. Among mental performance tasks, short-term memory appears unique in resisting sleep deprivation as well as melatonin administration (Reilly and Deykin, 1983).

The anatomical co-location of control centres for melatonin production and thermoregulation, the neural connections between the pineal gland and the pre-optic area of the hypothalamus, and the presence of melatonin receptors in the hypothalamus provide a basis for a relationship between body temperature regulation and melatonin. The circadian rhythm in melatonin production is related inversely to that of core temperature, with the downturn of the former at dawn closely coincident with the upturn of the latter. The relationship is not wholly causal since other factors are implicated in the rhythm of core temperature, about 25 per cent of the variation being common with metabolism (Reilly and Brooks, 1982). Hypothermic effects of exogenous melatonin have been extensively reported, reductions in core temperature ranging from 0.01°C to 0.30°C (Atkinson et al., 2003). Cagnacci et al. (1994) reported that exogenous melatonin restored the night time decline in core temperature after a B_1-adrenergic antagonist, atenolol, had suppressed it. It seems that small concentrations of melatonin can exert a maximal thermoregulatory effect, suggesting that effects of melatonin are related to a physiological threshold rather than a dose-response relationship. Central control mechanisms as well as peripheral signals from smooth muscle may be involved.

Melatonin increases peripheral blood flow, thereby increasing heat loss. This effect could be ergogenic when endurance exercise is conducted in hot conditions and performance is limited by a critical core temperature value. An increase in heat loss would delay hyperthermic fatigue and the time to reach this critical core temperature (Reilly et al., 2006). Atkinson et al. (2005) showed that performance of a cycling task was improved as a consequence of ingesting melatonin, due to retarding the rises in core temperature. Whether this ergogenic effect would overcome the negative influence of increased subjective fatigue caused by melatonin has not been explored in a competitive sport context.

Age and sex appear to mediate the hypothermic effects of melatonin. Cagnacci et al. (1995) found a blunted effect of exogenous melatonin on body temperature in older (54–62 years) compared to young (22–32 years) women despite similar serum melatonin levels in the two groups. Additionally, the phase of the menstrual cycle has been found to have a mediating effect. Following melatonin administration, the normal elevation of about 0.5°C during the luteal phase is still evident whereas the hypothermic effect is observed during the follicular phase (Cagnacci et al., 1997). This relative resistance to melatonin during the luteal phase has been attributed to either an inhibitory effect of progesterone on the actions of melatonin or an increase in its thermogenic properties (Cagnacci et al., 1996).

Apart from the favourable hypothermic effects of exogenous melatonin, other mechanisms may benefit endurance performance. A slow start due to drowsiness may be offset later by an increase in pace as the effects of ingested melatonin wear off. Such effects are possible in events of long duration, probably two hours or more; the beneficial effect of a lowered body temperature on the later stages of a prolonged exercise protocol have been demonstrated in a diurnal context

(Reilly and Garrett, 1995). Similarly, a glycogen-sparing effect of exogenous melatonin has been found (Mazepa *et al.*, 1999). A promotion of lipids as metabolic fuel during exercise would delay the onset of fatigue due to depleted glycogen stores in active muscles.

23.6   Melatonin and jet-lag

Jet-lag refers to a cluster of symptoms experienced after travelling across multiple meridians. The syndrome includes an inability to sleep at the right time, difficulty in concentrating, a feeling of disorientation and demotivation, and bowel irregularities (see Table 23.2). One symptom reliably associated with jet-lag is fatigue, but the perceived importance of the other symptoms depends upon the time of assessment. The amount of jet-lag is associated in the early morning with the poorer sleep the night before; during the daytime, there is decreased concentration and motivation; in the evening, someone with jet-lag does not feel ready for sleep (Waterhouse *et al.*, 2005). Symptoms of jet-lag are more marked after a flight to the east than to the west, and they increase in severity and duration with the number of time zones crossed.

The malaise of jet-lag results from desynchronised circadian rhythms while "body clock" time is out of harmony with local time in the new environment. Crossing one or two time zones presents no major problem for athletes but flying across three or more time zones leads to perceptible feelings of jet-lag (Reilly *et al.*, 2005; Waterhouse *et al.*, 2007). Symptoms regress as the body clock adjusts to the new time zone. During the period when the body clock adjusts to the new time zone, exercise performance may be adversely affected (Waterhouse *et al.*, 1997). Guidelines have been recommended to help accelerate the recovery processes and to ameliorate the adverse effects of jet-lag. These recommendations have incorporated position statements on behalf of the European College of Sport Science (Reilly *et al.*, 2007a) and the British Olympic Association (Reilly *et al.*, 1998). They take into account the direction of travel, number of meridians crossed, times of departure and arrival and the times to impending sports engagements.

Table 23.2 Common symptoms of jet-lag

Difficulty in sleeping at the correct time
Transient fatigue during the day
Lack of concentration
Poor motivation
Gastrointestinal disturbances
Temporary loss of appetite
Feelings of disorientation or "head-buzz"
Impaired mental and physical performance

Athletes at all levels of achievement show altered performance in the days after long-haul flights (Reilly and Waterhouse, 2005). This decrement is because aspects of physical performance retain a parallelism with body temperature and other markers of the body clock, which are inappropriately timed for the destination. Any decrement will be most marked if a sports event is held at a time corresponding to night time in the time zone just left. Mental performance and mood also deteriorate after a time-zone transition (Waterhouse et al., 2001). This deterioration is partly due to the inappropriate timing of the body temperature rhythm but there is the additional problem that performance is worse after poor sleep (due to the unadjusted temperature rhythm). This "double negative" effect (performance after sleep loss and too near to the trough of the temperature rhythm) can cause a substantial decrement in performance.

The subjective symptoms of jet-lag disappear, as do objective measurements of poorer sleep and performance, as the body clock adjusts to the new time zone. Therefore, there is an obvious premium on promoting this adjustment. Appropriate timing of exposure to light or light avoidance in the new time zone is required— this is the "behavioural" approach—and any trip should be planned to arrive a number of days before any important event, in order to accelerate this adjustment (see Table 23.3). Attempts can also be made to ameliorate the symptoms of jet-lag by using drugs including melatonin—this is the "pharmacological" approach. Even following the advice below, individuals will find that adjustment takes about one day per time zone crossed after an eastward transition, and slightly less after westward transitions.

Because the body clock is slow to change its phase, for sojourns of only a few days in a new time zone before returning home, adjustment is not possible. In these cases, the traveller is advised to time appointments in the new time zone to coincide with daytime, and to avoid times that coincide with night, on home time (Lowden and Akerstedt, 1998). In practice, after an eastward flight, the new afternoon is preferable to the new morning, and after westward flights, the new morning is preferable to the late afternoon and evening. Where adjustment to the new time zone can be achieved (sojourns lasting for several days), it is possible to give advice regarding the pre-flight days and the flight itself (Waterhouse et al., 2007). The guidelines offer specific advice according to direction of travel, times of departure and arrival and behaviour in the days following disembarkation. Other environmental aspects that might include altitude, heat and pollution can be included where appropriate.

A scheme for determining whether adjustment is necessary is required. For football teams participating in matches mid-week in Europe, for example, it may be possible to maintain a routine in tune with the normal circadian rhythm. In the case of travelling westward, a phase delay of the body clock is required, compared to a phase advance needed after travelling eastwards. Travel strategies encourage the use of either behavioural measures or pharmacological agents to help readjustment. Putative chronobiotic drugs include benzodiazepines, melatonin agonists (e.g. tasimelteon) and melatonin or central nervous stimulants,

Table 23.3 Bad and good times in local time for exposure to light after time-zone transitions to the east and west: a denotes promotion of a phase advance, b indicates a phase delay is promoted and c reflects that the body clock adjusts more easily to large phase delays than to large advances

Time zones to the east	Bad times for light exposure	Good times for light exposure
3	24:00–06:00[b]	08:00–14:00[a]
4	01:00–07:00[b]	09:00–15:00[a]
5	02:00–08:00[b]	10:00–16:00[a]
6	03:00–09:00[b]	11:00–17:00[a]
7	04:00–10:00[b]	12:00–18:00[a]
8	05:00–11:00[b]	13:00–19:00[a]
9	06:00–12:00[b]	14:00–20:00[a]
10	Can be treated as 14 hours to the west[c]	
11	Can be treated as 14 hours to the west[c]	
12	Can be treated as 14 hours to the west[c]	
Time zones to the west		
3	02:00–08:00[a]	18:00–24:00[b]
4	01:00–07:00[a]	17:00–23:00[b]
5	24:00–06:00[a]	16:00–22:00[b]
6	23:00–05:00[a]	15:00–21:00[b]
7	22:00–04:00[a]	14:00–20:00[b]
8	21:00–03:00[a]	13:00–19:00[b]
9	20:00–02:00[a]	12:00–18:00[b]
10	19:00–01:00[a]	11:00–17:00[b]
11	18:00–24:00[a]	10:00–16:00[b]
12	17:00–23:00[a]	09:00–15:00[b]

such as modafinil (which is on the list banned by WADA, the World Anti-Doping Agency) or caffeine. In general, the behavioural approach is favoured for athletes (Reilly *et al.*, 2005). It involves attending to lifestyle factors that include nutrition (Reilly *et al.*, 2007b) and the timing and intensity of training. In planning for international competition, it is clear that the hassles of travel must be accommodated in the preparations.

Melatonin has demonstrated positive effects in readjusting the body clock and in reducing the effects of jet-lag. It has been applied to help shift workers adjust to nocturnal shifts and to travellers cross multiple time zones (Arendt and Skeene, 2005). It has been administered to professional football players, along with behavioural measures, when travelling between Argentina and Japan (Cardinali *et al.*, 2002). In this instance, the light-dark cycle on board the aircraft was also manipulated in an approach that combined behaviour and drug treatment. The complete adjustment claimed by the authors has not been replicated in other studies where temazepam (Reilly *et al.*, 2001) and melatonin (Edwards *et al.*, 2000) have been used as putative chronobiotics (see Figure 23.1).

The frequent use of melatonin by athletes was acknowledged by the British Olympic Association (Reilly *et al.*, 1998); although not advocating either sleeping pills or melatonin as part of their travel strategy, the authors advised athletes who intended to use melatonin that only those with confidence from previous positive experiences with the compound should use it. In their study of travellers between the United Kingdom and Australia, Edwards *et al.* (2000) found that the rate of adjustment to the 10-hour phase shift and the severity of jet-lag did not differ between those using melatonin and those in a placebo group. Melatonin has also been used in combination with slow-release caffeine, a central nervous system stimulant, in a study of an eastward-bound flight across seven time zones (Lagarde *et al.*, 2001). Effects on performance were variable and while satisfactory levels of capability were maintained in the experimental subjects, this positive effect was evident only in grip strength of the dominant hand. In a follow-up report from the same group, caffeine had unwanted effects on recovery sleep (Beaumont *et al.*, 2004). The authors concluded that both drugs may have value in alleviating some symptoms related to jet-lag.

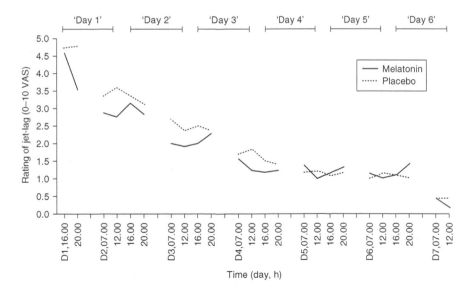

Figure 23.1 Melatonin had no significant effect in accelerating adjustment of the body clock in a long-haul flight by athletes across 10 time zones (data are from Edwards *et al.*, 2000).

23.7   Alternatives to melatonin: the benzodiazepines

The chronobiotic and soporific effects of melatonin are not disputed. The drugs known as benzodiazepines have a longer history as sleeping pills, the first drug to be produced in the mid-1950s. The best-known drugs were librium (chlordiazepoxide hydrochloride), introduced in the USA in 1960, and valium (diazepam), introduced in 1963. The benzodiazepines replaced barbiturates and propranediol derivatives as the drugs of clinical choice in treating stress and anxiety as the latter had a high rate of addiction.

Phenobarbitol is a 5-ethyl-5-phenyl substituted barbituric acid, first marketed in the USA in 1912 and the oldest of the currently available drugs for treating epilepsy. It enhances γ-aminobutyric acid (GABA) transmission by interacting with the $GABA_A$ receptor-chloride channel complex and it acts at glutamate receptors to decrease excitatory synaptic transmission. It is no longer a first-line treatment for epilepsy; nine new antiepileptic drugs have been approved in the USA since 1993. There is little evidence that the barbiturates had a major use amongst active athletes as an ergogenic aid in the years when they were being widely prescribed, although they may have been used more recently.

Benzodiazepines are widely employed as tranquillizers in the population at large and have been used for calming and anti-anxiety purposes in sports. They are listed among the drugs that may be taken by sports competitors. Now, more than two dozen benzodiazepine drugs form over 90 per cent of the tranquillizer market. More than 20 doses of these drugs per head of the US population are prescribed annually, giving an idea of the vast scale of consumption. Both barbiturates and benzodiazepines are among the top 10 of so-called street drugs used for leisure purposes. Benzodiazepines were celebrated as an antidote to stress by the Rolling Stones in 1966, in their song "Mother's Little Helper". Prescriptions for benzodiazepines peaked in the UK in 1979 before problems with addiction and withdrawal became evident. Withdrawal symptoms include anxiety, depression, diarrhoea, headache, insomnia, irritability, muscle and bone pain and vomiting. Benzodiazepines may be lethal when mixed with alcohol and methadone. They have been replaced in part by the so-called non-benzodiazepines.

Benzodiazepines decrease stress response indices, such as skin conductance and plasma corticosterone levels. They reduce anxiety in psychiatric and nonpsychiatric patients and demonstrate a superiority over barbiturates in clinical conditions. Their over-prescription has led to some patients being on long-term use and experiencing severe withdrawal symptoms when abruptly taken off them. The drugs affect various neurotransmitters, the cholinergic and serotonergic effects having importance in reducing the stress response.

The main anti-anxiety action of benzodiazepines seems to stem from the reduction in serotonergic activity, which the drugs produce. Serotonergic neurones are important in the experience of anxiety so this feeling is attenuated by the drugs. The effects of benzodiazepines on serotonergic neurones may be mediated by a primary action of the drugs on GABA. The GABA-releasing neurones are primarily inhibitory and it is possible that, when these are stimulated by the benzodiazepines, the release of serotonin is inhibited. The GABA system is recognized as playing a crucial role in anxiety: some anxiety-related states may be due to diminished transmission at the GABA receptors, which are functionally linked to benzodiazepine recognition sites (Corda *et al.*, 1986).

The benzodiazepines decrease the turnover in hemispheric cholinergic neurones by blocking the release of acetylcholine. By lowering the activity in cholinergic pathways, the drugs should have an adverse effect on human performance. Deterioration in detecting sensory signals and in reaction time in a rapid information-processing task with nightly doses of flurazepam and temazepam have been found the morning after taking the drugs (Figure 23.2). The carry-over effects are due to the long half-lives of these particular drugs. Other types of performance affected include the rate of tapping, motor manipulation and complex coordination tasks, as well as real and simulated driving.

The function of one particular cholinergic pathway is to trigger the release of corticotrophic-releasing factor from the hypothalamus into the pituitary blood vessels and to produce a spurt of adrenocorticotrophic hormone (ACTH) from the anterior pituitary. The benzodiazepines lower the emission of corticosteroid hormones from the adrenal cortex by affecting the ACTH release as a result of blocking cholinergic activity.

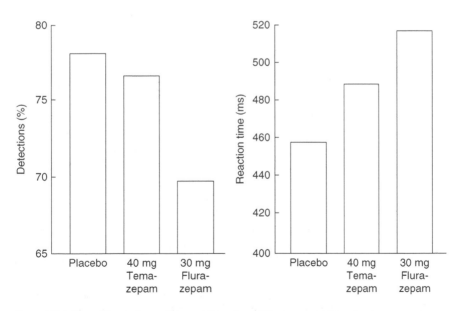

Figure 23.2 The effects of temazepam (40 mg) and flurazepam (30 mg) on correct detections and reaction time in a rapid information-processing task. The tasks were performed the morning after nightly administration of the drugs (from Wesnes and Warburton, 1983, with permission of John Wiley and Son Ltd.).

The benzodiazepines decelerate the turnover of noradrenaline. This effect is more apparent in conditions where noradrenaline levels have been increased by stress. This change is not the basis of the drug's anti-anxiety action, as repeated dosing with oxazepam results in a rapid tolerance to the decrease in noradrenaline turnover, whilst the drug maintains its anti-anxiety properties (Wesnes and Warburton, 1983). Similarly, dopamine turnover is retarded by benzodiazepines, but this effect is unrelated to the drugs' anti-anxiety properties.

Effects of benzodiazepines on human performance depend on the dosage and on the particular drug. Oxazepam, diazepam, nitrazepam, flurazepam and chlordiazepoxide are all 1,4-derivatives. Clobazam, a 1, 5-benzodiazepine derivative, does not seem to impair psychomotor performance but does retain its anti-anxiety properties (Wesnes and Warburton, 1983) and so may have more applications than the others in sport and exercise contexts.

Following the bans on alcohol overuse in the modern pentathlon, athletes at the 1972 Olympic Games in Munich were found to have used benzodiazepines and other tranquillizers, such as meprobamate, as anti-anxiety agents. Benzodiazepines are currently banned in the modern pentathlon though are not on the list banned by WADA. They were thought preferable to alcohol as they might reduce anxiety without the potential adverse effects on judgement and coordination associated with alcohol. Meprobamate acts as a mild tranquillizer without producing drowsiness. It is highly addictive and reduces tolerance to alcohol. The benzodiazepines are relatively safe in that they have low toxicity and few side effects apart from the dependence apparent upon withdrawal. Overdosing is a danger when benzodiazepines are combined with other central nervous system depressants, such as alcohol.

One of the primary effects of the GABA-mediated reaction to benzodiazepines is that the drugs act as muscle relaxants. They can therefore benefit recovery from muscle spasm and spastic-type muscle injuries. The effect is associated with feelings of relaxation and freedom from "nerves". The drugs cause drowsiness and could impair cognitive as well as muscle function in both submaximal and extreme efforts. Spontaneous activity of animals is reduced under the influence of these drugs. Cabri et al. (1988) demonstrated that the effects of alprazolam were dependent on the dose. Maximal torque on an isokinetic dynamometer was unaffected by a low dose (0.5 mg). Moderate doses of the drug (1.5 and 3.0 mg) reduced muscle performance during brief bouts of maximal effort, both 90 and 360 minutes after ingestion. The amplitude of the integrated electromyogram decreased, but the effect was reduced after 360 minutes. It was thought that GABA-ergic activity induced alterations both in central nervous system and in peripheral (neuromuscular) receptor sites for benzodiazepines.

Different benzodiazepines vary in their pharmacokinetic profiles and so their influence on muscle performance may also be variable. For this reason, Zinzen et al. (1994) compared the effects of therapeutic doses of flunitrazepam (plasma half-life of 31 hours) and triazolam (half-life of 8 hours) on performance, utilizing an isokinetic dynamometer. (Triazolam is banned from prescription in the

UK and in other European countries due to its potential for dependence.) No hangover effects were noted after eight hours of sleep with triazolam; in contrast, flunitrazepam was shown to impair muscle force production after the night's sleep, with subjects reporting a "sleepy impression" throughout the following day. Various stimulants, including caffeine, may offset the depressant effects of benzodiazepines on psychomotor skills. Caffeine interacts with the GABA-benzodiazepine system and so may reverse some adverse effects of these tranquillizers. Collomp *et al.* (1993) showed that moderate benzodiazepine intake (1 mg lorazepam) impaired performance on an all-out exercise test over 30 sec. Moderate caffeine intake (250 mg caffeine in combination with 1 mg lorazepam) antagonized the metabolic but not the performance effects of the tranquillizer.

The effects of benzodiazepines on sustained exercise performance are poorly documented. In a resting normal human, coronary blood flow is increased by 22.5 per cent by diazepam but more so (73 per cent) in persons with coronary artery disease. Whether the drugs are of benefit in the treatment of angina associated with effort is unknown (Powles, 1981). The benzodiazepines have been used for decades in the treatment of epilepsy.

Barbiturates and sedatives have long been used as sleeping pills. Such a use, to facilitate the sleep of athletes the night before competition, may be counterproductive because of a residual de-arousing effect the following day (Figure 23.2). The "hangover" effect of benzodiazepines was found to be greater for flurazepam (30 mg) than for temazepam (40 mg). Although the former produced better sleep, it resulted in less clearheadedness on waking and impaired performance on a rapid visual information-processing task (Wesnes and Warburton, 1984).

The "hangover" effect of sleeping tablets, including benzodiazepines, is likely to disturb complex skills more than simple motor tasks the following morning, and, depending on the sport, an increase in errors may increase injury risk. Alcohol can compound the adverse effects of other drugs on motor performance tasks (Kunsman *et al.*, 1992). Attention and reaction time tasks are impaired by a combination of temazepam and ethanol in doses that may be harmless when each is given alone. Subjects tend to be unaware of their reduced performance capabilities when taking these drugs in combination. There are likely to be increases also in injury risk. Of 402 victims of ski accidents, 20 per cent were positive for alcohol, 8.5 per cent for benzodiazepines and 2.5 per cent for both drugs together. Subjects positive for both tended to be older than the other persons examined (Barnas *et al.*, 1992).

Benzodiazepines were thought to help in adjusting circadian rhythms following time-zone transitions because of their promotion of sleep. Reilly *et al.* (2001) found temazepam had no effect in combating jet-lag in British athletes travelling over five time zones to the USA. There was no effect on the rate of adjustment to the new time zone, either in core temperature, performance measures or subjective symptoms. The ease of sleeping following travelling westwards and arriving in the evening local time probably rendered any sleep elixir superfluous in these circumstances. Low doses of benzodiazepines may benefit shift workers who have difficulty in sleeping during the day after a nocturnal shift. Wesnes and Warburton (1986) found that 10- to 20-mg doses of temazepam helped daytime sleep without detrimental residual effects on subsequent information processing during simulated shift work.

The circadian or 24-hour rhythm in arousal may have implications for the pharmacological effects of anti-anxiety drugs. The optimum dosage of drugs affecting the nervous system differs with the time of day at which they are administered. The barbiturate dose that is safe in the evening may have exaggerated effects the following morning. Benzodiazepine receptor binding also displays a circadian phase-dependent effect (Lemmer, 2007). The diurnal variation in responses to benzodiazepines and the implications this has for the dosage at different times of day for effective pre-contest tranquillization have not been thoroughly investigated.

The evolution of new benzodiazepines has been focused on reducing the half-life of drugs and thereby eliminating hangover effects (see Table 23.4). Effort has also been directed towards drugs that are anxiolytic without producing daytime sedation. The newer generation of related drugs include the non-benzodiazepines, differing in chemical structure from the benzodiazepines and from one another, and melatonin agonists.

The so-called non-benzodiazepines refer to benzodiazepine derivatives that bind more selectively to BZ1 receptors, which mediate sedation and have fewer side effects. They are now extensively used in the treatment of sleep disorders, the most important effects being to shorten sleep latency and reduce nocturnal awakenings. The drugs in this class include eszopiclone and the Z drugs: zaleplon, zolpidem and zopiclone (Terzano et al., 2008). They interfere less with homeostatic processes in the sleep-wake cycle and since 2000 have increased

Table 23.4 Sedative drugs and their elimination half-lives (hours)

Anxiolytic benzodiazepines:	Oxazepam	6–12
	Lorazepam	10–20
	Diazepam	30–60
Long-acting benzodiazepines:	Flunitrazepam	10–31
	Flurazepam	40–100
	Nitrazepam	25–35
Medium-acting benzodiazepines:	Lormetazepam	10–15
	Loprazolam	8–12
	Temazepam	10–15
Short-acting benzodiazepines:	Brotizolam	3–7
	Midazolam	1.5–2.5
	Triazolam	1.5–8
Non-benzodiazepines:	Zaleplon	1–1.5
	Zolpidem	1.5 to 2–4
	Zopiclone	4–6
Melatonin agonists:	Ramelteon	1.4
	Melatonin	1–2

prescription rates throughout the world at the expense of the classical benzodiazepines (Lemmer, 2007). Whereas diazepam and flunitrazepam bind to all subtypes of benzodiazepine receptor sites (BZ1–BZ3), non-benzodiazepines like zolpidem and zopiclone have an affinity for subtype BZ1. Zolpidem was shown to reduce the impairments in performance and mood disturbances due to shift work (Hart et al., 2003). Lemmer (2007) concluded that benzodiazepine receptor antagonists should not be used in addressing problems due to nocturnal shift work. Zopiclone has been reported to ease jet-lag, causing less fragmented sleep than a placebo on the first night after flying across five time zones (Daurat et al., 2000). Zolpidem and zopiclone act rapidly and do not affect short-term memory as does a classical benzodiazepine such as flunitrazepam. Nevertheless cognitive effects are likely, leading Lemmer (2007) to conclude that the air-cabin crew should never take sleeping pills to avoid impairment in cognitive function and reactivity to task demands. There is some evidence that diazepam and zolpidem reduce body temperature (Mailliet et al., 2001) but this effect has not been examined during exercise as it has for melatonin (Atkinson et al., 2003).

Melatonin agonists also have potential circadian phase-shifting properties. Tasimelteon (VEC 160) is a novel melatonin agonist developed for treatment of chronic insomnia and circadian sleep disorders (Doghranji, 2007). Its positive effects in shifting the circadian rhythm in melatonin has promoted its use in nocturnal shift work and travelling across multiple meridians (Rajaratnam et al., 2009). It is thought to have low potential for addiction and abuse and has minimal side effects. Its consequences for exercise performance and maintenance of training programmes are unknown.

Ramelteon also acts by mimicking the effects of melatonin. It combines with and activates melatonin's MT1 and MT2 receptors. Like melatonin, it does not interact with receptors for γ-aminobutyric acid or other neurotransmitters and does not seem to lead to substance abuse. There is, however, some evidence of residual effects the next day in insomniac patients using ramelteon (Wurtman, 2008) and it may therefore be inappropriate for athletes prior to competition.

23.8   Overview

Anxiety is common among athletes, most notably before competition. The anxiety may manifest as difficulty in sleeping, a good night's sleep being important for optimal exercise performance. A variety of anxiolytic measures may be called upon, including the use of pharmacological agents. Among these are melatonin, benzodiazepines, non-benzodiazepines and melatonin agonists.

Melatonin plays a central role in the regulation of the sleep-wake cycle. Synthetic analogues are available to the public in the USA but not in the European Union except by prescription. It has been used for a variety of nonspecific effects, including relaxation and health-related motives. It has been prescribed for correcting sleep disorders, to help shift workers adjust to nocturnal work and to travellers who cope with jet-lag.

Benzodiazepines replaced barbiturates as sleeping pills due to their lower toxicity and less addictiveness. Dependence and a rebound effect are evident if subjects are withdrawn rapidly from their use. The non-benzodiazepines act rapidly, have less hangover effects and have increased in prescription compared to the classic benzodiazepines. These drugs induce a pharmacological rather than a true physiological sleep. Although these hypnotic drugs have been advocated for correcting circadian rhythm disruptions associated with nocturnal shift work and travelling across multiple meridians, melatonin and the non-benzodiazepines seem to provide the best pharmacological option. Nevertheless, there is no convincing evidence that they are superior to a behavioural approach to combat jet-lag.

23.9   References

Arendt, J. and Skeene, D. (2005). Melatonin as a chronobiotic. *Sleep Medicine Reviews* **9**, 25–39.

Atkinson, G., Buckley, P., Edwards B., *et al.* (2001). Are there hangover effects on physical performance when melatonin is ingested by athletes before nocturnal sleep? *International Journal of Sports Medicine* **22**, 232–234.

Atkinson, G., Drust, B., Reilly, T. *et al.* (2003). The relevance of melatonin to sports medicine and science. *Sports Medicine* **33**, 808–831.

Atkinson, G., Holder, A., Robertson, C. *et al.* (2005). Effects of melatonin on the thermoregulatory responses to intermittent exercise. *Journal of Pineal Research* **39**, 353–359.

Barnas, L., Miller, G. H., Sperner, G. *et al.* (1992). The effects of alcohol and benzodiazepines on the severity of ski accidents. *Acta Psychiatrica Scandinavica* **86**, 296–300.

Bartsch, C., Bartsch, H. and Peschke, E. (2009) Light, melatonin and cancer: Current results and future perspectives. *Biological Rhythm Research* **40(1)**, 17–35.

Beaumont, M., Batejat, D. and Van Beers, P. (2004). Caffeine or melatonin effects on sleep and sleepiness after rapid eastward transmeridian flight. *Journal of Applied Physiology* **96**, 50–58.

Cabri, J., Clarys, J.P., DeWitte, B. *et al.* (1988). Circadian variation in blood pressure responses to muscular exercise. *Ergonomics* **31**, 1559–1566.

Cagnacci, A., Arangino, S., Angiolucci, M. *et al.* (1997). Potentially beneficial cardiovascular effects of melatonin administration in women. *Journal of Pineal Research* **22**, 16–19.

Cagnacci, A., Soldani, R., Laughlin, G.A. *et al.* (1996). Modification of circadian body temperature rhythm during the luteal phase: Role of melatonin. *Journal of Applied Physiology* **80**, 25–29.

Cagnacci, A., Soldani, R., Romagnolo, C. *et al.* (1994). Melatonin-induced decrease in body temperature in women: A threshold event. *Neuroendocrinology* **60**, 549–552.

Cagnacci, A., Soldani, R. and Yen, S.S.C. (1995). Hypothermic effect of melatonin and nocturnal core body temperature decline are reduced in aged women. *Journal of Applied Physiology* **78**, 314–317.

Cardinali, D.P., Bortman, G.P., Liotta, G. *et al.* (2002). A multifactorial approach employing melatonin to accelerate re-synchronisation of sleep-wake cycle after a 12 time-zone westerly transmeridian flight in elite soccer athletes. *Journal of Pineal Research* **32**, 41–46.

Carr, D.B. (1981). Plasma melatonin increase in women. *Journal of Clinical Endocrinology and Metabolism* **53**, 224–225.

Collomp, K.R., Ahmaidi, S.B., Caillaud, C.F. *et al.* (1993). Effects of benzodiazepine during a Wingate test: Interaction with caffeine. *Medicine and Science in Sports and Exercise* **25**, 1375–1380.

Corda, M.G., Concas, A. and Biggio, G. (1986). Stress and CABA receptors. In *Biochemical aspects of physical exercise*, ed G. Benzie, L. Packer and N. Siliprandi. Elsevier, Amsterdam. 399–409.

Cutolo, M. and Maestroni, G.J. (2005). The melatonin-cytokine connection in rheumatoid arthritis. *Annals of Rheumatic Diseases* **64**, 1109–1111.

Daurat, A., Benoit, O. and Buguet, A. (2000). Effects of zopiclone on the rest/activity rhythm after a westward flight across five time zones. *Psychopharmacology* **149**, 241–245.

Doghranji, K. (2007). Melatonin and its receptors: A new class of sleep promoting agents. *Journal of Clinical and Sleep Medicine* **3**, S17–S23.

Dollins, A.B., Lynch, H.J., Wurtman, R.J. *et al.* (1993). Effect of pharmacological daytime doses of melatonin on human mood and performance. *Psychopharmacology* **11**, 490–496.

Edwards, B. J., Atkinson, G., Waterhouse, J. *et al.* (2000). Use of melatonin in recovery from jet-lag following an eastward flight across 10 time-zones. *Ergonomics* **43**, 1501–1513.

Forsyth, J.J. and Reilly, T. (2005). The combined effect of time of day and menstrual cycle on lactate threshold. *Medicine and Science in Sports and Exercise* **37**, 2046–2053.

Fraschini, F., Cesarani, A., Alpini, D. *et al.* (1999). Melatonin influences human balance. *Biological Signals Reception* **8**, 111–119.

Hart, C.L., Ward, A.S., Haney, M. *et al.* (2003). Zolpidem-related effects on performance and mood during simulated night-shift work. *Experimental and Clinical Pharmacology* **11**, 259–268.

Kunsman, G.W., Manno, J.B., Przekop, M.A. *et al.* (1992). The effects of temazepam and ethanol on human psychomotor performance. *European Journal of Clinical Pharmacology* **43**, 603–611.

Lagarde, D., Chappuis, B., Billaud, P.F. *et al.* (2001). Evaluation of pharmacological aids on physical performance after a transmeridian flight. *Medicine and Science in Sports and Exercise* **33**, 628–634.

Lemmer, B. (2007). The sleep-wake cycle and sleeping pills. *Physiology and Behavior* **90**, 285–293.

Lewy, A., Emens, J.S., Sack, R.L. *et al.* (2002). Low, but not high, doses of melatonin entrained a free-running blind person with a long circadian period. *Chronobiology International* **19**, 649–658.

Lewy, A., Emens, J., Lefler, B. *et al.* (2005). Melatonin entrains free-running blind people according to a physiological dose-response curve. *Chronobiology International* **22**, 1093–1106.

Lieberman, H.R., Waldhauser, F., Garfield, G. *et al.* (1984). Effects of melatonin on human mood and performance. *Brain Research* **323**, 201–207.

Lowden, A. and Akerstedt, T. (1998). Retaining home-base sleep hours to prevent jet lag in connection with a westward flight across nine time zones. *Chronobiology International* **15**, 365–376.

Lucia, A., Diaz, B., Hoyos, J. *et al.* (2001). Hormone levels of world-class cyclists during the Tour of Spain stage race. *British Journal of Sports Medicine* **35**, 424–430.

Maestroni, G.J. (2001).The immunotherapeutic potential of melatonin. *Expert Opinion in Investigative Drugs* **10**, 467–476.

Mailliet, F., Galloux, P. and Poisson, D. (2001). Comparative effects of melatonin, zolpidem and diazepam on sleep, body temperature, blood pressure and heart rate measured by radio telemetry in Wistar rats. *Psychopharmacology* **156**, 417–426.

Mazepa, R.C., Cuevas, M.J., Collado, P.S. *et al.* (1999). Melatonin increases liver and muscle glycogen content in non-exercised and exercised rats. *Life Science* **66**, 153–160.

Montelone, P., Maj, M., Fusco, M. *et al.* (1990). Physical exercise at night blunts the nocturnal increase of plasma melatonin levels in healthy humans. *Life Science* **47**, 1989–1995.

Montelone, P., Fuschino, A., Nolfe, G. *et al.* (1992a). Temporal relationship between melatonin and cortisol responses to nighttime physical stress in humans. *Psychoendocrinology* **17**, 81–86.

Montelone, P., Maj, M., Fuschino, A. *et al.* (1992b). Physical stress in the middle of the dark phase does not affect light-depressed melatonin levels in humans. *Neuroendocrinology* **55**, 367–371.

Middleton, B., Arendt, J. and Stone, B. M. (1996). Human circadian rhythms in constant dim light (8 lux) with knowledge of clock time. *Journal of Sleep Research* **5(2)**, 69–76.

Peiser, B. (2009). Seasonal affective disorder and exercise treatment. *Biological Rhythm Research* **40(1)**, 85–97.

Powles, A.C.P. (1981). The effect of drugs on the cardiovascular response to exercise. *Medicine and Science in Sports and Exercise* **13**, 252–258.

Rajaratnam, S. M. W., Polymeropoulus, M. H., Fisher, D. M. *et al.* (2009). Melatonin agonist tasimelteon (VEC-162) for transient insomnia after sleep time shift, two randomised controlled multicentre trials. *Lancet*, **373**, 482–491. Available at http://www.thelancet.com/journals/lancet/article/PIIS0140-6736(08)61812-7/fulltext. (accessed 9 August 2010).

Reilly, T. and Brooks, G.A. (1982). Investigation of circadian rhythms in metabolic responses to exercise. *Ergonomics* **25**, 1093–1107.

Reilly, T. and Brooks, G.A. (1986). Exercise and the circadian variation in body temperature measures. *International Journal of Sports Medicine* **7**, 358–362.

Reilly, T. and Deykin, T. (1983). Effects of partial sleep loss on subjective states, psychomotor and physical performance tests. *Journal of Human Movement Studies* **9**, 157–170.

Reilly, T. and Garrett, R. (1995). The effects of time of day on self-paced performance of prolonged exercise. *Journal of Sports Medicine and Physical Fitness* **35**, 99–102.

Reilly, T. and Peiser, B. (2006). Seasonal variations in health-related human physical activity. *Sports Medicine* **36**, 473–485.

Reilly, T. and Waterhouse, J. (2005). *Sport, exercise and environmental physiology*. Elsevier, Edinburgh.

Reilly, T., Atkinson, G. and Budgett, R. (2001). Effect of low-dose temapzepam on physiological variables and performance tests following a westerly flight across five time-zones. *International Journal of Sports Medicine* **22**, 166–174.

Reilly, T., Drust, B. and Gregson, W. (2006). Thermoregulation in elite athletes. *Current Opinion in Clinical Nutrition and Metabolic Care* **9**, 666–671.

Reilly, T., Maughan, R. and Budgett, R. (1998). Melatonin: A position statement of the British Olympic Association. *British Journal of Sports Medicine* **32**, 99–100.

Reilly, T., Waterhouse, J. and Edwards, B. (2005). Jet lag and air travel: Implications for performance. *Clinics in Sports Medicine* **24**, 367–380.

Reilly, T., Atkinson, G., Edwards, B. *et al.* (2007a). Coping with jet-lag: A position statement for the European College of Sport Science. *European Journal of Sport Science* **7**, 1–7.

Reilly, T., Waterhouse, J., Burke, L. *et al.* (2007b). Nutrition for travel. *Journal of Sports Sciences* **25(Suppl. 1)**, S125–S134.

Rogers, N.L., Phan, O., Kennaway, D. *et al.* (1997). Effect of oral daytime melatonin administration on cognitive psychomotor performance in humans. *Sleep Research* **26**, 212.

Schernhammer, E.S., Laden, F., Speizer, F.E. *et al.* (2003). Night-shift-work and risk of colorectal cancer in the nurses' health study. *Journal of the National Cancer Institute* **95**, 825–828.

Slotten, H.A. and Krekling, S. (1997). Does melatonin have an effect on cognitive performance? *Psychoneuroendocrinology* **21**, 673–680.

Terzano, M.G., Milioli, G., De Paolis, F. *et al.* (2008). Z-drugs: Comparative tolerability. In *Sleep disorders, diagnosis and therapeutics*, ed. S.R. Pandi-Perumal, J.C. Verster, J.M. Monti, M. Lader and S.Z. Langer, Informa Healthcare, London. 364–378.

Theron, J.J., Oosthuizen, J.M.C. and Rautenbach, M.M. (1984). Effect of physical exercise on plasma melatonin levels in normal volunteers. *South African Medical Journal* **66**, 838–841.

Waterhouse, J., Minors, D., Akerstedt,T. *et al.* (2001). Rhythms of human performance. In *Handbook of behavioral neurobiology: Circadian clocks,* ed. J. Takahashi, F. Turek, R. Moore, Kluver Academic/Plenum, New York. 571–601.

Waterhouse, J., Nevill, A., Finnegan, J. *et al.* (2005). Further assessments of the relationship between jet lag and some of its symptoms. *Chronobiology International* **22**, 121–136.

Waterhouse, J., Reilly, T. and Atkinson, G. (1997). Jet-lag. *The Lancet* **350**, 1611–1616.

Waterhouse, J., Reilly, T., Atkinson, G. *et al.* (2007). Jet lag: Trends and coping strategies. *The Lancet* **369**, 1117–1129.

Wesnes, K. and Warburton, D.M. (1983). Stress and drugs. In *Stress and fatigue in human performance*, ed. R. Hockey, John Wiley, Chichester. 203–243.

Wesnes, K. and Warburton, D.M. (1984). A comparison of temazepam and flurazepam in terms of sleep quality and residual changes in performance. *Neuropsychobiology* **11**, 255–299.

Wesnes, K. and Warburton, D.M. (1986). Effects of temazepam on sleep quality and subsequent mental efficiency under normal sleeping conditions and following delayed sleep onset. *Neuropsychobiology* **15**, 187–191.

Wurtman, R.J. (2008). Ramelteon: A melatonin receptor agonist. In *Sleep disorders, diagnosis and therapeutics*, ed. S.R. Pandi-Perumal, J.C. Verster, J.M. Monti, M. Lader and S.Z. Langer, Informa Healthcare, London. 394–401.

Zinzen, E., Clarijs, J.P., Cabri, J. *et al.* (1994). The influence of triazolam and flunitrazepam on isokinetic and isometric muscle performance. *Ergonomics* **37**, 69–77.

Chapter 24

Hypoxic chambers and other artificial environments

David J. Armstrong

24.1   Introduction

Altitude training began after the 1968 Olympic Games in Mexico when athletes who lived at or trained at altitude were notably successful in endurance athletic events. Initially, limited availability of resources meant that the opportunity was only available to the elite athletes who had sufficient financial support. In order to broaden access and reduce the inconvenience inherent in prolonged sojourns to altitude training camps, sports scientists in Finland developed artificial hypoxic environments, which simulated high altitude. Most recently, the development of portable hypoxic tents and hypoxicators has opened access to athletes wishing to avail themselves of the technology. This poses questions to governing bodies about legitimacy, to end users about the risks to health and to the scientific community about their potential ergogenic value and indeed how that might be explained. This chapter will consider the development and range of artificial hypoxic environments, their ergogenic value, mode(s) of action, the ethics of their use and whether or not they constitute a risk to users' health.

24.2   Exercise at altitude

As altitude increases, the barometric pressure falls. At sea level the normal pressure is 760 mmHg; at 1000 m it is 680 mmHg; at 3000 m it is about 540 mmHg; and at the top of Mt. Everest (height 8848 m) it is 250 mmHg. So high-altitude conditions are referred to as low-pressure or hypobaric conditions.

The main problem associated with hypobaric environments is hypoxia. Although the proportion of oxygen in the air at any altitude is constant at 20.93 per cent, as ambient pressure decreases (with increase in altitude) the air is less dense. As a result there are fewer oxygen molecules in a given volume of air, and, if we were to inspire the same volume of air as at sea level, less oxygen would be inspired. Thus the uptake of oxygen into the body by the lungs is decreased and there is a decreased rate of oxygen delivery to the tissues where it is needed. However, the body is able to show some adaptive responses that compensate for the relative lack of oxygen in the air. Although these responses begin immediately on exposure to hypobaric conditions, for some people the full response is not manifested until weeks or months at altitude. However, even with complete acclimatization, the sea-level visitor to altitude is never as completely adapted as the individual born and bred at altitude. This becomes apparent with endurance sports events in particular.

The hypoxia of altitude is probably more widely recognised in mountaineering than in any other sporting activity. Mountaineers need to have very good aerobic fitness levels to climb the high peaks. The conventional practice has been to use oxygen to compensate for the reduced alveolar oxygen tension. In 1978, it was shown that Mt. Everest could be climbed without supplementary oxygen. This was possible with mountaineers who had a high VO_{2max}, were acclimatised and were favoured by the day-to-day variations in atmospheric pressure on the peak. At this level of altitude, prior acclimatization at medium altitude is essential. Nevertheless the ascents need to be planned so that the time above 6000 m is restricted to avoid inevitable high-altitude deterioration. Above an altitude of 5200 m (where the highest permanent settlement in the Andes is located) acclimatization is replaced by a steady deterioration. Appetite is suppressed, leading to a negative energy balance. Furthermore, there is an increased risk of "mountain sickness" and medical emergencies at these higher altitudes.

24.3   Adaptations to altitude

Physiological adaptations

An immediate physiological response to exercise in hypobaric conditions or lack of oxygen is respiratory compensation. This is achieved by an increased tidal volume (depth of breathing) or an increased respiratory frequency. An increase in depth of respiration is the main response, especially relevant during sports such as swimming and running where the breathing rate is synchronised with stroke or stride patterns.

The hyperventilation (increase in breathing) that occurs on exposure to altitude causes a problem in that more carbon dioxide is "blown off" from blood passing through the lungs. Elimination of carbon dioxide, which is a weak acid in solution in the blood, leaves the blood more alkaline than normal because of an excess of bicarbonate ions. The kidneys compensate by excreting bicarbonate over several days, which helps return the acidity of the blood towards normal. The outcome is that the alkaline reserve is decreased, and so the blood has a poorer buffering capacity for tolerating entry of additional acids into it. Consequently, lactic acid diffusing from muscle into blood during exercise at altitude will be more difficult to neutralise. High intensity performance will decline earlier than at sea level because of this, and the intensity of training will need to be reduced for exercise to be sustained.

The low oxygen tension (partial pressure) does not significantly affect the uptake of oxygen by the red blood cells until the oxygen pressure declines to a certain point. However, with adaptation to altitude the critical oxygen pressure falls. This results from increased production of 2,3-BPG (2,3-biphosphoglycerate) by the red blood cells and is beneficial in that it aids the unloading of oxygen from the red cells at the tissues. The oxygen-carrying capacity of the blood is enhanced by an increase in the number of red blood cells. This process begins within a few days of altitude and is stimulated by erythropoietin secreted by the kidneys, which later causes increased red blood cell production by the bone marrow. As a result, the bone marrow increases its iron uptake to form haemoglobin after about 48 hours at altitude. If the individual remains at high altitude, it takes two to three weeks to secure a true increase in total body haemoglobin and the red cell count continues to increase for a year or more but does not attain the values observed in high-altitude natives. The haemoglobin concentration also increases, and there is a rise in haematocrit, the percentage of blood volume occupied by red blood cells.

On first exposure to altitude, there is an increase in heart rate. Later, successful adaptation to altitude results in a reduction in the heart rate to a near normal level.

Within a few days of reaching an altitude location, a rise in haemoglobin concentration is apparent, but this initial increase in haemoglobin is a result of haemoconcentration due to the drop in plasma volume. Nevertheless, there is a gradual true increase in haemoglobin, which is mediated by stimulation of the bone marrow to overproduce red blood cells in the course of erythropoiesis. This requires that the body's iron stores are adequate and may, indeed, mean supplementation of iron intake prior to and during the stay at altitude.

Upon return to sea level it will take a few days for the acid-base status to be re-established. Hypoxia no longer stimulates erythropoiesis and the elevated red cell count will slowly come down. The decreased affinity of red blood cells for oxygen, which facilitated unloading to the active tissues by means of the activity of 2,3-BPG, is soon lost on return to sea level. Any exploitation of the haematological adaptation must be carefully timed to occur before the red blood cell count returns to normality: this may take up to six weeks. Otherwise, repeated sojourns to altitude are needed.

The use of altitude training camps for enhancement of sea-level performance received renewed interest in the 1990s amongst British coaches. A symposium convened by the British Olympic Association (1993) represented an attempt to coordinate the experiences of the various sports and provided an opportunity to consider the relevance of altitude training for its athletes.

The British middle and distance runners used a range of altitude locations from Albuquerque in the USA (1500 m) to Mexico City (2300 m). The difference in these two exposures was reflected in a significant increase in haemoglobin concentration at Mexico City and no change after Albuquerque. It does seem that an altitude in excess of 2000 m, when the reduction in ambient pressure takes the oxygen-saturation curve of haemoglobin into a steep decline, is needed to induce an appreciable effect on red cell mass.

The most comprehensive monitoring of athletes was of the rowers. Particular attention was given to reducing the training load on early exposure to avoid acute mountain sickness. Later, individuals were carefully programmed with increased training loads and metabolic responses were recorded (Grobler and Faulmann, 1993). The programme took into account the competitive schedule following the return to sea level. It has proved to be effective in the gold-medal winning men's teams at the 1996 and 2000 Olympic Games.

There is no complete consensus on the timing of this return to sea level before participation in major competition. A study of Swedish skiers was carried out for a three-week period at 1900 m with a subsequent long-term follow-up. Ingjer and Myhre (1992) reported that a strict liquid intake regimen was effective in reducing the fall in plasma volume associated with dehydration at altitude. The blood lactate response to a submaximal exercise test was lowered on an immediate return to sea level. This decrease was correlated with the improvement in haemoglobin and haematocrit that occurred at altitude. It seems that those who benefit most from altitude training are those with the greatest room for elevating oxygen-carrying capacity.

The level of altitude seemingly influences the stimulatory effect of erythropoietin. At about 1900 m the rise in serum erythropoietin is about 30 per cent higher than at sea level after two to three days, but at 4500 m this increase is about 300 per cent. Serum erythropoietin concentrations decrease after approximately one week at altitude, and this may be associated with increased oxygenation of the tissues due to an increase in red cell 2,3-BPG. The average true rise in haemoglobin approximates to 1 per cent each week, at least at altitudes between 1.8 and 3 km (Berglund, 1992).

Best estimates are that optimal haematological adaptations to altitude take around 80 days. This may be accelerated by periodic visits to higher altitudes (up to about 3 km) but not by training there. The inability to tolerate high training loads at altitude may lead to a drop in aerobic fitness, which offsets the positive effects of the altitude sojourn. The answer may be a combination of living at altitude for a sustained period but frequently returning to near-sea level (locally if possible) for strenuous exercise training. This strategy has been referred to as "live high, train low" (Levine, 1995).

Altitude simulation

Altitude training to enhance subsequent performance capability at sea level has been practised since the 1960s and is still widely used by sea-level natives in a range of sports. Such a manoeuvre is legal and has spawned the development of training camps based at altitude resorts. It even encouraged many professional endurance athletes to reside at altitude. Thus, access to altitude training depended upon either an accident of birth or the access to sufficient resources to be able to travel to and live at a suitable venue. This could entail considerable travel and disruption to the life of an athlete. Even then, exposure to altitude demanded careful attention to physiological detail so that adverse effects (such as acute mountain sickness) were avoided. Of greater significance was the key physiological disadvantage that altitude limits the intensity of the training that an athlete can undertake. Indeed, one of the first studies of altitude training reported that there was 3–8 per cent deterioration in 800 yd, 1 mile and 2 mile times in collegiate athletes following 63 days of living and training at 4000m altitude (Buskirk *et al.*, 1967).

Because of the advantages conferred by place of birth and the disadvantages of training at altitude, sports scientists sought to develop alternative methods that would combine the benefits of living at altitude with those of training at sea level. Two quite different approaches to this challenge were developed in the 1990s. The first approach simply asked the question "What if the athlete lives and/or sleeps at altitude but trains at or near sea-level?" Levine and Stray-Gundersen's resulting study (1997) was seminal and resulted in a sea change in altitude training and the creation of the concept of living high and training low. The second approach was developed out of the need to increase access to altitude training for Finnish athletes. It involved the same principle of living at altitude and training at sea level but achieved it by simulation because Finland did not offer the same geographical opportunities as those available to Levine and Stray-Gundersen in Utah in the USA. Simulation of altitude was achieved by the creation of hypoxic apartments using a nitrogen-dilution technique. The first report about this was published by Rusko *et al.* in 1995.

National provision of altitude-training facilities has increased enormously over the last couple of decades. For example, in China, altitude training for athletes from sea-level locations began in the 1960s. From the 1980s, 20 different sports events involving sports teams from about 20 provinces have taken part in altitude training. In 2004, China had 18 bases available for altitude training. These bases offer the facilities for live low, train high (LL-TH: low-pressure chambers); live high, train low (LH-TL: altitude houses); live high, train high (LH-TH: low-pressure chambers); and live low, train low (IHE: intermittent hypoxic exposure) (Weng, 2004). In the UK, the English Institute of Sport has nine regional centres that offer a range of artificial hypoxic training environments including LH-TL, using oxygen filtration and normobaric hypoxia. In June 2009, Lord Coe opened the first of six Perform centres in Rossendale, Lancashire, UK. These centres offer simulated hypoxic training facilities. Wilber (2007b) includes summary information about the types of artificial hypoxic training environments and modalities that are provided by different nations. As well as national facilities, many sports clubs and universities offer "local" provision of artificial hypoxic training environments. In addition, amateur and recreational athletes can simply buy their own hypoxicators for use at home.

In order to distinguish between the original training modality of living and training at altitude and the new modality of living at altitude but training at sea level, the acronyms LH-TH and LH-TL became commonplace. The approaches to altitude training, together with the subsequent list of acronyms, have burgeoned over the last decade with the advent of technological advances. If altitude is simulated by reducing the fractional concentration of oxygen without reducing the barometric pressure below that of sea level, it is referred to as normobaric hypoxia. In addition to the original method of diluting the fractional concentration of oxygen with 100 per cent nitrogen, normobaric hypoxia can also be created by oxygen filtration. A more recent variation on the theme of LH-TL is to live at natural altitude (hypobaric hypoxia) but to simulate training at sea level by inspiring supplemental oxygen ($F_iO_2 \approx 0.26$). This is referred to as LH-TLO$_2$. Obviously, the altitude exposure time varies both with the method used and the experimental design but on average, it can be anything up to 22 h/d for natural/terrestrial altitude and 12–16 h/d for simulated altitude in the various LH-TL models. Most recently, there has been much research into physiological and ergogenic effects of frequently repeated, brief periods of exposure to normobaric or hypobaric hypoxia. If these exposures are introduced at rest, then this is referred to as intermittent hypoxic exposure (IHE) or, if introduced during training, it are referred to as intermittent hypoxic training (IHT). These latest methods have been facilitated by the development of portable devices (hypoxicators and face masks) that can deliver a hypoxic stimulus. There is also the antithesis of this approach, which involves intermittent hypoxic training or live low, train high (LL-TH).

Does it work?

The answer to this question is not as simple and as straightforward as might be expected because whether altitude training or simulated altitude training works or not depends upon what it is meant to achieve. Thus, if it is to prepare the athlete for competition at altitude, then there seems to be little doubt that the answer is that it does. However, if the purpose of the altitude training or simulated altitude training is to improve sea level performance, then the answer is contentious (Wilber, 2007b; Gore et al., 2007). Moreover, whether there is benefit or not also depends upon the model of altitude training and the nature of the hypoxic stimulus that is being used (e.g. LH-TL, LL-TH, IHE, IHT or IHIT). The issue is further compounded by the use of different technologies to achieve the same hypoxic stimulus (e.g. whether normobaric hypoxia produced by diluting the oxygen with nitrogen or by using an oxygen-filtering membrane to reduce the inspired oxygen) and what is meant by "does it work". A full literature review of the effects of altitude training upon performance at sea level is beyond the scope of this chapter, which will, instead, attempt to summarise the findings to date and highlight some of the controversies that exist. There are numerous comprehensive literature reviews (e.g. Wilber, 2001: Hahn et al., 2001; Rusko et al., 2004; Loffredo and Glazer, 2006).

The raison d'être for altitude training was to mimic the effects of living at altitude, which are considered to cause adaptive changes to the oxygen-carrying capacity of the blood by increasing erythropoiesis. Therefore, studies of altitude training were designed to test the hypothesis that altitude training increased erythropoiesis and hence aerobic capacity (as measured by VO_{2max}). The hypothesis therefore defined the experimental design and the variables that were measured. However, conflicting results were obtained with some studies showing an increase in erythopoietic markers and/or VO_{2max} whilst others did not, as detailed in recent reviews (Wilber, 2007b; Gore et al., 2007). The Finnish studies reported an increase in EPO (31 per cent) and in reticulocytes (50 per cent) (Rusko et al., 1995) and EPO (84 per cent) and RBC Mass (7 per cent) (Laitinen et al., 1995). A later study confirmed the increases in EPO and RBC mass adding an increase in VO_{2max} compared to sea level controls (Rusko et al., 1999). It is of interest, though, that the increase in EPO did not correlate with the increase in RBC mass. The Swedish investigators Piehl-Aulin et al. (1998) also reported an increase in EPO and reticulocyte count but without an increase in haemoglobin mass, haematocrit or VO_{2max}. Data from the Australian studies confirmed an increase in EPO but not in reticulocytes (Ashenden et al., 2000) or haemoglobin mass (Ashenden et al., 1999).

The observant reader will have noticed the absence of detail about the ability of the subjects (i.e. trained, well-trained, elite); whether the study was pre-season, during season or post-season; whether iron status was monitored and/or supplemented; what variables were recorded (haematological, physiological, metabolic, ergonomic); the methods used to record those variables; the nature of the hypoxic stimulus; the inclusion or not of sea-level control subjects, etc. Indeed these are some of the explanations suggested for the discrepancies in the results and conclusions. However, some of these criticisms are implicit in the design of studies of this nature. For example, it is difficult to recruit significant numbers of elite athletes from the same discipline who are prepared to act as either subject or control for a period of at least one month in a year when perhaps they need to prepare for Olympic competition.

However, the important question from the athletes' point of view is not "Does it work scientifically?" but "Does it improve performance?" The answers to the latter question were reviewed recently by Wilber (2007b) in an altitude/hypoxic training symposium. In a pioneering study involving collegiate distance runners (Levine and Stray-Gundersen, 1997), utilising LH-TL via natural/terrestrial altitude, a 1 per cent improvement in 5000-m running time in the altitude-trained group compared to the sea-level control group was observed. This was equivalent to a 13.4 sec improvement. The original study of the LH-TL model demonstrated that exposure for >20 hr/day to 2500 m altitude caused an increase in erythrocyte volume, VO_{2max} and improved performance in a 5000-m time trial (Levine and Stray-Gundersen, 1997). Although the group response in the aforementioned study showed a mean improvement, there was a wide variability in the individual responses. This led to the subclassification of athletes into "responders" and "nonresponders" on the basis of the 5000-m times before and after 28 days of LH-TL (Chapman et al., 1998). A subsequent study involving elite US NT distance runners showed a 1 per cent (5.8 sec) improvement in a 3000-m time-trial performance (Stray-Gundersen et al., 2001). Improvements in performance have also been reported in Swiss NT orienteers, US NT long-track speedskaters and US NT marathon runners (cited in Wilber, 2007b). Studies using LH-TL via nitrogen dilution have demonstrated improvements in performance in Australian NT cyclists (Martin *et al.*, 2002), Finnish NT 400-m runners (Nummela and Rusko, 2000) and in running economy of Australian NT runners (Saunders *et al.*, 2004). The consistently positive findings of these studies are in contrast with those using LH-TL via oxygen filtration, which have produced conflicting reports (Wilbur, 2007b). Whilst they have demonstrated improvements in cycling peak power output and cycling power at respiratory compensation point in French NT endurance athletes (Schmitt *et al.*, 2006) they have failed to demonstrate improvements in 2000-m swim TT in French NT swimmers (Robach *et al.*, 2006a) or VO_{2max} and time to exhaustion in French NT Nordic skiers (Robach *et al.*, 2006b)

Studies using LH-TLO$_2$ have produced improvements in performance (as measured by 100 kJ work interval and increments in power output equivalent) in trained endurance athletes and in US NT junior cyclists (as measured by 120 kJ cycling time trial). Sixteen studies that used IHE and IHT and included either recreational or elite athletes and fitness or training matched controls were reviewed by Wilber (2007b). More studies reported no improvement in performance than reported improvements in performance following intermittent exposure to hypoxia. This may be a consequence of the variety of protocols (IHE or IHT; normobaric or hypobaric hypoxia) that were used and the variation in exposure to hypoxia (from 2 h/d @ 2500m for 10 d to 3 h/d @ 4000–5000 m for 28 d). The latter would be expected to be particularly important because the "dose" of hypoxia is considered to be critical to any response to altitude training (Wilber *et al.*, 2007). Current opinion is that a minimum effective exposure to natural altitude is 22 h/d for four weeks at 2000–2500 m (Wilber *et al.*, 2007) and at simulated altitude is >12 h/d for more than three weeks at 2100–2500 m (Rusko *et al.*, 2004).

In addition to the anticipated benefits of altitude training upon aerobic parameters and performance, there have been reports of improvement in anaerobic performance. Thus 12 well-trained triathletes completed a sea level–controlled, cross-over study involving exposure of 2 h/d for 10 days to hypobaric IHT at a simulated altitude of 2500 m (Hendriksen and Meeuwsen, 2003). There were significant increases (P < 0.05) in anaerobic mean power (4.1 per cent) and anaerobic peak power (3.8 per cent) in the test group versus the sea-level controls. Nummela and Rusko (2000) investigated the effects of LH-TL on eight Finnish National Team 400-m runners. Athletes lived at a simulated normobaric hypoxia of 2200 m for 16–17 h/d for 10 days and trained at sea level. Seven days after completion of the LH-TL regimen, they undertook a 400-m time trial. Compared with pre-aptitude values, the test group was 1 per cent faster than the sea-level control group. This would correspond to a 0.4 sec improvement. Maximal anaerobic run tests (MART) were significantly faster at 5.0 mmol/l and 7.0 mmol/l blood lactate levels than the sea-level controls. The studies are of interest in view of the revelation by Dwain Chambers that he used IHT, under the coaching supervision of Victor Conte (formerly of BALCO), from October 2008 in preparation for the 2009 season. Chambers became the European Indoor 60m Champion and went on to finish sixth in the final of the 2009 World Championships in Berlin.

If we accept that LH-TL does increase performance, is this increase sufficient to justify inclusion in the training programme of an elite athlete? Several authors have argued that it is. A relative improvement in performance of 0.5 per cent improves the chance of a top athlete winning a medal in international competition (Hopkins and Hewson, 2001). In the 10000-m final of the 2000 Sydney Olympics, the difference between the winning time of Haile Gebreselassie (27:18:20 min:sec) and that of second place Paul Tergat (27:18:29 min:sec) was just 0.005 per cent (Wilber, 2007a). A sample selection of just two studies taken from internationally respected laboratories demonstrates that the changes in performance are of the order of magnitude that would improve the chances of an athlete winning a medal. First, the original study of the effect of LH-TL upon elite US National Team distance runners demonstrated a 1 per cent (5.8 sec) improvement in a 3000-m time trial (Stray-Gundersen et al., 2001). Second, a six-study analysis of LH-TL (Hahn et al., 2001) reported a 1.0 per cent improvement in supramaximal effort lasting $\approx$ 4 min. This improvement would have been more than sufficient to increase the athlete's chance of winning by 10–20 per cent (Hopkins, 1999).

How does it work?

As described above, it is generally accepted that training at altitude will improve performance at sea level provided that the "dose" of altitude is sufficient. However, the causal link between altitude and improved performance is unresolved and remains contentious. Levine and Stray-Gundersen (2005) have modestly proposed the "Levine and Stray-Gundersen's Postulates", which are based upon the Nobel Laureate Robert Koch's Henle-Koch Postulates relating to causation and disease (cited in Evans, 1976). Levine and Stray-Gundersen contend that the causative link between intermittent hypoxia and improvement in VO_{2max} and performance is an increase in erythrocyte volume. Based upon their initial studies in 1997 and 1998, the test groups showed an increase in erythrocyte volume, VO_{2max} and performance. The control group, who lived and trained at sea level, showed no increase in erythrocyte volume and no subsequent increase in VO_{2max} and performance. Furthermore, the key distinguishing feature between the responders and the nonresponders was the greater increase in erythropoietin in the former as opposed to the latter. Since exposure to altitude has been shown to increase erythropoietic activity, and direct stimulation of erythropoiesis, using erythropoietin, has been shown to increase VO_{2max} in laboratory-based tests and performance in competition, the causal link would seem to be irrefutable. Moreover, Levine and Stray-Gundersen (2005) state that in a large number of runners (n > 100), running economy never changed, anaerobic capacity never changed and muscle biopsies did not manifest an increase in buffer capacity or oxidative enzymes. It is perhaps of interest to note the following caveat in the discussion by Evans (1976), "The Henle-Koch Postulates are a useful historical reference point but were not regarded as rigid criteria by Koch himself and should not be today".

At the molecular level, the link between hypoxia and increased erythropoiesis is explained by hypoxia-inducible factor-1α (HIF-1α), which is present in every cell in the body and is the global regulator of oxygen homeostasis (Semenza, 2004). Hypoxia-inducible factor-1 consists of α- and β- subunits. In normoxia, HIF-1α is rapidly degraded, having a half-life of five to eight minutes. In hypoxia, HIF-1α is stabilised and transported into the nucleus where it is dimerised with HIF-1β, which is independent of O_2 regulation. HIF-1 binds to hypoxia-responsive elements of HIF-1 target genes that stimulate the synthesis of a number of proteins, including erythropoietin, which stimulates erythropoiesis; vascular endothelial growth factor, which stimulates angiogenesis; nitric oxide synthetase, which causes vasodilation; glycolytic enzymes, which increase anaerobic metabolism (Rusko et al., 2004); glucose transporters 1 and 3, and monocarboxylate transporters 1 and 4, which are critical for glucose uptake and lactate metabolism within muscle; carbonic anhydrase, which is needed for pH regulation; and tyroxine hydroxylase, which increases dopamine synthesis and accelerates ventilation (Gore et al., 2007). This might explain why altitude and exposure to hypoxia can affect all the major systems of the body (e.g. central nervous, respiratory, cardiovascular and muscular) rather than simply the erythropoietic system.

This plethora of responses at the tissue, cellular and molecular levels would appear to make it unlikely that the effects of altitude/hypoxic training can be explained simply by an increase in red cell mass (Levine and Stray-Gundersen, 2005). This has led to the proposal of an alternative to the erythropoiesis paradigm and which embraces non-haematological mechanisms. These include improved economy of exercise and mitochondrial efficiency, muscle pH regulation and muscle buffering capacity (βM) (Gore et al., 2007). In a recent review of factors affecting VO_{2max}, Levine significantly extended the discussion beyond the Fick equation, which states that cardiac output multiplied by the a-vO_2 difference explains VO_{2max} (Levine, 2008). Levine states that "defining the link between metabolic demand, cardiovascular control and fatiguing exercise including muscle receptors, neural pathways and central integration will be an important direction for future research". This suggestion, taken together with the "non-haematological theory" of Gore et al. (2007), indicates that progress in understanding the effects of hypoxic training upon athletic performance will likely come from a multifaceted, interdisciplinary approach that will no longer be restricted by postulates and paradigms.

24.4   WADA attitude to artificially induced hypoxic conditions

Consequent upon concerns about the purported widespread use of artificially induced hypoxic conditions, WADA undertook a consultation process amongst stakeholders to decide whether to prohibit or not. For a substance or method to be included in the prohibited list, it must fulfil two out of three of the following criteria:

- It must be performance enhancing.
- It must pose a threat to the health of the athlete.
- It must violate the spirit of sport.

In September 2006, the WADA executive committee published the 2007 prohibited list. In so doing, they had accepted the recommendations of their scientific and ethics committees and had not included artificially induced hypoxic conditions on the list. This was despite being informed by the committees that "the method was performance enhancing, raised some concerns but was inconclusive about the method's threat to athlete health, and determined that the method was contrary to the spirit of sport". WADA added the caveat that "a substance or method may, but is not required to, be added to the Prohibited List if it meets two of these three criteria". Moreover, WADA (2006) expressed the concern that "in addition to the results varying individually from case to case, use of this method may pose health risks if not properly implemented and under medical supervision".

The decision not to ban the method was widely approved. UK Sport (2006) was included in the consultation process and recommended a cautious and pragmatic approach. It did not support the inclusion of hypoxic conditions on the prohibited list and recommended further investigation into the safety and efficacy of the devices used. UK Sport stated that "on a more practical level, there is currently no realistic solution for the regulatory control of hypoxic chambers so there would be no way of monitoring its use or misuse if it was added to the List. This, we believe, would threaten the credibility of the List at a time when we are making great strides in further improving the confidence athletes and support staff have in the anti-doping system".

Others disagreed with the justification for not banning artificial hypoxic environments whilst agreeing with the decision. Thus, in an editorial in the *Scandinavian Journal of Medical Science and Sport*, Levine (2006), writing on behalf of and with the approval of the panel of 76 physicians, bioethicists and sports scientists who had advised WADA, asserted that the majority of members of the international scientific community strongly urged WADA not to place artificial hypoxic devices on the banned list for 2007. The editorial addressed the three criteria for inclusion of a substance or method. The first criterion (i.e. ergogenic benefit) was not fulfilled because the effects of real or simulated altitude training are uncertain, controversial and quite variable between individuals. This alone would distinguish it from either ESAs or blood doping.

This is supported by the results of a study published in 2001 by Ashenden *et al.* who had made a direct comparison of the physiological responses to simulated altitude exposure and r-HuEpo administration. Twenty-three well-trained athletes were exposed to a simulated altitude of 2650–3000 m for 11–23 nights using nitrogen-dilution, normobaric hypoxia and were compared to control, healthy volunteers who received r-HuEpo (150 IU/kg) for 25 days. The group mean increase in serum erythropoietin (422 per cent for r-HuEpo vs 59 per cent for simulated altitude), percent reticulocytes (89 per cent vs 30 per cent) and VO_{2max} (6.6 per cent versus – 2.0 per cent) indicated the changes induced by simulated altitude were relatively modest compared with those obtained with r-HuEpo. Based on the different magnitude of these responses, the authors concluded that simulated altitude facilities should not be considered unethical based on the tenet that they provide an alternative means of obtaining the benefits sought by illegal r-HuEpo doping. Within each group—test, control and placebo—there was considerable variation in response as indicated by standard deviation and range.

Ashenden et al. strongly disagreed with the scientific and ethical aspects of the "passivity" argument that had been opined by the WADA Ethical Issues Advisory Panel (WADA, 2006) as being contrary to the spirit of sport and hence fulfilling WADA's third criterion. Finally, they contended that real or simulated altitude was quite safe and unlikely to injure an athlete, thus not fulfilling the second criterion for inclusion. The rebuttals of the criteria for inclusion have deliberately been presented out of sequence in this chapter in order to finish with a consideration of the safety of the athletes, which should be of paramount importance. Contrary to the view proposed by Levine (2006), the scientific community has expressed concerns about the safety of artificial hypoxic environments. On announcing the prohibited list for 2007, the WADA executive committee stated that its scientific committees found that the method raised some concerns but was inconclusive about the method's threat to athletes' health. The recommendation of UK Sport (2006) was for further investigation into the safety of hypoxia-inducing devices. Lippi et al. (2007) stated that the scientific community had been warned that hypoxia may be thrombogenic and that recent studies had suggested a variety of mechanisms, including endothelial injury, a procoagulant response, raised haematocrit and blood viscosity following prolonged exposure to hypoxia. Concerns have also been expressed by the Fédération Internationale de Mèdecine du Sport about the side effects and safety of sleeping high and training low in normobaric hypoxia (Niess et al., 2006). Finally, in a totally different context (i.e. that of air travel), Dine and Kreider (2008) have actually proposed using a hypoxia altitude simulation test (HAST) to identify those patients at risk of cardiopulmonary events when exposed to oxygen concentrations of 17.1 to 15.1 per cent in the cabin of an airplane. This is the range of oxygen concentrations that can be provided by commercial hypoxicators that are readily available to athletes.

The issue of safety of artificial hypoxic environments therefore bears comparison with that of the safety of erythropoietin. As WADA (2006) stated in its justification for not prohibiting the use of artificial hypoxic environments, "use of this method may pose health risks if not properly implemented and under medical supervision". No doubt many coaches, sports scientists and sports physicians would argue that under the appropriate supervision and when used "scientifically" and cautiously, EPO is safe. Indeed, Dr. Michele Ferrari, an Italian sports physician and coach, once famously asserted that EPO was no more dangerous than orange juice (depending on the quantity used or consumed). The danger then might not be to the elite athlete who benefits from expert supervision but to the amateur or recreational athlete who is unsupervised and who erroneously believes that more is better. It was precisely these conditions (i.e. the lack of supervision and unfettered use) that were thought to have been responsible for the deaths of the Belgian and Dutch cyclists in the early days of EPO abuse. Therefore, perhaps it is incumbent upon sports' leading anti-doping agency, WADA, to learn from history and to take a lead in highlighting the possible health risks of artificial hypoxic environments. According to Wilber (2007b), hypobaric/hypoxic practices are currently prohibited by the Italian Health Ministry and this takes judicial precedence over WADA regulations in areas of Italian jurisprudence (hence applying to participants in the Giro d'Italia). This may possibly have been instituted because of concerns that athletes were using the method as an excuse for raised haemoglobin and/or haematocrit induced by abuse of ESAs, which was of concern to WADA (Wilber, 2007b). Whatever the reason, it may be sending out the right message and leading by example through elite athletes who are, after all, the role models for amateur and recreational athletes.

24.5 Conclusion

Altitude training began as an accident of birth and became the prerogative of the athlete fortunate enough to have sufficient financial backing. In the 1990s, the advent of simulated altitude widened access through the development of hypoxic houses, apartments and tents. Most recently, the development of portable hypoxicators has brought down the cost of access to artificial hypoxia environments from that of a small car to that of a pair of carbon skis or wheels. This "open access" must raise concerns for the risks to health of amateur or recreational users. Whilst the governing bodies of sport and their scientific advisers are rightly preoccupied with the ergogenic value, mode(s) of action and ethics of artificial hypoxic environments, they should not lose sight of the potential health risks that they may pose to unsupervised athletes.

24.6 References

Ashenden, M.J., Gore, C.J. and Martin, G.P. (1999). Effects of a 12-day "live high, train low" camp on reticulocyte production and haemoglobin mass in elite female road cyclists. *European Journal of Applied Physiology* **80**, 5, 472.

Ashenden, M.J., Gore, C.J., Dobson, G.P. *et al.* (2000). Simulated moderate altitude elevates serum erythropoietin but does not increase reticulocyte production in well-trained runners. *European Journal of Applied Physiology* **81**, 428–435.

Ashenden, M.J., Hahn, A.G., Martin, D.T. *et al.* (2001). A comparison of the physiological response to simulated altitude exposure and r-HuEpo administration. *Journal of Sports Sciences* **19**, 831–837.

Berglund, B. (1992). High altitude training: Aspects of haematological adaptations. *Sports Medicine* **14**, 289–303.

British Olympic Association. (1993). The altitude factor in athletic performance. *Proceedings of International Symposium (Lilleshall), 13–15 December,* BOA, London.

Buskirk, E.R., Kollias, J., Akers, R.F. *et al.* (1967). Maximal performance at altitude and on return from altitude in conditioned runners. *Journal of Applied Physiology* **23**, 259–266.

Chapman, R.F., Stray-Gundersen, J. and Levine, B.D. (1998). Individual variation in response to altitude training. *Journal of Applied Physiology* **85**, 1448–1456.

Dine, C.J. and Kreider, M.E. (2008). Topics in practice management. Hypoxia altitude simulation test. *Chest* **133**, 1002–1005.

Evans, A.S. (1976). Causation and disease: The Henle-Koch postulates revisited. *Yale Journal of Biological Medicine* **49(2)**, 175–195.

Gore, C.J., Clark, S.A. and Saunders, P.U. (2007). Nonhematological mechanisms of improved sea-level performance after hypoxic exposure. *Medicine and Science in Sports and Exercise* **39(9)**, 1600–1609.

Grobler, J. and Faulmann, L. (1993). The British experience. *BOA Technical News* **1(5)**, 3–5.

Hahn, A.G., Gore, C.J., Martin, D.T. *et al.* (2001). An evaluation of the concept of living at moderate altitude and training at sea level. *Comparative of Biochemistry and Physiology* **128**, 777–789.

Hendriksen, I.J. and Meeuwsen, T. (2003). The effect of intermittent training in hypobaric hypoxia on sea-level exercise: A cross-over study in humans. *European Journal of Applied Physiology* **88**, 396–403.

Hopkins, W.G. (1999). *Reliability of competitive performance of elite track and field athletes.* 5th IOC World Congress on Sports Science, Sydney, Australia, abstract 126.

Hopkins, W.G. and Hewson, D.J. (2001). Variability of performance of distance runners. *Medicine and Science in Sports and Exercise* **33**, 1588–1592.

Ingjer, F. and Myhre, K. (1992) Physiological effects of altitude training on young elite male cross-country skiers. *Journal of Sports Science* **10**, 49–63.

Laitinen, H., Alopaeus, K., Heikkinen, H. *et al.* (1995). Acclimatization to living in normobaric hypoxia and training in normoxia at sea level in runners. *Medicine and Science in Sports and Exercise* **27(Suppl. 1)**, 109.

Levine, B. D. (1995). Training and exercise at high altitudes. In *Sport, leisure and ergonomics*, ed. G. Atkinson and T. Reilly, E. and F.N. Spon, London. 74–92.

Levine, B.D. and Stray-Gundersen, J. (1997). "Living high-training low": Effect of moderate-altitude acclimatization with low-altitude training on performance. *Journal of Applied Physiology* **83**, 102–112.

Levine, B. and Stray-Gundersen, J. (2005). Point: Positive effects of intermittent hypoxia (live high:train low) on exercise performance are mediated primarily by augmented red cell volume. *Journal of Applied Physiology* **99**, 2053–2055.

Levine, B.D. (2006). Should "artificial" high altitude environments be considered doping? *Scandinavian Journal of Medicine and Science in Sports* **16**, 297–301.

Levine, B.D. (2008). VO_{2max}: What do we know, and what do we still need to know? *Journal of Physiology* **586**, 25–34.

Lippi, G., Franchini, M. and Guidi, G.C. (2007). Prohibition of artificial hypoxic environments in sports: Health risks rather than ethics. *Applied Physiology Nutrition and Metabolism* **32**, 1206–1207.

Loffredo, B.M. and Glazer, J.L. (2006). The ergogenics of hypoxia training in athletes. *Current Sports Medicine Reports* **5**, 203–209.

Martin, D.T., Hahn, A.G., Lee, H. *et al.* (2002). Effects of a 12-day "live high, train low" cycling camp on 4-min and 30-min performance. *Medicine and Science in Sports and Exercise* **34(Suppl.5)**, S274.

Niess, A., Dickhuth, H-H. and Bärtsch, P. (2006). FIMS position statement. The sleep-high–train low concept as performed in altitude simulation facilities. *The International Federation of Sports Medicine*. Available at http://www.fims.org (accessed 14 September 2009).

Nummela, A. and Rusko, H. (2000). Acclimatization to altitude and normoxic training improve 400-m running performance at sea level. *Journal of Sports Science* **18**, 411–419.

Piehl-Aulin, K., Svedenhag, J. Wide, L. *et al.* (1998). Short-term intermittent normobaric hypoxia-haematological, physiological and mental effects. *Scandinavian Journal of Medicine and Science in Sports* **8**, 132–137.

Robach, P., Schmitt, L, Brugniaux, J.V. *et al.* (2006a). Living high–training low: Effect on erythropoiesis and aerobic performance in highly-trained swimmers. *European Journal of Applied Physiology* **96(4)**, 423–433.

Robach, P., Schmitt, L, Brugniaux, J.V. *et al.* (2006b). Living high–training low: Effect on erythropoiesis and maximal aerobic performance in elite Nordic skiers. *European Journal of Applied Physiology* **97**, 695–705.

Rusko, H.K., Leppavuori, A., Makela, P. *et al.* (1995). Living high, training low: A new approach to altitude training at sea level in athletes. *Medicine and Science in Sports and Exercise* **27(5)**, S6.

Rusko, H. K., Tikkanen, H., Paavolainen, L. *et al.* (1999). Effect of living in hypoxia and training in normoxia on sea level VO_{2max} and red cell mass. *Medicine and Science in Sports and Exercise* **31(5)**, S86.

Rusko, H.K., Tikkanen, H.O. and Peltonen, J.E. (2004). Altitude and endurance training. *Journal of Sports Science* **22**, 928–945.

Saunders, P.U., Telford, R.D., Pyne, D.B. *et al.* (2004). Improved running economy in elite runners after 20 days of simulated moderate-altitude exposure. *Journal of Applied Physiology* **96**, 931–937.

Schmitt, L., Millet, G., Robach, P. *et al.* (2006). Influence of "living high–training low" on aerobic performance and economy of work in elite athletes. *European Journal of Applied Physiology* **97**, 627–636.

Semenza, G.L. (2004). O_2-regulated gene expression: Transcriptional control of cardiorespiratory physiology by HIF-1. *Journal of Applied Physiology* **96**, 1173–1177.

Stray-Gundersen, J., Chapman, R.F. and Levine, B.D. (2001). "Living high-training low" altitude training improves sea level performance in male and female elite runners. *Journal of Applied Physiology* **91**, 1113–1120.

UK Sport. (2006). More research needed on hypoxic chambers. Available at http://www.uksport.gov.uk/news/more_research_needed_on_hypoxic_chambers/ (accessed 22 July 2009).

Weng, Q. (2004). The recent development of altitude training in China. High Altitude Training Symposium, Hong Kong.

Wilber, R.L. (2001). Current practices in altitude training. *Sports Medicine* **31**, 249–265.

Wilber, R.L. (2007a). Introduction to altitude/hypoxic training symposium. *Medicine and Science in Sports and Exercise* **39(9)**, 1587–1589.

Wilber, R.L. (2007b). Application of altitude/hypoxic training to elite athletes. *Medicine and Science in Sports and Exercise* **39(9)**, 1610–1624.

Wilber, R.L., Stray-Gundersen, J. and Levine, B.D. (2007). Effect of hypoxic "dose" on physiological responses and sea-level performance. *Medicine and Science in Sports and Exercise* **39(9)**, 1590–1599.

World Anti-Doping Agency (WADA). (2006). WADA executive committee approves the 2007 prohibited list. Available at http://www.wada-ama.org/en/newsarticle.ch2?articleId=3115325 (accessed 22 July 2009).

Section 4

The extent of doping in sport

Chapter 25

Prevalence of drug misuse in sport

David R. Mottram

25.1 Introduction

Meaningful data on the prevalence of use of performance-enhancing drugs in sport are difficult to obtain. Evidence may be as diverse as statistics on positive dope tests, results of surveys of athletes (of either their self-reported use or of their perceptions of drug use by others), through to anecdotal reports and investigative journalism (Yesalis *et al.*, 2001). These sources of evidence are inconsistent, leading to speculation of levels of prevalence of drug use ranging from less than 1 per cent to more than 90 per cent. A number of studies have been undertaken to evaluate the prevalence of doping within individual countries or sports. However, it has been suggested that such studies generally underestimate the problem due to small sample populations (Lippi *et al.*, 2008). The purpose of this chapter is to evaluate the published evidence and to comment on the validity and accuracy of this evidence.

25.2 Statistics on doping control in sport

Statistics from WADA-accredited laboratories

Statistics on doping control are available from the World Anti-Doping Agency (WADA), which assumed responsibility for anti-doping in 2003. Prior to this date, responsibility lay with the International Olympic Committee's (IOC's) Medical Commission. Statistical results from the IOC were reviewed in a previous edition of this book (Mottram, 2005).

The statistical data since 2003 are derived from results from WADA-accredited laboratories (n = 34 in 2008). Overall, the percentage of positive test results has remained consistently low, despite a steady increase in the number of tests conducted annually (Table 25.1).

An adverse analytical finding is defined by WADA, in their World Anti-Doping Code, as "a report from a laboratory or other WADA-approved entity that, consistent with the International Standard for laboratories and related technical documents, identifies in a sample the presence of a prohibited substance or its

Table 25.1 Adverse analytical findings by WADA-accredited laboratories from 2003 to 2008

	A-samples analysed	Number of adverse findings	% of adverse findings
2008	274,615	5,061	1.84
2007	223,898	4,402	1.97
2006	198,143	3,887	1.96
2005	183,337	3,909	2.13
2004	169,187	2,909	1.72
2003	151,210	2,447	1.62

metabolites or markers (including elevated quantities of endogenous substances) or evidence of the use of a prohibited method". These figures include findings from athletes who had received approval to take a drug, having applied successfully for a Therapeutic Use Exemption.

Variations exist in the extent of analytical findings both between laboratories and between sports. Generally, there have been few consistent patterns. However, in terms of laboratories, Tokyo consistently recorded a low percentage of adverse findings (0.25 per cent to 0.61 per cent) between 2003 and 2008, whereas the Paris laboratory (4.95 per cent to 6.00 per cent) and Ghent laboratory (3.80 per cent to 4.72 per cent) recorded consistently high findings over the same period. This variation may be accounted for by the extent to which individual laboratories conduct no-notice, out-of-competition testing (OOCT) and the types of sport within the population for which the laboratory conducts tests.

Certain sports exhibited percentage adverse findings consistently above the annual, average WADA figures. These are shown in Table 25.2.

Table 25.2 Sports that exhibited consistently high adverse analytical findings by WADA-accredited laboratories from 2003 to 2008

	% of adverse findings					
	2003	*2004*	*2005*	*2006*	*2007*	*2008*
All sports	1.62	1.72	2.13	1.96	1.97	1.84
Baseball	2.47	2.86	3.69	2.32	2.69	1.11
Billiard sports	0.91	4.50	9.96	7.36	6.03	2.42
Boxing	3.68	3.17	3.41	2.39	3.16	2.21
Cycling	3.93	4.60	3.78	4.17	3.91	1.89
Golf	2.92	1.82	5.21	2.67	3.90	0.92
Motorcycle racing	2.37	4.21	3.23	2.72	3.92	2.59
Weightlifting	2.06	3.02	2.50	2.86	3.02	2.05

Table 25.3 Number of adverse findings of WADA-prohibited substances identified by WADA-accredited laboratories from 2003 to 2008 (some findings correspond to multiple measurements on the same athlete, such as longitudinal studies on testosterone)

	2003	2004	2005	2006	2007	2008
Anabolic agents	872	1191	1864	1966	2322	3259
Stimulants	516	382	509	490	793	472
Cannabinoids	378	518	503	553	576	496
Beta-2 agonists	297	381	609	631	399	350
Glucocorticosteroids	286	548	325	282	288	316
Diuretics and other masking agents	142	157	246	290	359	436
Hormones and related substances	79	78	162	42	41	106
Beta blockers	30	25	42	28	27	31
Narcotics	26	15	17	16	21	28
Agents with anti-oestrogenic activity*	6	8	21	30	8	29
Enhancement of oxygen transfer	–	2	–	–	3	–
Chemical and physical manipulation	2	–	–	4	3	–
Total	2634	3305	4298	4332	4850	5523

* Agents with anti-oestrogenic activity were renamed hormone antagonists and modulators in 2008.

For each year, the highest number of adverse findings recorded from all laboratories in all sports were related to anabolic agents (Table 25.3).

Tables 25.4 to 25.9 show the incidence of positive test results from WADA-accredited laboratories for the more commonly misused drugs, including stimulants, anabolic agents, beta-2 agonists (β_2-agonists), glucocorticosteroids, diuretics and other masking agents and peptide hormones.

Table 25.4 WADA statistics for the number of positive results for substances classed as stimulants from 2003 to 2008

	2003	2004	2005	2006	2007	2008
Stimulants						
Pseudoephedrine*	189	–	–	–	–	–
Ephedrine	100	102	93	66	50	54
Amphetamine	43	112	194	199	430	166
Cocaine	48	75	85	85	101	77
Caffeine*	39	–	–	–	–	–
Methylphenidate	9	7	17	32	38	40
Others	88	86	120	108	174	135
Total	516	382	509	490	793	472

* Pseudoephedrine and caffeine were removed from the WADA prohibited list and placed on a monitoring list in 2004. Pseudoephedrine was reinstated on the WADA prohibited list in 2010.

Stimulants, such as pseudoephedrine, ephedrine and caffeine, that are available without a prescription and present in over-the-counter (OTC) medicines, created particular problems for athletes. Most of these over-the-counter drugs, with the exception of ephedrine, methylephedrine and cathine were removed from the prohibited list in 2004. They were placed on a monitoring list and continue to be tested for by WADA laboratories to establish their continued pattern of use by athletes. Partly as a result of this monitoring programme, pseudoephedrine was reinstated on the WADA prohibited list in 2010.

Testosterone is the most frequently identified anabolic steroid (Table 25.5), although some of the positive results occur as a result of multiple measurements performed on the same athlete during longitudinal studies.

The adverse findings for anabolic agents are unlikely to reflect the true prevalence of anabolic steroid use for a number of reasons (Mottram, 1999). Athletes are adept at tailoring their anabolic steroid regimes to avoid detection. The drugs are taken during training and the doping regime is stopped prior to competition. The extent of out-of-competition testing has increased but is not universal.

There has been a rise in the number of "positive" test results for β_2-agonists (Table 25.6). The majority of these results were, however, deemed permissible by WADA as the drugs were administered by inhalation and Therapeutic Use Exemptions had been granted to the athletes prior to competing.

Results on glucocorticosteroids (Table 25.7) include adverse findings for which the athletes may have been granted Therapeutic Use Exemptions under WADA regulations.

In addition to their use as masking agents, diuretics are also used by athletes to achieve short-term weight loss in sports where weight categories apply, such as boxing and wrestling, and by jockeys in horse racing (see Table 25.8).

Table 25.5 WADA statistics for the number of positive results for substances classed as anabolic agents from 2003 to 2008

	2003	2004	2005	2006	2007	2008
Anabolic steroids						
Testosterone	304	392	1132	1124	1607	2166
Nandrolone	256	339	298	237	203	266
Stanozolol	159	226	233	222	172	259
Methandienone	59	63	56	126	98	136
Boldenone	16	19	28	37	40	93
Metenolone	11	22	28	30	23	28
Methyltestosterone	12	32	7	33	26	34
Others	55	98	82	104	100	204
Other anabolic agents						
Clenbuterol	–	–	–	53*	53	73
Totals	872	1191	1864	1966	2322	3259

* Clenbuterol statistics moved from β_2-agonists to anabolic agents in 2006.

Table 25.6 WADA statistics for the number of positive results for substances classed as β₂-agonists from 2003 to 2008

	2003	2004	2005	2006	2007	2008
Beta₂-agonists						
Salbutamol	189	251	357	391	60	56
Terbutaline	76	78	171	175	182	163
Clenbuterol*	31	46	52	–	–	–
Formoterol	–	4	18	42	107	91
Salmeterol	–	1	4	16	37	30
Others	1	1	7	7	13	10
Total	297	381	609	631	399	350

Results on β₂-agonists include adverse findings for which the athletes may have been granted Therapeutic Use Exemptions under WADA regulations.
* Clenbuterol has been recorded under anabolic agents from 2006.

Table 25.7 WADA statistics for the number of positive results for substances classed as glucocorticosteroids from 2003 to 2008

	2003	2004	2005	2006	2007	2008
Glucocorticosteroids						
Triamcinolone	131	246	25	18	18	20
Betamethasone	80	121	47	45	42	39
Prednisolone	52	61	35	30	16	37
Methylprednisolone	12	25	22	9	10	14
Dexamethasone	7	17	13	9	6	14
Budesonide	4	50	116	142	154	151
Prednisone	–	28	23	20	7	28
Others	–	–	44	9	35	13
Total	286	548	325	282	288	316

Table 25.8 WADA statistics for the number of positive results for substances classed as diuretics and other masking agents from 2003 to 2008

	2003	2004	2005	2006	2007	2008
Diuretics and other masking agents						
Furosemide	48	62	91	90	111	104
Hydrochlorothiazide	42	44	67	88	103	137
Epitestosterone	10	6	5	15	14	8
Finasteride	1	–	28	44	53	84
Others	41	45	55	53	78	103
Total	142	157	246	290	359	436

Table 25.9 WADA statistics for the number of positive results for substances classed as peptide hormones from 2003 to 2008

	2003	2004	2005	2006	2007	2008
Peptide hormones						
Erythropoietin	51	38	15	17	22	51
Human chorionic gonadotropin	14	24	143	22	15	46
Darbepoetin	7	–	1	1	2	2
Leutinizing hormone	7	16	3	2	2	1
Mircera	–	–	–	–	–	5
Insulin	–	–	–	–	–	1
Total	79	78	162	42	41	106

Most peptide hormones (Table 25.9) are endogenous within the body and proof that an athlete has taken such hormones can be difficult to obtain. With respect to erythropoietin (EPO), the product taken by athletes is recombinant-EPO, which has characteristics that allow it to be distinguished from endogenous EPO using an electrophoretic testing technique.

With respect to other drugs on the WADA prohibited list, it had previously been observed (Mottram, 2005) that the number of positive test results for cannabinoids (marijuana, cannabis) had increased dramatically reflecting the increased use of this "recreational" drug in society, but this probably did not indicate an increasing trend in its use for performance enhancement because the pharmacological properties of cannabinoids are likely to have adverse, rather than positive, effects on performance in most sports. The number of positive test results for cannabinoids has continued to increase since 2003 (Table 25.3).

Statistics derived from national surveys

A few studies have been undertaken into the extent of drug misuse within specific countries. These are listed in Table 25.10.

Table 25.10 Published statistics on doping control in specific countries

Author	Country	Years data collected	No. of samples	% positive test results
Bahr and Tjornhom (1998)	Norway	1977–1995	12,870	1.2
Ueki et al. (1998)	Japan	1985–1996	~14,000	~1.0
Mottram et al. (1997)	UK	1991–1995	17,193	1.0–1.5
Delbeke (1996)	Belgium	1987–1994	4374	7.8 in cyclists
Benzi (1994)	Italy	1988–1992	N/A	0.29–0.59
Van der Merwe and Kruger (1992)	S. Africa	1986–1991	2066	5.2–5.9 in most years

Bahr and Tjornhom (1998) collected data about Norwegian athletes from four accredited laboratories in Germany, Norway, Sweden and the UK. The drugs identified in the tests were anabolic agents (75 per cent) (almost half of which were testosterone), stimulants (17 per cent), narcotic analgesics (8 per cent), diuretics (5 per cent) and 4 per cent manipulation attempts. The majority were unannounced tests. A gradual decrease in the percentage of positive samples was recorded among Norwegian athletes as the frequency of testing, in high-prevalence sports, such as powerlifting, weightlifting and athletics, was increased from 1987 to 1995. The authors commented on the beneficial effects of unannounced OOCT.

Japan (Ueki *et al.*, 1998) have conducted tests both in competition and OOCT since 1985. In line with international trends, the drugs abused the most were stimulants and anabolic steroids. Ephedrine, methylephedrine and phenyl-propanolamine, all available over the counter, were the main stimulants, and nandrolone and testosterone the main steroids. The authors noted the value of testing agencies being independent from sports federations.

A review of data from the UK (Mottram *et al.*, 1997) showed that anabolic steroids and stimulants are the two main drugs of abuse, with narcotic analgesics also frequently detected. The authors commented on the fact that competitors may have been taking drugs that were undetectable at the time.

In the Belgian study (Delbeke, 1996), the percentage of positive results was higher than most other countries, as reported earlier in this chapter under statistics from WADA laboratories. However, this study was confined to cyclists, as this was the most popular sport in that country, and cycling has a long-standing repu-tation for being associated with drug misuse. The most frequently used drugs were stimulants, including OTC products and amphetamines. There were also many positive results for nandrolone. The tests were all conducted unannounced, which may also account for the high level of positive results.

In an Italian study in 1992, stimulants (55 per cent), anabolic agents (32 per cent), beta blockers (10 per cent) and narcotics (3 per cent) were the main drugs identified (Benzi, 1994). Amphetamines were the most frequently identified stimulant, being associated with cyclists' use. However, the percentage of posi-tive results overall decreased from 0.59 per cent in 1988 to 0.29 per cent in 1992. The author commented on the low number of accredited laboratories, worldwide. Few tests are therefore conducted relative to the number of athletes participating in sport. The author concluded that the data generated from the laboratories is only the "tip of the iceberg".

In the South African study (Van der Merwe and Kruger, 1992) samples were taken from athletes from a wide range of sports. The percentage of positive results over the study period was very consistent each year, being relatively high (average 5.5 per cent). The main drugs identified were stimulants (50.4 per cent) and anabolic steroids (41.6 per cent).

These national studies, in general, reflect international trends, with anabolic agents and stimulants being the most frequently identified drugs, although the principal class identified varied from country to country. National differences exist where particular sports dominate the scene or where a more extensive regime of OOCT exists.

WADA has concluded that OOCT is the most effective means of detection and deterrence. Under the World Anti-Doping Code, WADA requires international sports federations to have out-of-competition testing programmes in addition to in-competition testing. Furthermore, WADA conducts around 3000 independent out-of-competition tests a year on elite athletes.

25.3   Surveys into drug misuse in sport

There have been many survey-based studies published on the prevalence of drug misuse. Unfortunately, few have been based on surveys conducted with athletes and even fewer with elite athletes. Surveys are broadly divided into those that ask about self-use of drugs and those that seek information on perceived use by others. Results from the former type of study tend to under-report (Thevis *et al.*, 2008) whilst those on perceived use tend to produce exaggerated claims.

Evidence such as that presented by Franke and Berendonk (1997), relating to the systematic approach to the misuse of drugs in sport by the government of the German Democratic Republic, is rare. The logistical, social and ethical problems associated with obtaining such data are immense, hence the scarcity of such studies in the literature.

This section of the chapter reviews some of the more recently published surveys on drug misuse in athletes (Table 25.11).

University students who participated in intercollegiate athletics were the subjects in the Spence and Gauvin (1996) study. Painkillers (17.7 per cent), alcohol (94.1 per cent), anabolic steroids (0.9 per cent), amphetamines (0.7 per cent), marijuana (19.8 per cent) and cocaine (0.8 per cent) were the main drugs from the IOC prohibited list cited as being used by respondents.

La Torre *et al.* (2001) conducted a study using amateur athletes from a number of sports. Doping was considered to be widespread at high-level sport (27.8 per cent of participants). The percentage of athletes who declared using amino acids

Table 25.11 Surveys on drug misuse in sport by athletes

Author	Year	Country	Subjects
Spence and Gauvin	1996	Canada	754
La Torre *et al.*	2001	Italy	1056
Chester *et al.*	2003	UK	112
Alaranta *et al.*	2006	Finland	446
Thevis *et al.*	2008	Germany	964
Tscholl *et al.*	2008	International	2944

and/or creatine was 16.5 per cent. Of the respondents, 28.6 per cent of them considered it acceptable to use drugs in order to improve performance.

The Chester *et al.* (2003) study looked specifically at OTC stimulants and surveyed regional, national and international track and field athletes. Results showed that 3.4 per cent of respondents declared that they had used OTC stimulants specifically for performance enhancement.

Alaranta *et al.* (2006) described a self-reported survey of elite athletes in Finland. Thirty per cent reported that they personally knew an athlete who used banned substances. Fifteen per cent had been offered banned substances, particularly speed, and power athletes, of which stimulants were the most frequently offered, followed by anabolic steroids.

Thevis *et al.* (2008) conducted a survey of sports science students but also carried out urine chemical analysis for anabolic steroids, stimulants and selected drugs covered by doping control regulations. In total, 11.2 per cent of the urine samples contained drugs subject to doping control. Surprisingly, no anabolic steroids were detected. The most frequently detected substance was the major metabolite for tetrahydrocannabinol in cannabis (9.8 per cent), followed by stimulants related to cocaine and amphetamines (1.0 per cent). Cannabis use had not been reported by any participants in the study, highlighting the issue of underreporting where self-use questionnaire surveys are employed.

Tscholl *et al.* (2008) examined medication use in players during FIFA World Cups in 2002 and 2006. Each team physician documented all medication and nutritional supplements taken in the 72 hours prior to each match. Results recorded 1.8 substances/player/match, of which 42.9 per cent were medicinal and 57.1 per cent nutritional supplements. The most frequently prescribed medicines were non-steroidal anti-inflammatory drugs, β_2-agonists and corticosteroids. The high intake of these substances led the authors to conclude that it was unclear whether the medications were taken solely for therapeutic purposes.

As previously stated, published work on drug use by athletes is scarce. The few studies reported above indicate that results are highly variable. They are based on surveys with widely differing aims and protocols; some surveys sought information on self-use, while others gauged predicted use by fellow athletes. Other variables included the type of sport undertaken by respondents and the specificity, or otherwise, of drugs under investigation.

25.4   A perspective on the prevalence of drug misuse in sport through medical practitioners

In this section of the chapter, the role and views of those who currently or who are likely to prescribe performance-enhancing drugs to athletes are considered.

Dawson (2001) observed that patients who should concern the physician most are not the high-profile, elite athletes but young members of society who are being increasingly drawn to the use of performance-enhancing drugs.

In general, medical practitioners lack knowledge about drug misuse in sport (Greenway and Greenway, 1997; Rosano *et al.*, 2005). Consequently, some doctors may prescribe banned substances to athletes, not knowing about the prohibited list (Laure, 1997). However, drugs may be prescribed in the full knowledge of the purpose for which they may be used (Laure, 1997). Either way, this study reported that 61 per cent of performance-enhancing drug supplies for amateur athletes was obtained from medical practitioners. A study by Green *et al.* (2001) in Canada found that 32.1 per cent of national collegiate student athletes who took anabolic steroids obtained them from physicians other than their institutions' team physicians.

A study by Gupta and Towler (1997) indicated that 53 per cent of medical practitioners had reported that they had seen at least one patient in the previous year who had wanted anabolic steroids for nonmedical purposes. Of these practitioners, 6 per cent reported that they had seen more than 20 patients who mentioned steroid use. Moreover, a small minority of these doctors were prepared to prescribe anabolic steroids for body-building purposes. Dawson (2001) has identified four general groups of patients that use performance-enhancing drugs. These are:

1   those who are seriously involved in sport and see the use of drugs as a tool to achieve their ultimate goal;
2   those who have recently become involved in sport or started to attend a gymnasium;
3   occupational users who take drugs to overcome feelings of being threatened at work;
4   "recreational users" who use these drugs in an effort to enhance aspects of personal well-being.

Drugs prescribed for sporting injuries, some of which are subject to prohibition restrictions, provide a difficult prescribing dilemma in the treatment of sports injuries. The issue is also raised with respect to providing harm minimisation advice to known anabolic steroid users, as highlighted in the study by Gupta and Towler (1997) where 40 per cent of medical practitioners surveyed indicated a willingness to provide such advice. Dawson (2001) suggested that the policy of drug prohibition causes an increased ethical pressure on physicians. When advising patients on the use of performance-enhancing drugs, are physicians being complicit in their patients' drug use or simply upholding their oath to do their best to protect their patients' health?

Dean (2000) discusses the professional dilemma faced by medical practitioners with regard to treating athletes who are involved in drug misuse. It is unethical for a doctor to withhold treatment from a patient on the basis of a moral judgement that the patient's activities or lifestyle might have contributed to the condition for which treatment is sought. On the other hand, doctors who prescribe or collude in the provision of drugs or treatment, with the intention of improperly enhancing performance in sport, are equally acting unethically. This was highlighted in the case of six Finnish skiers who tested positive for the masking agent hydroxy ethyl starch at the World Nordic Skiing Championships in 2001. It transpired that their head coach and two national team doctors had assisted the athletes with the intravenous administration of the drug (Seiler, 2001).

As Dean (2000) surmises, when it comes to therapeutic treatment for athletes, involving banned drugs, practitioners are damned if they do and damned if they don't. This argument applies particularly in the case of those drugs, such as β_2-agonists and glucocorticosteroids, that medical practitioners may be required to complete Therapeutic Use Exemption forms for athletes who claim to suffer from asthma or who have inflammatory sports injuries (Orchard et al., 2006).

There is little accurate information on the prevalence of drug misuse in sport from evidence derived from medical practitioners. This does highlight an area of concern regarding the ready availability of drugs for performance enhancement through medical practitioners. There is certainly scope for improved education, for medical practitioners, on prohibited substances in sport (Greenway and Greenway, 1997) because general practitioners and sport physicians have particular responsibility in addressing the issue of doping in sport (Lippi et al., 2008).

25.5 General discussion

The number of tests conducted annually by accredited laboratories has steadily increased over the years (Table 25.1). Despite this increase, the percentage of positive results has remained consistently low, at below 2 per cent. Few people would regard the figures for positive test results as being an indication of the true prevalence of drug misuse in sport. These reasons are:

- too few tests are conducted relative to the number of athletes competing in sport;
- a large proportion of the drugs do not need to be taken at the time of competing and the extent of out-of-competition testing is inconsistent between sports federations and between national anti-doping organisations; and
- athletes continue to be adept at using drugs only during times when they are least likely to be tested.

Another factor that leads one to believe that statistics are misleading with regard to prevalence is the increasing use of drugs that naturally occur in the body. It is extremely difficult to determine what would be a "normal" level of such substances in an "average" athlete. Indeed, in the case of human growth hormone we do not yet have a validated test procedure. There must, therefore, be innumerable instances of the use of these drugs that remain undetected. The introduction by WADA of steroid profiling and athlete "passports" goes some way towards addressing this problem (Mareck et al., 2008).

What is needed is good, quality research on athletes' drug use at all levels of ability from junior to elite. Unfortunately, ethical constraints and the reluctance of athletes to divulge true and accurate information on the subject make this an unachievable goal. We are therefore left in the position of mere speculation. This encourages the media to publish unsubstantiated conjecture and rumour. In turn, this fuels misconceptions and fears in the minds of competitors, which itself encourages further drug use in sport.

25.6   References

Alaranta, A., Alaranta, H., Holmila, J. *et al.* (2006). Self-reported attitudes of elite athletes towards doping: Differences between type of sport. *International Journal of Sports Medicine* **27**, 842–846.

Bahr, R. and Tjornhom, M. (1998). Prevalence of doping in sports: Doping control in Norway, 1977–1995. *Clinical Journal of Sports Medicine* **8**, 32–37.

Benzi, G. (1994). Pharmacoepidemiology of the drugs used in sports as doping agents. *Pharmacological Research* **29(1)**, 13–26.

Chester, N., Reilly, T. and Mottram, D.R. (2003). Over-the-counter drug use amongst athletes and non-athletes. *Journal of Sports Medicine and Physical Fitness* **43**, 111–118.

Dawson, R.T. (2001). Hormones and sport. Drugs in sport—The role of the physician. *Journal of Endocrinology* **170**, 55–61.

Dean, C. (2000). Performance enhancing drugs; damned if you do and damned if you don't. *British Journal of Sports Medicine* **34**, 154.

Delbeke, F.T. (1996). Doping in cyclism: Results of unannounced controls in Flanders (1987–1994). *International Journal of Sports Medicine* **17(6)**, 434–438.

Franke, W.W. and Berendonk, B. (1997). Hormonal doping and androgenization of athletes: A secret program of the German Democratic Republic government. *Clinical Chemistry* **43(7)**, 1262–1279.

Green, G.A., Uryasz, F.D., Petr, T.A. *et al.* (2001). NCAA study of substance use and abuse habits of college student-athletes. *Clinical Journal of Sports Medicine* **11(1)**, 51–56.

Greenway, P. and Greenway, M. (1997). General practitioner knowledge of prohibited substances in sport. *British Journal of Sports Medicine* **31**,129–131.

Gupta, L. and Towler, B. (1997). General practitioners' views and knowledge about anabolic steroid use—Survey of GPs in a high prevalence area. *Drug and Alcohol Review* **16**, 373–379.

La Torre, G., Limongelli, F., Masala, D. *et al.* (2001). Knowledge, attitudes and behaviour towards doping and food supplementation in a sample of athletes of central-southern Italy. *Medicina Dello Sport* **54(3)**, 229–233.

Laure, P. (1997). Doping in sport: Doctors are providing drugs. *British Journal of Sports Medicine* **31**, 258–259.

Lippi, G., Franchini, M. and Guidi, G.C. (2008). Doping in competition or doping in sport? *British Medical Bulletin* **86**, 95–107.

Mareck, U., Geyer, H., Opfermann, G. *et al.* (2008). Factors influencing the steroid profile in doping control analysis. *Journal of Mass Spectrometry* **43**, 877–891.

Mottram, D.R. (1999). Banned drugs in sport: Does the International Olympic Committee (IOC) list need updating? *Sports Medicine* **27(1)**, 1–10.

Mottram, D.R. (2005). Prevalence of drug misuse in sport. In *Drugs in Sport*, 4th ed., ed. D.R. Mottram, Routledge, London. 357–380.

Mottram, D.R., Reilly, T. and Chester, N. (1997). Doping in sport: The extent of the problem. In *Esteve Foundation symposium. Vol.7: The clinical pharmacology of sport and exercise*, ed. T. Reilly and M. Orme, Excerpta Medica, Amsterdam. 3–12.

Orchard, J.W., Fricker, P.A., White, S.C. *et al.* (2006). The use and misuse of performance-enhancing substances in sport. *Medical Journal of Australia* **184**, 132–136.

Rosano, A., Carletti, M., Donini, L.M. *et al.* (2005). Doping and supplements: Awareness and knowledge by the Italian general practitioners. *Medicina Dello Sport* **58(4)**, 265–272.

Seiler, S. (2001). Doping disaster for Finnish Ski Team: A turning point for drug testing? *Sportscience* **5(1)**, 1–3.

Spence, J.C. and Gauvin, L. (1996). Drug and alcohol use by Canadian university athletes: A national survey. *Journal of Drug Education* **26(3)**, 275–287.

Thevis, M., Sauer, M., Geyer, H. *et al.* (2008). Determination of the prevalence of anabolic steroids, stimulants and selected drugs subject to doping controls among elite sport students using analytical chemistry. *Journal of Sports Sciences* **26(10)**, 1059–1065.

Tscholl, P., Junge, A. and Dvorak, J. (2008). The use of medication and nutritional supplements during FIFA World Cups 2002 and 2006. *British Journal of Sports Medicine* **42**, 725–730.

Ueki, M. Hiruma, T., Ikekita, A. *et al.* (1998) Trends in drug abuse in competitive sports, and the international anti-doping movement. *Journal of Toxicology: Toxin Reviews* **17(1)**, 73–83.

Van der Merwe, P.J. and Kruger, H.S.L. (1992). Drugs in sport—Results of the past 6 years of dope testing in South Africa. *South African Medical Journal* **82**, 151–153.

Yesalis, C.E. Kopstein, A.N. and Bahrke, M.S. (2001). Difficulties in estimating the prevalence of drug use among athletes. In *Doping in elite sport: The politics of drugs in the Olympic movement*, ed. W. Wilson and E. Derse, Human Kinetics, Champaign, Illinois. 43–62.

Synopsis of drugs used in sport

David R. Mottram

In Section 1 of this synopsis an overview of the more commonly used classes of drugs and methods on the 2010 WADA prohibited list is presented under the headings:

- WADA category
- use in sport
- pharmacological action
- adverse effects

Section 2 of this synopsis presents information on drugs that are not prohibited and are commonly used by athletes. The adverse effects of these drugs and the implications for their use in sport are described.

Section 1. WADA-prohibited drugs and methods

Anabolic androgenic steroids

WADA category

I. Substances and methods prohibited at all times (in and out of competition). S1. Anabolic agents 1. Anabolic androgenic steroids.

Use in sport

Anabolic androgenic steroids (AASs) are used to improve strength by increasing lean body mass, decreasing body fat, prolonging training by enhancing recovery time and increasing aggressiveness.

Pharmacological action

AASs have two major effects: (i) an androgenic or mascularizing action and (ii) an anabolic or tissue building effect. They may be taken orally or by deep intramuscular injection. Injectable preparations may be water- or oil-based. In general, oil-based preparations have a longer biological half-life. AASs produce their effect through an action on endogenous androgen receptors. They increase protein synthesis and possibly have an anticatabolic effect by antagonizing the effect of glucocorticoid hormones such as cortisol, released during intense exercise.

Adverse effects

Acne and water retention are common, reversible side effects. Prolonged use may lead to male-pattern baldness. Cardiovascular side effects associated with AAS use include hypertension and alteration of cholesterol levels. The liver is a target tissue for androgens and it is the principal site for steroid metabolism, especially after oral administration. A number of effects on the liver have been described, including hepatocyte hypertrophy and, at high doses, cholestasis and peliosis hepatis. Androgens also increase the risk of liver tumours. Psychological effects with AASs, such as mania, hypomania and depression, have been reported. In females, the extent of AAS use is less well known. The risks of steroid misuse in women are greater than in men, with some irreversible side effects. Females prefer oral steroids, which are shorter acting than the oil-based injectable steroids, such as testosterone, which are more likely to produce side effects such as acne, unwanted facial hair, cliteromegaly and a change in the shape of the face, with squaring of the jaw line. In males, AAS misuse is commonly associated with testicular atrophy and reduced sperm production. Gynaecomastia is a common side effect among male body builders and may be associated with steroid misuse.

Erythropoietin

WADA category

I. Substances and methods prohibited at all times (in and out of competition). S2. Peptide hormones, growth factors and related substances.

Use in sport

The increase in production of erythrocytes by erythropoietin (EPO) improves the oxygen-carrying capacity of the blood. This effect is particularly useful in endurance sports. Misuse normally involves synthetic, recombinant EPO. More recently, the erythropoietin derivative Darbepoetin and the erythropoietin receptor activator, CERA, have been used, both of which are prohibited by WADA.

Pharmacological action

EPO is a glycoprotein hormone, produced primarily in the kidney. The stimulus for its production is reduced oxygen delivery to the kidney. Its effect is to increase the number of erythrocytes that are produced from the bone marrow and to increase the rate at which they are released into the circulation.

Adverse effects

EPO can, initially, produce flu-like symptoms, such as headaches and joint pain, but these usually resolve spontaneously, even with continued use. Up to 35 per cent of patients on EPO develop hypertension and the risk of thrombosis is increased. In sport, the misuse of EPO poses a significant potential risk to health since the raised haematocrit increases blood viscosity, which may be further exacerbated through dehydration.

Human growth hormone and insulin-like growth factor

WADA category

I. Substances and methods prohibited at all times (in and out of competition). S2. Peptide hormones, growth factors and related substances.

Use in sport

Human growth hormone (hGH) is used to increase muscle mass, allow users to train harder, longer and more frequently, and to promote faster recovery after training.

Pharmacological action

Human GH is a polypeptide hormone produced by the pituitary gland, to maintain normal growth from birth to adulthood. It has a short half-life (about 20 minutes), during which time it activates hepatic GH receptors, mediating the production of insulin-like growth factor 1 (IGF-1). It is IGF-1 that is responsible for most of the anabolic action of hGH.

Adverse effects

Overuse of hGH in children can lead to "gigantism", in adults it can lead to "acromegaly". Features of acromegaly include skeletal deformities, arthritis and enlargement of organs such as the heart, lungs, liver, intestines and spleen. Hypertension, diabetes mellitus, peripheral neuropathy and muscle weakness, despite an increase in size, may develop. Increased protein synthesis also produces thickening and coarsening of the skin. Association between the use of hGH and leukaemia has been reported.

Where athletes use IGF-1, adverse effects are the same as for hGH. IGF-1 commonly produces hypoglycaemia, as it promotes the uptake of glucose into cells.

The use of hGH has become more popular among female athletes, because there is no risk of developing the androgenic side effects associated with AASs.

β_2-agonists

WADA category

I. Substances and methods prohibited at all times (in and out of competition). S3. β_2-agonists and S1 anabolic agents 2. Other anabolic agents.

Salbutamol and salmeterol, when administered by inhaler, are permitted in sport provided their use is declared.

Other drugs used in the treatment of asthma, including corticosteroids (subject to restriction, see below), anticholinergics, methyl xanthines and cromoglycate, are permitted in sport.

Use in sport

All β_2-agonists are potent bronchodilators and may, therefore, improve performance in aerobic exercise. β_2-agonists, particularly clenbuterol, possess anabolic activity and are used as an alternative or in addition to anabolic steroids.

For salbutamol, even though permitted, a positive test result is determined by a concentration in urine greater than 1000 ng/ml.

Pharmacological action

Bronchodilation is mediated through stimulation of the β_2-adrenoreceptors in the smooth muscle of the respiratory tract. β_2-adrenoreceptors are also found in skeletal muscle, the stimulation of which induces muscle growth. β_2-agonists are also capable of reducing subcutaneous and total body fat.

Adverse effects

At the higher doses likely to be experienced by misusers in sport, these drugs lose their selectivity, leading to stimulation of β_1-adrenoreceptors. This commonly produces fine tremor, usually of the hands, and may produce tachycardia, arrhythmias, nausea, insomnia and headaches.

When clenbuterol is used in doses producing anabolic effects, additional side effects such as generalized myalgia, asthenia, periorbital pain, dizzy spells, nausea, vomiting and fever have been reported.

Diuretics

WADA category

I. Substances and methods prohibited at all times (in and out of competition).
S5. Diuretics and other masking agents.

Use in sport

Diuretics do not have performance-enhancing effects but have been used to increase urine production in an attempt to dilute other doping agents and/or their metabolites. Diuretics are also used to reduce weight in sports where weight classification applies. In this context they are subject to testing at the time of the weigh-in.

Diuretics are used by body builders to counteract the fluid-retentive effects of androgenic anabolic steroids.

Pharmacological action

Diuretics variably exert their pharmacological effect on the kidneys, to produce an increased loss of fluid.

Adverse effects

The primary adverse effect results from induced hypohydration, although concomitant electrolyte disturbances compromise the heart and muscles. These effects are exacerbated where hyperthermia and dehydration accompany fatigue and glycogen depletion.

Blood doping

WADA category

I. Substances and methods prohibited at all times (in and out of competition).
M1. Enhancement of oxygen transfer.

Use in sport

Blood doping increases the oxygen-carrying capacity of the blood.

Adverse effects

Blood doping may lead to adverse effects associated with hyperviscocity of the blood, as discussed under EPO. Otherwise, autologous blood doping carries no more risk than any other procedure involving invasive techniques. However, risks due to cross-infection and non-matched blood may occur where non-autologous infusion is carried out.

Amphetamines

WADA category

II. Substances and methods prohibited in competition. S6. Stimulants a: Non-specified stimulants.

Use in sport

Amphetamines are used, during competition, to reduce fatigue and to increase reaction time, alertness, competitiveness and aggression. Amphetamines may be used out of competition to intensify training.

Amphetamines and derivatives such as ecstasy are recreational drugs; therefore, competitors may test positive for amphetamines having not intended to use them for performance enhancement.

Pharmacological action

There are four mechanisms: (i) by releasing neurotransmitters, such as noradrenaline, dopamine and serotonin, from their respective nerve terminals; (ii) inhibition of neurotransmitter uptake; (iii) direct action on neurotransmitter receptors; and (iv) inhibition of monoamine oxidase activity. Of these, neurotransmitter release is the most important.

Adverse effects

The adverse effects of amphetamines include restlessness, irritability, tremor and insomnia with an increase in aggressive behaviour and the potential for addiction. At higher doses, amphetamines may produce sweating, tachycardia, pupillary dilation, increased blood pressure and heat stroke. Effects on the heart may lead to arrhythmias, of which ventricular arrhythmia is potentially fatal.

Cocaine

WADA category

I. Substances and methods prohibited in competition. S6. Stimulants a: Non-specified stimulants.

Cocaine possesses local anaesthetic properties. Other local anaesthetics are permitted in sport.

Use in sport

Studies on the ergogenic effects of cocaine are inconclusive. Cocaine is a "recreational" drug and many instances of positive doping results have arisen from residual levels remaining in the body after recreational use, rather than an attempt by the athlete to enhance performance. Cocaine is notable for distorting the user's perception of reality; therefore the athlete may perceive enhanced performance where, in reality, a decrease in endurance and strength, due to the drug, exists.

Pharmacological action

The pharmacological effects of cocaine on the brain are complex and include inhibition of the uptake of various central neurotransmitters, particularly dopamine.

Adverse effects

The complex pharmacology of cocaine leads to a wide spectrum of adverse effects, including a negative effect on glycogenolysis, paranoid psychosis, seizures, hypertension and myocardial toxicity, which could lead to ischaemia, arrhythmias and sudden death, especially following intense exercise. Smoked "crack" cocaine is more dangerous as the rate of absorption is greater, leading to a more intense effect on the cardiovascular system.

Ephedrine and other sympathomimetics available in over-the-counter (OTC) medicines

This group includes drugs such as ephedrine, methylephedrine and l-methylamphetamine. In 2010, the sympathomimetic, pseudoephedrine, was re-introduced to the prohibited list.

WADA category

I. Substances and methods prohibited in competition. S6. Stimulants b: Specified stimulants.

WADA regulations define a positive result for these substances if they appear in the urine at concentrations above specified threshold levels.

Competitors should be aware of the fact that even the manufacturers' recommended doses may result in exceeding permitted levels.

Other drugs that are found, commonly, in OTC medicines, such as antihistamines (e.g. triprolidine, astemizole), analgesics (e.g. paracetamol), imidazole decongestants (e.g. xylometazoline), cough suppressants (e.g. pholcodine) and expectorants (e.g. ipecacuanha) are not prohibited by WADA.

Use in sport

Sympathomimetics produce central stimulant effects.

Pharmacological action

These drugs produce decongestion by decreasing mucus secretion. They are structurally related to amphetamine and therefore produce a similar, though weaker, effect as central stimulants.

Adverse effects

OTC sympathomimetics variably produce side effects such as headache, tachycardia, dizziness, hypertension, irritability and anxiety.

Narcotics

WADA category

II. Substances and methods prohibited in competition. S7. Narcotics.
   Some less potent narcotics, such as codeine, dihydrocodeine, dextropropoxyphene and dextromethorphan, are permitted by WADA.

Use in sport

Potent narcotic analgesics are misused in sport for their pain-relieving properties.

Pharmacological action

Alkaloids from the opium poppy and their synthetic analogues interact with brain receptors that are normally acted upon by the endogenous endorphin transmitters. Narcotics have the capacity to moderate pain but also affect emotions. Frequent use may induce tolerance and dependency, the extent of which is variable depending on the narcotic used.

Adverse effects

In high doses, narcotic analgesics can cause stupor and coma, with the possibility of death due to respiratory depression. Where dependency has occurred, withdrawal symptoms include craving, anxiety, sweating, insomnia, nausea and vomiting, muscle aches and potential cardiovascular collapse.

Cannabinoids

WADA category

II. Substances and methods prohibited in competition. S8. Cannabinoids.
   Passive smoking of cannabinoids has been cited as the reason for a positive test result on a number of occasions.

Use in sport

Cannabinoid effects are incompatible with most sports; therefore tests are only conducted in certain sports.

Pharmacological action

The active constituent of marijuana is 1–5–9-tetrahydrocannabinol (THC). When smoked, 60–65 per cent is absorbed and effects are noted within 15 minutes and last for three hours or so. It produces a sedating and euphoric feeling of well-being.

Adverse effects

The central depressant effects of THC decrease the motivation for physical effort, and motor co-ordination, short-term memory and perception are impaired. In addition to its psychological effects, THC induces tachycardia, bronchodilation and an increased blood flow to the limbs.

Glucocorticosteroids

WADA category

II. Substances and methods prohibited in competition. S9. Glucocorticosteroids.
   Glucocorticosteroids are prohibited when administered orally, rectally or by intravenous or intramuscular injection. Glucocorticosteroids are permitted, subject to Therapeutic Use Exemption, if the route of administration is limited to inhalation or by intra-articular, periarticular, peritendinous, epidural or intradermal injection. Topical preparations when used for auricular, buccal, dermatological, gingival, nasal, ophthalmic and perianal disorders are not prohibited.

Use in sport

Glucocorticosteroids are important in the management of sports injuries, due to their potent anti-inflammatory properties.

Pharmacological action

These drugs are related to the adrenocorticosteroid hormone released from the adrenal cortex. They have a widespread effect on the body including glucocorticoid effects on carbohydrate, protein and fat metabolism and on electrolyte and water balance, as well as their anti-inflammatory effect. As anti-inflammatory agents they reduce the swelling, tenderness and heat associated with injury.

Adverse effects

Local damage may be produced at the site of injection due to dosage volume and subcutaneous atrophy, with associated depigmentation. Corticosteroids produce a catabolic effect on skeletal muscle, leading to muscle weakness soon after treatment has begun, even with modest doses.

Alcohol

WADA category

III. Substances prohibited in particular sports. P1. Alcohol.

Use in sport

Alcohol (ethanol) may be used, potentially, as a performance-enhancing drug due to its anti-anxiety effect. In some team sports, where alcohol is part of a social convention, peer pressure may lead to an overindulgence with consequences for the partaker and for fellow competitors.

Pharmacological action

Alcohol affects neural transmission in the CNS by altering the permeability of axonal membranes and thereby slowing nerve conductance. Alcohol also decreases glucose utilization in the brain. Overall, alcohol impairs concentration, reduces anxiety and induces depression and sedation.

Adverse effects

The adverse effects of alcohol have been extensively documented over many centuries.

Beta blockers

WADA category

III. Substances prohibited in particular sports. P2. Beta blockers.

Use in sport

Beta blockers have a use in sport where motor skills can be affected by muscle tremor, caused by anxiety. Beta blockers are therefore prohibited in certain sports, such as archery and other shooting events and in high-risk sports, such as ski jumping, bobsleigh and motorcycling.

Pharmacological action

Beta blockers are first-line drugs in the management of angina pectoris, hypertension, some cardiac arrhythmias, hyperthyroidism and glaucoma and are used occasionally for migraine and essential tremor.

Adverse effects

The adverse effects of beta blockers vary according to the properties of the individual drug. Beta blockers may produce bronchoconstriction, fatigue, cold extremities, sleep disturbances and nightmares.

Section 2. Drugs used in sport that are not on the WADA prohibited list

In this section, consideration is given to the use of therapeutic drugs in the management of illnesses that athletes may experience and for which they may self-medicate or seek medical advice from a general practitioner, pharmacist or other health professional.

Non-steroidal anti-inflammatory drugs (NSAIDs)

Use in sport

NSAIDs, such as aspirin and indomethacin, are widely used as analgesic and anti-inflammatory drugs for the treatment of sports injuries.

Pharmacological action

The analgesic, anti-inflammatory and antipyretic activity of NSAIDs is based on their ability to inhibit prostaglandin synthesis.

Adverse effects

The most common adverse effects associated with NSAIDs are gastrointestinal, including nausea, dyspepsia and ulcers.

Topical administration of NSAIDs may offer an effective and possibly safer alternative route of administration.

Benzodiazepines and other anxiolytics

Use in sport

A number of classes of drugs have been used as anxiolytics, including alcohol, beta blockers and benzodiazepines. The first two classes have been described above, as they are restricted in certain sports.

Pharmacological action

Benzodiazepines variously reduce the activity of a number of central neurotransmitters, such as acetylcholine, serotonin and noradrenaline. The anti-anxiety effect is primarily through release of gamma-aminobutyric acid, which inhibits the release of serotonin.

Adverse effects

Benzodiazepines are relatively free of adverse effects. However, they are liable to produce dependency if used for extended periods. Benzodiazepines may also be used by athletes for insomnia. Under these circumstances, athletes need to be aware of the "hangover" effect of these drugs.

Caffeine

Use in sport

Caffeine was removed from the prohibited list by WADA in January 2004. However, WADA continues to monitor for its misuse in sport.

Caffeine may be used primarily for its central stimulant effect to improve alertness, reaction time and attention span. In addition, caffeine may increase the mobilization and utilization of fatty acids, leading to a sparing of muscle glycogen.

Pharmacological action

Caffeine inhibits the phosphodiesterase group of enzymes, which activate second messengers such as cyclic AMP. They act as one of the links between receptor activation and cellular responses. Caffeine also directly antagonizes adenosine receptors.

Adverse effects

Mild side effects associated with caffeine include irritability, insomnia and gastrointestinal disturbances. More severe effects include peptic ulceration, delirious seizures, coma and superventricular and ventricular arrhythmias.

Cough and cold preparations

Use in sport

The use of these medications for self-limiting conditions is questionable. The only potential use for drugs is for the control of symptoms such as headache, fever, runny nose and cough. However, many of the drugs found in OTC cough and cold remedies are sympathomimetics used as decongestants. Some of these, such as ephedrine and pseudoephedrine, are banned by WADA, although there are cut-off concentrations in the urine for these drugs.

Pharmacological action

Apart from the sympathomimetic decongestants discussed previously, cough and cold medicines may contain analgesics (paracetamol, codeine), antihistamines (e.g. triprolidine, astemizole), imidazole decongestants (e.g. xylometazoline) cough suppressants (e.g. pholcodine) and expectorants (e.g. ipecacuanha), all of which are permitted by WADA.

Adverse effects

In general, cough and cold preparations are taken for short periods of time and therefore side effects are limited. However, nasal decongestants are liable to produce rebound congestion if used for more than one week. Sedating antihistamines may have adverse effects on performance in most sports.

Antidiarrhoeals

Use in sport

First-line treatment for diarrhoea is oral rehydration therapy (ORT). Antimotility drugs may be used for short-term symptomatic relief of acute diarrhoea if it is likely to affect performance.

Pharmacological action

ORT enhances the absorption of water and replaces electrolytes. Antimotility drugs (codeine, diphenoxylate, loperamide) are opioids with a direct relaxant effect on the smooth muscle of the gastrointestinal tract.

Adverse effects

Tolerance and dependence may develop with prolonged use of antimotility drugs. Loperamide may produce abdominal cramps, drowsiness and skin reactions.

Nutritional supplements

Use in sport

Nutritional supplements are used by many athletes to maintain a "balanced" diet. However, many athletes have used supplements in an attempt to enhance performance through ergogenic aids, without contravening WADA regulations.

The manufacture and sale of nutritional supplements is not as closely regulated as that for drugs. Nutritional supplements may therefore contain banned substances or their precursors, which produce the same metabolites as banned substances in the urine. The use of nutritional supplements may therefore lead to a positive dope test result.

Pharmacological action

Manufacturers may make exaggerated claims regarding the ergogenic properties of their products. There is little, if any, evidence that nutritional supplements possess ergogenic properties in athletes consuming a balanced diet.

Adverse effects

Some nutritional supplements have the potential for harm. Creatine has been the subject of many studies, but results are equivocal as to whether it produces ergogenic effects. There are few reliable scientific data on possible adverse effects of creatine, but its potential effect on renal dysfunction and electrolyte imbalance, leading to a predisposition to dehydration and heat-related illness, suggests caution in its use.

Index